HARRY BLUMENTHAL, M.A., M.F.C.C.
Washington-Whittier Medical Building
12468 East Washington Blvd.
Whittier, California 90602

D1554456

RENÉ A. SPITZ: DIALOGUES FROM INFANCY

RENÉ A. SPITZ: DIALOGUES FROM INFANCY

Selected Papers

Edited by

ROBERT N. EMDE

INTERNATIONAL UNIVERSITIES PRESS, INC.
New York

Library of Congress Cataloging in Publication Data

Spitz, René A. (René Arpad), 1887–1974.
   Dialogues from infancy.

   Bibliography: p.
   Includes index.
   1. Infant psychiatry — Addresses, essays, lectures.
I. Emde, Robert N.   II. Title.
RJ502.5.S65   1983   618.92'89   83-26461
ISBN 0-8236-5787-6

Contents

Contents

Contents

Preface

The First World Congress of Infant Psychiatry, held in Portugal in April 1980, was dedicated to the memory of René Spitz in recognition of his pioneering observations and generative theory. This event also indicated the widespread influence of Spitz's work. The current volume is intended to increase the availability of many of Spitz's papers, which are frequently cited among health care professionals and developmental psychologists.

René Spitz was born in Vienna in 1887 and died in Denver in 1974. In between he led a rich and varied life in many of the cities of the Western world, practicing psychoanalysis, teaching, and carrying on his research. It is remarkable to realize (especially for those of us who knew him) that when he undertook his research and set about making his observations and movies of infants and their mothers, Spitz was already in his late forties. In a way, this collection of his papers gives testimony to the extent to which research and development are possible at mid-life.

To enhance their relevance to today's theories and clinical formulations, the papers are grouped by topic. Within each topic, papers appear chronologically. I hope this format will also serve to highlight the developmental rather than fixed nature of Spitz's ideas.

A major function of the editorial comments is to let the reader know why papers were selected and grouped in a particular way as well as to indicate something of their historical and current interest. Thus informed, the reader can then better set his or her own priorities for reading. Since the intended audience for this collection is multidisciplinary, I have also attempted in the editorial comments to provide keys to today's scientific and clinical literature. This will allow the interested reader to pursue areas where Spitz's work has been especially generative, and where hypotheses suggested by Spitz still remain to be tested.

The motion picture films of René Spitz are discussed in a section coauthored by Emde and Harmon. These films are still available, and many original film and manuscript sources can be studied in the René Spitz film archives. Since many inquiries are being received about these materials, a description has been included.

The seven commentaries that close the book are brief statements by leaders of a number of disciplines that have been influenced by Spitz's contributions. Although neither their commentaries nor mine are intended to be eulogies, obviously I have made selections that will indicate the usefulness of Spitz's work. I have not interpreted my editorial function to include the search for balanced criticism, a task that is more appropriate for historians and future scientists.

A special acknowledgement is due to my editorial assistant, Michelle Lampl, whose help in all phases of assembling this volume has been invaluable. An anthropology graduate student reading Spitz for the first time, she offered thoughtful reactions and fresh views that were invaluable in the selection and grouping of papers, and her comments also helped me formulate what should be said in the editorial commentary. She also administered many editorial details in the preparation of the manuscript. I also wish to acknowledge the Research Scientist Award Program of the National Institute of Mental Health, which gave me partial salary support during my work on this volume (Grant No. 5KO5MH3680804), and the University of London, Institute of Psychiatry, Department of Child and Adolescent Psychiatry, which provided office facilities for me while I finished this task during a work-study year. Among the many who were close to René and who encouraged me in this ''labor of love,'' I wish to give a special thanks to his daughter, Eva Blum, and to David Metcalf and Herbert Gaskill. Finally, I would like to acknowledge the unusual encouragement of Martin V. Azarian, President of International Universities Press and the diligence of Ellen Bilofsky as copy editor.

ROBERT N. EMDE

PART 1

DEPRIVATION OF MOTHERING

Editor's Introduction

Of all Spitz's work, these first four papers are probably the best known worldwide. They contain classic observations of deprived infants, observations that Spitz also documented in films illustrating the suffering and depression of these children. (See especially, *Grief: A Peril in Infancy* and *Somatic Consequences of Emotional Starvation in Infants*. These and other available films, are discussed in Part 7.)

A historical note is important. Strange as it may seem to today's health care professionals, it used to be considered the best practice for a baby awaiting adoption to be in an institution for a prolonged period. This waiting period was thought necessary to provide sufficient time for the developmental unfolding of the baby's intellectual and personality features that would allow an appropriate match with adoptive parents and avoid the awkward problems of "mismatching." The fact that so many institutionalized infants did not come up to the standards of many adoptive parents for intellect and sociability was considered a reflection of the "morally inferior" nature of women conceiving out of wedlock. Indeed, some of these women (and their "paramours") may have been suspected "constitutional psychopathic inferiors." This diagnostic label, used in the United States in the 1930s, crystallized the prevailing attitude that this kind of misery was to a large extent constitutional, fixed, and not subject to (or deserving of) amelioration. That the progeny of these women were sickly, in spite of good institutional hygienic care, fit in not only with the doctrine of the Protestant ethic regarding the products of sinfulness but also with a still-influential social Darwinism, which held that humanity was naturally evolving toward a state of social and moral betterment. The sickly infants were confirmation of an evolutionary process at work; they were constitutionally less equipped for adaptation and survival.

Into this climate entered Spitz and his writings. Based on his observations, he offered a counterview: it was the *experience* of the institutionalized infants

3

that, in large part, led to developmental and physical retardation; moreover, much of this experience had to do with deficits in mothering, with separation, and with depression. Spitz's observations and this counterview ultimately became compelling. As a result of these papers and Bowlby's (1951) report reviewing them and adding more evidence, adoption procedures were changed around the world. The goal became early adoption whenever feasible, and "waiting" ceased to be valued. The counterview was hopeful: improvement of development through environmental change was possible.

These papers are also important in understanding history in still another sense, namely, in following the development of Spitz's thinking. In rereading them, we become aware that, as he focused on the institutional experience, Spitz was not just writing about babies deprived of their mothers. He became increasingly interested in understanding the *mothering process* to find out what was essential about early ego development. One sees Spitz being drawn to the importance of affective reciprocity as well as to his better-known psychoanalytic concepts of early development.

Many of the observations and inferences found in these early papers reappear throughout the other papers in this volume. Throughout his productive lifetime, Spitz continually integrated these early findings into his ideas about the emergence of dialogue, about ego development, and about infant psychiatry. His experience in the "foundling home" and "nursery" environments became, in a sense, the foundations for much of his later developmental and clinical theorizing. To appreciate the later Spitz, the reader must also have shared in this early experience.

Hospitalism: An Inquiry into the Genesis of Psychiatric Conditions in Early Childhood

> En la Casa de Ninos Expositos el nino se va poniendo
> triste y muchos de ellos mueren de tristeza.
> *(1760, from the diary of a Spanish bishop.)*

I. THE PROBLEM

The term *hospitalism* designates a vitiated condition of the body due to long confinement in a hospital, or the morbid condition of the atmosphere of a hospital. The term has been increasingly preempted to specify the evil effect of institutional care on infants placed in institutions from an early age, particularly from the psychiatric point of view. This study is especially concerned with the effect of continuous institutional care of infants under one year of age, for reasons other than sickness. The model of such institutions is the foundling home.

Medical men and administrators have long been aware of the shortcomings of such charitable institutions. At the beginning of our century one of the great foundling homes in Germany had a mortality rate of 71.5 percent in infants in the first year of life (Schlossman, 1920). In 1915 Chapin (1915a) enumerated ten asylums in the larger cities of the United States, mainly on the Eastern seaboard, in which the death rates of infants admitted during their first year of life varied from 31.7 percent to 75 percent by the end of their second year. In a discussion in the same year before the American Pediatric Association, Dr. Knox of Baltimore stated that in the institutions of that city 90 percent of the infants died by the end of their first year (reported in Chapin, 1915b). He believed that the remaining 10 percent probably were saved because they had been taken out of the institution in time. Dr. Shaw of Albany remarked in the same discussion that the mortality rate of Randalls Island Hospital was probably 100 percent.

Conditions have since greatly changed. At present the best American institutions, such as Bellevue Hospital, New York City, register a mortality rate of less than 10 percent (Bakwin, 1942), which compares favorably with the

Reprinted from *The Psychoanalytic Study of the Child*, Vol. 1. New York: International Universities Press, 1945, pp. 53–74.

mortality rate of the rest of the country. While these and similar results were being achieved both here and in Europe, physicians and administrators were soon faced with a new problem: they discovered that institutionalized children practically without exception developed subsequent psychiatric disturbances and became asocial, delinquent, feeble-minded, psychotic, or problem children. Probably the high mortality rate in the preceding period had obscured this consequence. Now that the children survived, the other drawbacks of institutionalization became apparent. They led in this country to the widespread substitution of institutional care by foster home care.

The first investigation of the factors involved in the psychiatric consequences of institutional care of infants in their first year was made in 1933 in Austria by H. Durfee and K. Wolf. Further contributions to the problem were made by L. G. Lowrey (1940), L. Bender and H. Yarnell (1941), H. Bakwin (1942), and W. Goldfarb (1943, 1944a, 1944b; Goldfarb and Klopfer, 1944). The results of all these investigations are roughly similar.

Bakwin found greatly increased susceptibility to infection in spite of high hygienic and nutritional standards. Durfee and Wolf found that children under three months show no demonstrable impairment in consequence of institutionalization; but that children who had been institutionalized for more than eight months during their first year show such severe psychiatric disturbances that they cannot be tested. Bender, Goldfarb, and Lowrey found that after three years of institutionalization, the changes effected are irreversible. Lowrey found that whereas the impairment of children hospitalized during their first year seems irremediable, that of children hospitalized in the second or third year can be corrected.

Two factors, both already stressed by Durfee and Wolf, are made responsible by most of the authors for the psychological injury suffered by these children.

First: Lack of stimulation. The worst offenders were the best equipped and most hygienic institutions, which succeeded in sterilizing the surroundings of the child from germs but which at the same time sterilized the child's psyche. Even the most destitute of homes offers more mental stimulation than the usual hospital ward.

Second: The presence or absence of the child's mother. Stimulation by the mother will always be more intensive than even that of the best trained nursery personnel (Ripin, 1930). Those institutions in which the mothers were present had better results than those where only trained child nurses were employed. The presence of the mothers could compensate even for numerous other shortcomings.

We believe that further study is needed to isolate clearly the various factors operative in the deterioration subsequent to prolonged care in institutions.

The number of infants studied by Bakwin, Durfee and Wolf, and Lowrey in single institutions is very small, and Bender and Yarnell and Goldfarb did not observe infants in the first 12 months of life. We are not questioning here whether institutions should be preferred to foster homes, a subject now hardly ever discussed—the decision can by implication be deduced from the results of the studies of the Iowa group in their extensive research on the "nature versus nurture" controversy (Updegraff, 1932; Skeels, 1938, 1940; Skeels, Updegraff, Wellman, and Williams, 1938; Skodak, 1939; Stoddard, 1940). It may seem surprising that in the course of this controversy no investigation has covered the field of the first year of life in institutions.[1] All Iowa investigators studied either children in foster homes or children over one year of age, using their findings for retrospective interpretations.[2] They did not have at their disposal a method of investigation that would permit the evaluation and quantification of development, mental or otherwise, during the first year of life. Their only instrument is the I.Q., which is unreliable (Simpson, 1939), and not applicable during the first year. However, the baby tests worked out by Hetzer and Wolf (1928) fill the gap, providing not only a quotient for intelligence but also quantifiable data for development as a whole, such as indication of developmental age and of a developmental quotient. They provide, furthermore, quantifiable data on six distinct sectors of personality, namely: development of perception, body mastery, social relations, memory, relations to inanimate objects, and intelligence (which in the first year is limited to understanding of relations between and insight into the functions of objects).

With the help of these data ("dimensions"), a profile (personality curve) is constructed, from which relevant conclusions can be drawn and with the help of which children can be compared with one another. Averages of development in any one sector or in all of them can be established for given environments. Finally, the relevant progresses of one and the same child in the several sectors of its personality can be followed up. The profiles present a cross-section of infantile development at any given moment; but they also can be combined into longitudinal curves of the developmental progress of the child's total personality as well as of the various sectors of the personality.

[1] Woodworth (1941) in discussing the results of the Child Welfare Research Station of the State University of Iowa makes the following critical remarks: "The causes of the inferior showing of orphanage children are obviously open to debate. . . . It would seem that a survey and comparative study of institutional homes for children would be instructive . . ." (p. 71).

[2] Jones (1940) takes exception to this method as follows: "It seems probable that we shall turn from retrospective surveys of conditions assumed to have had a prior influence, and shall prefer to deal with the current and cumulative effects of specific environmental factors. It may also be expected that our interest will shift to some extent from mass statistical studies . . . to investigations of the dynamics of the growth process in individuals" (p. 455).

The aim of my research is to isolate and investigate the pathogenic factors responsible for the favorable or unfavorable outcome of infantile development. A psychiatric approach might seem desirable; however, infant psychiatry is a discipline not yet existent: its advancement is one of the aims of the present study.

II. Material[3]

With this purpose in mind a long-term study of 164 children was undertaken.[4] In view of the findings of previous investigations this study was largely limited to the first year of life, and confined to two institutions, in order to embrace the total population of both (130 infants). Since the two institutions were situated in different countries of the Western hemisphere, a basis of comparison was established by investigating noninstitutionalized children of the same age group in their parents' homes in both countries. A total of 34 of these were observed. We thus have four environments. (See Table 1.)

III. Procedure

In each case an anamnesis was made which whenever possible included data on the child's mother; and in each case the Hetzer-Wolf baby tests were administered. Problems cropping up in the course of our investigations for which the test situation did not provide answers were subjected to special experiments elaborated for the purpose. Such problems referred, for instance, to attitude and behavior in response to stimuli offered by inanimate objects,

---

[3] It is interesting to note that independently of our approach to this problem (mapped out and begun in 1936) Woodworth (1941) recommends a research program on extremely similar lines as being desirable for the better understanding of the problem of heredity and environment:

> Orphanages. Present belief based on a certain amount of evidence regards the orphanages as an unfavorable environment for the child but the causes are not well understood. Two general projects may be suggested.
>
> (a) A survey of institutional homes for children with a view to discovering the variations in their equipment and personnel and in their treatment of the children, with some estimate of the results achieved.
>
> (b) Experimental studies in selected orphanages which retain their children for a considerable time, with a view to testing out the effects of specific environmental factors. For example, the amount of contact of the child with adults could be increased for certain children for the purpose of seeing whether this factor is important in mental development. It is conceivable that an orphanage could be run so as to become a decidedly favorable environment for the growing child, but at present we do not know how this result could be accomplished [pp. 90–91].

[4] I wish to thank K. Wolf, Ph.D., for her help in the experiments carried out in "Nursery" and in private homes, and for her collaboration in the statistical evaluation of the results.

TABLE 1.

Environment	Institution No. 1[a]	Corresponding private background[b]	Institution No. 2	Corresponding private background
Number of children	69	11	61	23

by social situations, etc. All observations of unusual or unexpected behavior of a child were carefully protocolled and studied.

A large number of tests, all the experiments and some of the special situations were filmed on 16 mm. film. A total of 31,500 feet of film preserve the results of our investigation to date. In the analysis of the movies the following method was applied: Behavior was filmed at sound speed, i.e., 24 frames per second. This makes it possible to slow action down during projection to nearly one-third of the original speed so that it can be studied in slow motion. A projector with additional hand drive also permits study of the films frame by frame, if necessary, to reverse action and to repeat projection of every detail as often as required. Simultaneously the written protocols of the experiments are studied and the two observations compared.

IV. RESULTS

For the purpose of orientation we established the average of the developmental quotients for the first third of the first year of life for each of the environments investigated. We contrasted these averages with those for the last third of the first year. This comparison gives us a first hint of the significance of environmental influences for development. (See Table 2.)

Thus the children in the first three environments were at the end of their first year on the whole well developed and normal, whether they were raised in their progressive middle-class family homes (where obviously optimal circumstances prevailed and the children were well in advance of average development), or in an institution or a village home, where the development was not brilliant but still reached a perfectly normal and satisfactory average.

---

[a] Institution No. 1 will from here on be called "Nursery"; institution No. 2, "Foundling Home."

[b] The small number of children observed in this particular environment was justified by the fact that it has been previously studied extensively by other workers; our only aim was to correlate our results with theirs. However, during the course of one year each child was tested at least at regular monthly intervals.

TABLE 2.

Type of Environment	Cultural and Social Background	Developmental Quotients	
		Average of first four months	Average of last four months
Parental Home	Professional	133	131
	Village Population	107	108
Institution	"Nursery"	101.5	105
	"Foundling Home"	124	72

The children in the fourth environment, though starting at almost as high a level as the best of the others, had spectacularly deteriorated.

The children in Foundling Home showed all the manifestations of hospitalism, both physical and mental. In spite of the fact that hygiene and precautions against contagion were impeccable, the children showed, from the third month on, extreme susceptibility to infection and illness of any kind. There was hardly a child in whose case history we did not find reference to otitis media, or morbilli, or varicella, or eczema, or intestinal disease of one kind or another. No figures could be elicited on general mortality; but during my stay an epidemic of measles swept the institution, with staggeringly high mortality figures, notwithstanding liberal administration of convalescent serum and globulins, as well as excellent hygienic conditions. Of a total of 88 children up to the age of 2½, 23 died. It is striking to compare the mortality among the 45 children up to 1½ years, to that of the 43 children ranging from 1½ to 2½ years: Usually, the *incidence* of measles is low in the younger age group, but among those infected the mortality is higher than that in the older age group; since in the case of Foundling Home every child was infected, the question of incidence does not enter; however, contrary to expectation, the mortality was much higher in the older age group. In the younger group, 6 died, i.e., approximately 13 percent. In the older group, 17 died, i.e., close to 40 percent. The significance of these figures becomes apparent when we realize that the mortality from measles during the first year of life in the community in question, outside the institution, was less than .5 percent.

In view of the damage sustained in all personality sectors of the children during their stay in this institution we believe it licit to assume that their vitality (whatever that may be), their resistance to disease, was also progressively sapped. In the ward of the children ranging from 18 months to 2½ years, only 2 of the 26 surviving children speak a couple of words. The same 2 are able to walk. A third child is beginning to walk. Hardly any of them can eat alone. Cleanliness habits have not been acquired and all are incontinent.

In sharp contrast to this is the picture offered by the oldest inmates in Nursery, ranging from 8 to 12 months. The problem here is not whether the children walk or talk by the end of the first year; the problem with these 10-month-olds is how to tame the healthy toddlers' curiosity and enterprise. They climb up the bars of the cots after the manner of South Sea Islanders climbing palms. Special measures to guard them from harm have had to be taken after one 10-month-old actually succeeded in diving right over the more than two-foot railing of the cot. They vocalize freely and some of them actually speak a word or two. And all of them understand the significance of simple social gestures. When released from their cots, all walk with support and a number walk without it.

What are the differences between the two institutions that result in the one turning out normally acceptable children and the other showing such appalling effects?

A. SIMILARITIES[5]

1. Background of the children

Nursery is a penal institution in which delinquent girls are sequestered. When, as is often the case, they are pregnant on admission, they are delivered in a neighboring maternity hospital, and after the lying-in period their children are cared for in Nursery from birth to the end of their first year. The background of these children provides for a markedly negative selection since the mothers are mostly delinquent minors as a result of social maladjustment or feeble-mindedness, or because they are psychically defective, psychopathic,

---

[5] Under this heading we enumerate not only actual similarities but also differences that are of no etiological significance for the deterioration in Foundling Home. These differences comprise two groups: differences of no importance whatever, and differences that actually favor the development of children in Foundling Home.

or criminal. Psychic normalcy and adequate social adjustment is almost excluded.

The other institution is a foundling home pure and simple. A certain number of the children housed have a background not much better than that of the Nursery children; but a sufficiently relevant number come from socially well-adjusted, normal mothers whose only handicap is inability to support themselves and their children (which is no sign of maladjustment in women of Latin background). This is expressed in the average of the developmental quotients of the two institutions during the first four months, as shown in Table 2.

The background of the children in the two institutions does therefore not favor Nursery; on the contrary, it shows a very marked advantage for Foundling Home.

2. Housing Conditions

Both institutions are situated outside the city, in large spacious gardens. In both, hygienic conditions are carefully maintained. In both, infants at birth and during the first six weeks are segregated from the older babies in a special newborns' ward, to which admittance is only permitted in a freshly sterilized smock after hands are washed. In both institutions infants are transferred from the newborns' ward after 2 or 3 months to the older babies' wards, where they are placed in individual cubicles, which in Nursery are completely glass enclosed; in Foundling Home, glass enclosed on three sides and open at the end. In Foundling Home the children remain in their cubicles up to 15 to 18 months; in Nursery they are transferred after the sixth month to rooms containing four to five cots each.

One-half of the children in Foundling Home are located in a dimly lighted part of the ward; the other half, in the full light of large windows facing southeast, with plenty of sun coming in. In Nursery, all the children have well-lighted cubicles. In both institutions the walls are painted in a light neutral color, giving a white impression in Nursery, a gray-green impression in Foundling Home. In both, the children are placed in white painted cots. Nursery is financially the far better provided one: We usually find here a small metal table with the paraphernalia of child care, as well as a chair, in each cubicle; whereas in Foundling Home it is the exception if a low stool is to be found in the cubicles, which usually contain nothing but the child's cot.

3. Food

In both institutions adequate food is excellently prepared and varied according to the needs of the individual child at each age; bottles from which children are fed are sterilized. In both institutions a large percentage of the younger children are breast-fed. In Nursery this percentage is smaller, so that in most cases a formula is soon added, and in many cases weaning takes place early. In Foundling Home all children are breast-fed as a matter of principle as long as they are under three months, unless disease makes a deviation from this rule necessary.

4. Clothing

Clothing is practically the same in both institutions. The children have adequate pastel-colored dresses and blankets. The temperature in the rooms is appropriate. We have not seen any shivering child in either setup.

5. Medical Care

Foundling Home is visited by the head physician and the medical staff at least once a day, often twice, and during these rounds the chart of each child is inspected as well as the child itself. For special ailments a laryngologist and other specialists are available; they also make daily rounds. In Nursery no daily rounds are made, as they are not necessary. The physician sees the children when called.

Up to this point it appears that there is very little significant difference between the children of the two institutions. Foundling Home shows, if anything, a slight advantage over Nursery in the matter of selection of admitted children, of breast-feeding, and of medical care. It is in the items that now follow that fundamental differences become visible.

B. DIFFERENCES

1. Toys

In Nursery it is the exception when a child is without one or several toys. In Foundling Home my first impression was that not a single child had a toy. This impression was later corrected. In the course of time, possibly in reaction to our presence, more and more toys appeared, some of them quite intelligently fastened by a string above the baby's head so that he could reach it. By the time we left, a large percentage of the children in Foundling Home had a toy.

2. Visual Radius

In Nursery the corridor running between the cubicles, though rigorously white and without particular adornment, gives a friendly impression of warmth. This is probably because trees, landscape and sky are visible from both sides and because a bustling activity of mothers carrying their children, tending them, feeding them, playing with them, chatting with each other with babies in their arms, is usually present. The cubicles of the children are enclosed but the glass panes of the partitions reach low enough for every child to be able at any time to observe everything going on all around. He can see into the corridor as soon as he lifts himself on his elbows. He can look out of the windows, and can see babies in the other cubicles by just turning his head; witness the fact that whenever the experimenter plays with a baby in one of the cubicles the babies in the two adjoining cubicles look on fascinated, try to participate in the game, knock at the panes of the partition, and often begin to cry if no attention is paid to them. Most of the cots are provided with widely spaced bars that are no obstacle to vision. After the age of six months, when the child is transferred to the wards of the older babies, the visual field is enriched as a number of babies are then together in the same room, and accordingly play with each other.

In Foundling Home the corridor into which the cubicles open, though full of light on one side at least, is bleak and deserted, except at feeding time when five to eight nurses file in and look after the children's needs. Most of the time nothing goes on to attract the babies' attention. A special routine of Foundling Home consists in hanging bed sheets over the foot and the side railing of each cot. The cot itself is approximately 18 inches high. The side railings are about 20 inches high; the foot and head railings are approximately 28 inches high. Thus, when bed sheets are hung over the railings, the child lying in the cot is effectively screened from the world. He is completely separated from the other cubicles, since the glass panes of the wooden partitions begin 6 to 8 inches higher than even the head railing of the cot. The result of this system is that each baby lies in solitary confinement up to the time when he is able to stand up in his bed, and that the only object he can see is the ceiling.

3. Radius of Locomotion

In Nursery the radius of locomotion is circumscribed by the space available in the cot, which up to about 10 months provides a fairly satisfactory range.

Theoretically the same would apply to Foundling Home. But in practice this is not the case for, probably owing to the lack of stimulation, the babies lie supine in their cots for many months and a hollow is worn into their mattresses. By the time they reach the age when they might turn from back to side (approximately the seventh month) this hollow confines their activity to such a degree that they are effectively prevented from turning in any direction. As a result we find most babies, even at 10 and 12 months, lying on their backs and playing with the only object at their disposal, their own hands and feet.

4. Personnel

In Foundling Home there is a head nurse and five assistant nurses for a total of 45 babies. There nurses have the *entire* care of the children on their hands, except for the babies so young that they are breast-fed. The latter are cared for to a certain extent by their own mothers or by wet nurses; but after a few months they are removed to the single cubicles of the general ward, where they share with at least seven other children the ministrations of *one* nurse. It is obvious that the amount of care one nurse can give to an individual child when she has eight children to manage is small indeed. These nurses are unusually motherly, baby-loving women; but of course the babies of Foundling Home nevertheless lack all human contact for most of the day.

Nursery is run by a head nurse and her three assistants, whose duties do not include the care of the children, but consist mainly in teaching the children's mothers in child care, and in supervising them. The children are fed, nursed, and cared for by their own mothers or, in those cases where the mother is separated from her child for any reason, by the mother of another child, or by a pregnant girl who in this way acquires the necessary experience for the care of her own future baby. Thus in Nursery each child has the full-time care of his own mother, or at least that of the substitute which the very able head nurse tries to change about until she finds someone who really likes the child.

V. Discussion

To say that every child in Nursery has a full-time mother is an understatement, from a psychological point of view. However modern a penal institution may be, and however constructive and permissive its reeducative policies, the deprivation it imposes upon delinquent girls is extensive. Their opportunities for an outlet for their interests, ambitions, activity, are very much impoverished. The former sexual satisfactions as well as the satisfactions of competitive activity in the sexual field, are suddenly stopped: regulations prohibit flashy dresses, vivid nail polish, or extravagant hairdos. The kind of social life in which the girls could show off has vanished. This is especially traumatic as these girls become delinquent because they have not been able to sublimate their sexual drives, to find substitute gratifications, and therefore do not possess a pattern for relinquishing pleasure when frustrated. In addition, they do not have compensation in relations with family and friends, as formerly they had. These factors, combined with the loss of personal liberty, the deprivation of private property and the regimentation of the penal institution, all add up to a severe narcissistic trauma from the time of admission; and they continue to affect the narcissistic and libidinal sectors during the whole period of confinement.

Luckily there remain a few safety valves for their emotions: the relationships (1) with wardens, matrons, and nurses; (2) with fellow prisoners; (3) with the child. In the relationship with the wardens, matrons, and nurses, who obviously represent parent figures, much of the prisoner's aggression and resentment is bound. Much of it finds an outlet in the love and hate relationship to fellow prisoners, where all the phenomena of sibling rivalry are revived.

The child, however, becomes for them the representative of their sexuality, a product created by them, an object they own, which they can dress up and adorn, on which they can lavish their tenderness and pride, and of whose accomplishments, performance and appearance they can boast. This is manifested in the constant competition among them as to who has the better dressed, more advanced, more intelligent, better looking, the heavier, bigger, more active—in a word, the better baby.[6] For their own persons they have more or less given up the competition for love, but they are intensely jealous of the attention given to their children by the matrons, wardens, and fellow prisoners.

It would take an exacting experimenter to invent an experiment with conditions as diametrically opposed in regard to the mother-child relationship as they are in these two institutions. Nursery provides each child with a mother to the *n*th degree, a mother who gives the child everything a good mother does and, beyond that, everything else she has.[7] Foundling Home does not give the child a mother, nor even a substitute mother, but only an eighth of a nurse.

We are now in a position to approach more closely and with better understanding the results obtained by each of the two institutions. We have already cited a few: we mentioned that the developmental quotient of Nursery achieves a normal average of about 105 at the end of the first year, whereas that of the Foundling Home sinks to 72; and we mentioned the striking difference of the children in the two institutions at first sight. Let us first

---

[6] The psychoanalytically oriented reader of course realizes that for these girls in prison the child has become a hardly disguised phallic substitute. However, for the purposes of this article I have carefully avoided any extensive psychoanalytic interpretation, be it ever so tempting, and limited myself as closely as possible to results of direct observations of behavior. At numerous other points it would be not only possible but natural to apply analytic concepts; that is reserved for future publication.

[7] For the nonpsychoanalytically oriented reader we note that this intense mother-child relationship is not equivalent to a relationship based on love of the child. The mere fact that the child is used as a phallic substitute implies what a large part unconscious hostility plays in the picture.

consider the point at which the developments in the two institutions deviate.

On admission the children of Foundling Home have a much better average than the children of Nursery; their hereditary equipment is better than that of the children of delinquent minors. But while Foundling Home shows a rapid fall of the developmental index, Nursery shows a steady rise. They cross between the fourth and fifth months, and from that point on the curve of the average developmental quotient of the Foundling Home drops downward with increasing rapidity, never again to rise. (See Fig. 1.)

The point where the two curves cross is significant. The time when the children in Foundling Home are weaned is the beginning of the fourth month. The time lag of one month in the sinking of the index below normal is explained by the fact that the quotient represents a cross-section including all sectors of development, and that attempts at compensation are made in some of the other sectors.

However, when we consider the sector of Body Mastery, which according to Wolf[8] is most indicative for the mother-child relationship, we find that the curves of the children in Nursery cross the Body Mastery curve of the Foundling Home children between the third and fourth month. The inference is obvious. As soon as the babies in Foundling Home are weaned the modest human contacts which they have had during nursing at the breast stop, and their development falls below normal.

One might be inclined to speculate as to whether the further deterioration of the children in Foundling Home is not due to other factors also, such as the perceptual and motor deprivations from which they suffer. It might be argued that the better achievement of the Nursery children is due to the fact that they were better provided for in regard to toys and other perceptual stimuli. We shall therefore analyze somewhat more closely the nature of deprivations in perceptual and locomotor stimulation.

First of all it should be kept in mind that the nature of the inanimate perceptual stimulus, whether it is a toy or any other object, has only a very minor importance for a child under 12 months. At this age the child is not yet capable of distinguishing the real purpose of an object. He is only able to use it in a manner adequate to his own functional needs (C. Bühler, 1928). Our thesis is that perception is a function of libidinal cathexis and therefore the result of the intervention of an emotion of one kind or another.[9] Emotions are provided for the child through the intervention of a human partner, i.e.,

[8] K. M. Wolf, "Body Mastery of the Child as an Index for the Emotional Relationship between Mother and Child." Unpublished manuscript.

[9] This is stating in psychoanalytic terms the conviction of most modern psychologists, beginning with Compayré (1893) and shared by such familiar authorities in child psychology as Stern (1930) and K. Bühler (1918), and in animal psychology, Tolman (1932).

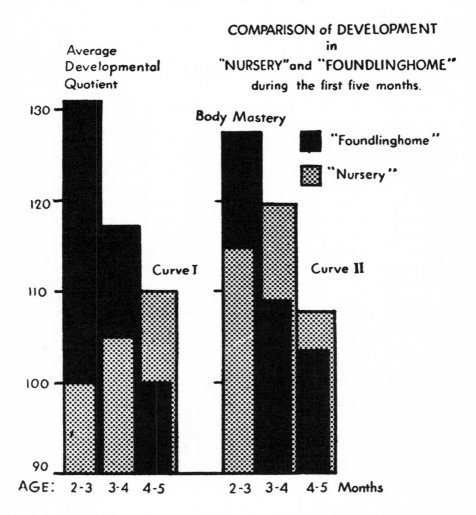

FIGURE 1. COMPARISON OF DEVELOPMENT IN "NURSERY" AND
"FOUNDLING HOME"

by the mother or her substitute. A progressive development of emotional interchange with the mother provides the child with perceptive experiences of its environment. The child learns to grasp by nursing at the mother's breast and by combining the emotional satisfaction of that experience with tactile perceptions. He learns to distinguish animate objects from inanimate ones by the spectacle provided by his mother's face (Gesell & Ilg, 1937) in situations fraught with emotional satisfaction. The interchange between mother and child is loaded with emotional factors and it is in this interchange that the child learns to play. He becomes acquainted with his surroundings through the mother's carrying him around; through her help he learns security in locomotion as well as in every other respect. This security is reinforced by her being at his beck and call. In these emotional relations with the mother the child is introduced to learning, and later to imitation. We have previously mentioned that the motherless children in Foundling Home are unable to speak, to feed themselves, or to acquire habits of cleanliness: it is the security provided by the mother in the field of locomotion, the emotional bait offered by the mother calling her child, that "teaches" him to walk. When this is lacking, even children two to three years old cannot walk.

The children in Foundling Home have, theoretically, as much radius of locomotion as the children in Nursery. They did not at first have toys, but they could have exerted their grasping and tactile activity on the blankets, on their clothes, even on the bars of the cots. We have seen children in Nursery without toys; they are the exception—but the lack of material is not enough to hamper them in the acquisition of locomotor and grasping skills. The presence of a mother or her substitute is sufficient to compensate for all the other deprivations.

It is true that the children in Foundling Home are condemned to solitary confinement in their cots. But we do not think that it is the lack of perceptual stimulation *in general* that counts in their deprivation. We believe that they suffer because their perceptual world is emptied of human partners, that their isolation cuts them off from any stimulation by any persons who could signify mother representatives for the child at this age. The result, as Figure 1 shows, is a complete restriction of psychic capacity by the end of the first year.

This restriction of psychic capacity is not a temporary phenomenon. It is, as can be seen from the curve, a progressive process. How much this deterioration could have been arrested if the children were taken out of the institution at the end of the first year is an open question. The fact that they remain in Foundling Home probably furthers this progressive process. By the end of the second year the developmental quotient sinks to 45, which corresponds to a mental age of approximately ten months, and would qualify these children as imbeciles.

The curve of the children in Nursery does not deviate significantly from the normal. The curve sinks at two points, between the sixth and seventh, and between the tenth and twelfth months. These deviations are within the normal range; their significance will be discussed in a separate article. It has nothing to do with the influence of institutions, for the curve of the village group is nearly identical.

VI. PROVISIONAL CONCLUSIONS

The contrasting pictures of these two institutions show the significance of the mother-child relationship for the development of the child during the first year. Deprivations in other fields, such as perceptual and locomotor radius, can all be compensated by adequate mother-child relations. "Adequate" is not here a vague general term. The examples chosen represent the two extremes of the scale.

The children in Foundling Home do have a mother—for a time, in the beginning—but they must share her immediately with at least one other child, and from three months on, with seven other children. The quantitative factor here is evident. There is a point under which the mother-child relations cannot be restricted during the child's first year without inflicting irreparable damage. On the other hand, the exaggerated mother-child relationship in Nursery introduces a different quantitative factor. To anyone familiar with the field it is surprising that Nursery should achieve such excellent results, for we know that institutional care is destructive for children during their first year; but in Nursery the destructive factors have been compensated by the increased intensity of the mother-child relationship.

These findings should not be construed as a recommendation for overprotection of children. In principle the libidinal situation of Nursery is almost as undesirable as the other extreme in Foundling Home. Neither in the nursery of a penal institution nor in a foundling home for parentless children can the normal libidinal situation that obtains in a family home be expected. The two institutions have here been chosen as experimental setups for the purpose of examining variations in libidinal factors ranging from extreme frustration to extreme gratification. That the extreme frustration practiced in Foundling Home has deplorable consequences has been shown; the extreme gratification in Nursery can be tolerated by the children housed there for two reasons: (1) The mothers have the benefit of the intelligent guidance of the head nurse and her assistants, and the worst exaggerations are thus corrected. (2) Children during their first year of life can stand the ill effects of such a situation much better than at a later age. In this respect Nursery has wisely limited the duration of the children's stay to the first 12 months. For children older than this we should consider a libidinal setup such as that in Nursery very dangerous indeed.

VII. Further Problems

This is the first of a series of publications on the results of a research project on infancy that we are conducting. As such it is a preliminary report. It is not intended to show more than the most general outline of the results of early institutional care, giving at the same time a hint of the approach we use. The series of other problems on which this investigation has shed some light, as well as the formulation of those problems that could be recognized as such only in the course of the investigation, have not been touched upon in our present study and can only summarily be touched upon; they are headings, as it were, of the chapters of our future program of publication.

Apart from the severe developmental retardation, the most striking single factor observed in Foundling Home was the change in the pattern of the reaction to strangers in the last third of the first year (Gesell & Thompson, 1934). The usual behavior was replaced by something that could vary from extreme friendliness to any human partner combined with anxious avoidance of inanimate objects, to a generalized anxiety expressed in bloodcurdling screams which could go on indefinitely. It is evident that these deviant behavior patterns require a more thorough and extensive discussion than our present study would have permitted.

We also observed extraordinary deviations from the normal in the time of appearance and disappearance of familiar developmental patterns; and certain phenomena unknown in the normal child, such as bizarre stereotyped motor patterns distinctly reminiscent of the stereotypy in catatonic motility. These and other phenomena observed in Foundling Home require an extensive discussion in order to determine which are to be classified as maturation phenomena (which appear even under the most unfavorable circumstances, and which appear with commensurate retardation when retardation is general); or which can be considered as the first symptoms of the development of serious psychiatric disturbances. In connection with this problem a more thorough discussion of the rapidity with which the developmental quotients recede in Foundling Home is intended.

Another study is to deal with the problems created by the enormous overprotection practiced in Nursery.

And finally the rationale of the one institutional routine as against that of the other will have to be discussed in greater detail. This study will offer the possibility of deciding how to compensate for unavoidable changes in the environment of children orphaned at an early age. It will also shed some light on the social consequences of the progressive disruption of home life caused by the increase of female labor and by the demands of war; we might state that we foresee in the course of events a corresponding increase in asociality, in the number of problem and delinquent children, of mental defectives, and of psychotics.

It will be necessary to take into consideration in our institutions, in our charitable activities, in our social legislation, the overwhelming and unique importance of adequate and satisfactory mother-child relationship during the first year, if we want to decrease the unavoidable and irreparable psychiatric consequences deriving from neglect during this period.

Hospitalism:
A Follow-up Report

I

The striking picture of the infants studied in Foundling Home encouraged us to make every effort to get whatever information we could on the further development of the individual children. Distance made it impossible for the author to attend to this personally. The investigator who assisted in the original study was therefore directed to ascertain, at regular intervals, certain objectively observable facts on all those infants who were still available. He visited Foundling Home during the two years following our own study, at four-monthly intervals. On these occasions, equipped with a questionnaire prepared by the author, he asked the nursing personnel a series of questions. He observed each child's general behavior, and tried to make contact with each. He took some motion pictures of them, and a set of stills at the end of the two years. Finally, some bodily measurements, namely, weight, height, and occipital circumference, were taken.

The questions referred to three principal sectors of personality:

1. Bodily performance: the gross indicator used was whether the child could sit, stand, or walk.

2. Intellectual capacity to handle materials: the gross indicator used was whether the child was capable of eating food alone with the help of a spoon, and whether he could dress alone.

3. Social relations: these were explored by ascertaining the number of words spoken by each child, and by finding out whether he was toilet trained.

We are only too well aware that the resulting information is inadequate for a thorough study. As will be seen, however, even this inadequate follow-up yields a number of instructive data.

As is usually the case in follow-up investigations, only a relatively small number of the children originally seen could be checked on. Two years ago, when we first visited the ward reserved for the children from birth to 1½ years, and the ward for children from 1½ to 3 years, a total of 91 children were present. In the course of the first year, 27 of these died of various

Reprinted from *The Psychoanalytic Study of the Child*, Vol. 2. New York: International Universities Press, 1946, pp. 113–117.

causes, among which were an epidemic of measles, intercurrent sickness, and cachexia; by the end of the second year, another 7 of those originally seen had died; this represents a total mortality of over 37 percent in a period of two years.

Thirty-six children could not be learned about because 23 had been taken back to their families; 7 had been adopted (mostly by their own illegitimate parents); 2 had been placed in children's institutions; and 4 could not be accounted for.

At the time of this writing[1] 21 children of those originally seen are still at the institution. Of these the youngest is two years of age, the oldest four years and one month. The data on their development are as follows:

1. Bodily development:

Incapable of any locomotion		5
Sit up unassisted (without walking)		3
Walk assisted		8
Walk unassisted		5
	Total	21

2. Handling materials:

Cannot eat alone with spoon		12
Eat alone with spoon		9
	Total	21
Cannot dress alone		20
Dresses alone		1
	Total	21

3. Adaptation to demands of environment:

Not toilet trained in any way		6
Toilet trained, partially[2]		15
	Total	21

4. Speech development:

Cannot talk at all		6
Vocabulary: 2 words		5
Vocabulary: 3 to 5 words		8
Vocabulary: a dozen words		1
Uses sentences		1
	Total	21

[1] June 12, 1946.

[2] These children are trained "to a certain extent." According to my observer many of the so-called "toilet trained" children were found to soil in their beds; their training appears to be limited to their making use of the toilet when put on it.

As seen from these data, the mental development of these 21 children is extraordinarily retarded, compared to that of normal children between the ages of two and four, who move, climb, and babble all day long, and who conform to or struggle against the educational demands of the environment. This retardation, which amounts to a deterioration, is borne out by the weights and heights of these children, as well as by their pictures.

Normal children, by the end of the second year weigh, on the average, 26½ pounds, and the length is 33½ inches. At the time of this writing, 12 of the children in Foundling Home range in age between 2.4 and 2.8; 4, between 2.8 and 3.2; and 5, between 3.2 and 4.1. But of all of these children, only 3 fall into the weight range of a normal *2-year-old* child, and only 2 have attained the length of a normal child of that age. All others fall below the normal 2-year-level—in one case, as much as 45 percent in weight and 5 inches in length. In other words, the physical picture of these children impresses the casual observer as that of children half their age.

In our previous article on the subject (Spitz, 1945b) we expressed the suspicion that the damage inflicted on the infants in Foundling Home by their being deprived of maternal care, maternal stimulation, and maternal love, as well as by their being completely isolated, is irreparable. Our follow-up confirms this assumption. After their fifteenth month, these children were put into more favorable environmental conditions than before, i.e., in the ward for the older children. This is a large room, sunny, without the partitions which in the ward for the younger children isolated the infants from each other and from every environmental stimulus. Three to five nurses are constantly in the room, and they chat with each other and with the children. The children are also taken out of their cots and placed on the floor. Thus they have infinitely more active stimulation than they previously experienced in the ward for younger children. Notwithstanding this improvement in environmental conditions, the process of deterioration has proved to be progressive. It would seem that the developmental imbalance caused by the unfavorable environmental conditions during the children's first year produces a psychosomatic damage that cannot be repaired by normal measures. Whether it can be repaired by therapeutic measures remains to be investigated.

We have advisedly spoken of psychosomatic damage. From the figures given above it can be seen that quite apart from the inadequate psychic and physical development, all these children showed a seriously decreased resistance to disease, and an appalling mortality. Those who survived were all far below the age-adequate weight reached by normal children of comparable age.

II

In view of these findings we once again examined the data on Nursery, the institution compared to Foundling Home in our previous article. The organization of Nursery did not permit a follow-up extended to the fifth year, as did that of Foundling Home. As a rule children leave Nursery when they are a full year old. However, a certain number of exceptions are made in this rule, and in the course of our study of Nursery, which now covers a period of 3½ years, 29 children were found who stayed longer than a year. The age at which these left varied from the thirteenth to the eighteenth month (1.1 to 1.6). This means that the *oldest* of them was *half a year younger* than the youngest child in our follow-up in Foundling Home, and *2½ years younger than the oldest*. In spite of this enormous difference in age, the Nursery children all ran lustily around on the floor; some of them dressed and undressed themselves; they fed themselves with a spoon; nearly all spoke a few words; they understood commands and obeyed them; and the older ones showed a certain consciousness of toilet requirements. All of them played lively social games with each other and with the observers. The more advanced ones imitated the activities of the nurses, sweeping the floor, carrying and distributing diapers, etc. In all these children, tests showed that the developmental quotients which in the eleventh and twelfth months had receded somewhat,[3] not only came up to the normal age level, but in most cases surpassed it by far.

But the gross physical picture alone, as expressed by the figures on morbidity and mortality of the children in Nursery, is sufficiently striking. During the 3½ years of our study of Nursery we had occasion to follow 122 infants, each for approximately a full year.[4] During this time *not a single child died*. The institution was visited by no epidemic. Intercurrent sickness was limited, on the whole, to seasonal colds, which in a moderate number developed into mild respiratory involvement; there was comparatively little intestinal disturbance; the most disturbing illness was eczema. The unusually high level of health maintained in Nursery impelled us to look into its past record. We investigated the files of Nursery for 10 years prior to the beginning of our work there. We found that during the whole of the last 14 years a total of three children have died: one of pneumonia at the age of three months; and two of pyloric stenosis, the first at the age of one month, the second after several operations at the age of nine months.

---

[3] The average retardation in the developmental quotient was approximately 12 points during the eleventh and twelfth months.

[4] Exceptions to this are 6 children who because of circumstances in their families left before their tenth month. This is more than counterbalanced by the group of 29 children who stayed longer than one year.

It is in the light of these findings, which show what can be achieved in an institution under favorable circumstances and adequate organization, that the consequences of the methods used in Foundling Home should be evaluated.

Anaclitic Depression:
An Inquiry into the Genesis of Psychiatric
Conditions in Early Childhood, II

with the assistance of KATHERINE M. WOLF, Ph.D.

I. OBSERVATION

A. A CIRCUMSCRIBED PSYCHIATRIC SYNDROME

In the course of a long-term study of infant behavior in a nursery (Spitz, 1945b) where we observed 123 unselected infants, each for a period of 12 to 18 months, we encountered a striking syndrome. In the second half of the first year, a few of these infants developed a weepy behavior that was in marked contrast to their previously happy and outgoing behavior. After a time this weepiness gave way to withdrawal. The children in question would lie in their cots with averted faces, refusing to take part in the life of their surroundings. When we approached them we were ignored. Some of these children would watch us with a searching expression. If we were insistent enough, weeping would ensue and, in some cases, screaming. The sex of the approaching experimenter made no difference in the reaction in the majority of cases. Such behavior would persist for 2 to 3 months. During this period some of these children lost weight instead of gaining; the nursing personnel reported that some suffered from insomnia, which in one case led to segregation of the child. All showed a greater susceptibility to intercurrent colds or eczema. A gradual decline in the developmental quotient was observed in these cases.

This behavior syndrome lasted three months. Then the weepiness subsided, and stronger provocation became necessary to provoke it. A sort of frozen rigidity of expression appeared instead. These children would lie or sit with wide-open, expressionless eyes, frozen, immobile face, and a faraway expression as if in a daze, apparently not perceiving what went on in their envi-

Reprinted from *The Psychoanalytic Study of the Child*, Vol. 2. New York: International Universities Press, 1946, pp. 313–342.

ronment. This behavior was in some cases accompanied by autoerotic activities in the oral, anal, and genital zones. Contact with children who arrived at this stage became increasingly difficult and finally impossible. At best, screaming was elicited.

Among the 123 unselected children observed during the whole of the first year of their life we found this clear-cut syndrome in 19 cases. The gross picture of these cases showed many, if not all, of these traits. Individual differences were partly quantitative: i.e., one or the other trait, as for instance weeping, would for a period dominate the picture, and thus would impress the casual observer as the only one present; and partly qualitative: i.e., there was an attitude of complete withdrawal in some cases, as against others in which, when we succeeded in breaking through the rejection of any approach, we found a desperate clinging to the grown-up. But apart from such individual differences the clinical picture was so distinctive that once we had called attention to it, it was easily recognizable by even untrained observers. It led us to assume that we were confronted with a psychiatric syndrome, which we illustrate in the three case histories following.

B. CASE HISTORIES

Case 1. Colored female. No significant events or behavior during the first half year. She is a particularly friendly child who smiles brilliantly at the approach of the experimenter.

When she was 7½ months old we noticed that her radiant smiling behavior had ceased. During the following two weeks it was impossible to approach her, as she slept heavily during the total of 12 hours we were there. After this period a change of behavior took place, which was protocolled as follows:

"She lay immobile in her crib. When approached she did not lift her shoulders, barely her head, to look at the experimenter with an expression of profound suffering sometimes seen in sick animals. With this expression she examined the observer. As soon as the observer started to speak to her or to touch her she began to weep. This was not the usual crying of babies which is always accompanied by a certain amount of vocalization going into screaming. It was a soundless weeping, tears running down her face. Speaking to her in soft comforting tones only resulted in the weeping becoming more intense, intermingled with moans and sobs, shaking her whole body.

"In the course of a two months' observation it was found that this reaction deepened. It was more and more difficult to make contact with the child. In our protocols there is a note seven weeks later to the effect that it took us almost an hour to achieve contact with her. In this period she lost weight and developed a serious feeding disturbance, having great difficulties in taking any food and in keeping it down."

After two months a certain measure was taken. The syndrome disappeared.

Case 2. White female. Intelligent, friendly child who smiles easily and ecstatically at the approaching observer. No notable event in the course of the first seven months. At this time a change occurred in the child. The observers got the feeling that the child was apprehensive. A week or two later the change was accentuated. The temper of the child had become unequal. She still was mostly friendly to the observer, but as often as not broke out crying when the observer approached closer. After another two weeks she could no longer be approached. No amount of persuasion helped. Whenever approached she sat up and wailed. Two weeks later, she would lie on her face, indifferent to the outside world, not interested in the other children living in the same room. Only strong stimulation could get her out of her apathy. She would then sit up and stare at the observer wide-eyed, a tragic expression on her face, silent. She would not accept toys, in fact she withdrew from them into the farthest corner of her bed. If the approach was pressed she would break into tears. This went on until the child was nine months old.

At this point a certain measure was taken. The syndrome disappeared.

Case 3. White female. This is a moderately intelligent, unusually beautiful child with enormously big blue eyes and golden curls. At the end of the eleventh month the child, who never had been very active, began to lose interest in playing with the experimenter, so that testing became difficult. In the following two weeks this behavior was more marked. The child was not only passive, but refused to touch any toys offered to her. She sat in a sort of daze, by the hour, staring silently into space. She did not even show the apprehensiveness in the presence of the approaching observer that was shown by other children. If a toy was put into contact with her she would withdraw into the farthest corner of her bed and there sit wide-eyed, absent, and without contact, with an immobile rigid expression on her beautiful face. When the toys were left with her she did not touch them until the experimenter had left the room. Then she immediately threw them out of her bed, where one would find them five or ten minutes later, forming a half-circle around the child, who would be sitting again in the same posture as before, or lying on her face. At 11 months, 25 days (0; 11 + 25) she was observed to alternate playing with her feces with genital masturbation, still in the same position described above. The fecal play would consist in her pulling a small pellet of feces the size of a very small pea out of her soiled diaper. With the same rigid immobile expression and rigid immobile body, she would roll this pellet on the sheet, pick it up, roll it between thumb and forefinger without looking at it, lose it from her fingers, and eagerly seek it again on the sheet. The time when she was seeking it on the sheet was the only moment when the rigid expression disappeared; and a near smile appeared when she had found it again. Alternately, she would rub her genitals.

As in the other cases, a certain measure was taken, in this case when the child was 11 months, 30 days (0; 11 + 30). The syndrome disappeared.

In all three cases the measure taken was the restitution of the mother, from whom the child had been separated approximately three to four months earlier.

II. Discussion of the Syndrome

In the three case histories the principal symptoms composing the syndrome are manifest. These symptoms fall into several categories; within each category we have grouped them on a scale of increasing severity. They are not all necessarily present at the same time, but most of them show up at one point or another in the clinical picture. They are:

Apprehension, sadness, weepiness.
Lack of contact, rejection of environment, withdrawal.
Retardation of development, retardation of reaction to stimuli, slowness of movement, dejection, stupor.
Loss of appetite, refusal to eat, loss of weight.
Insomnia.

To this symptomatology should be added the physiognomic expression in these cases, which is difficult to describe. This expression would in an adult be described as depression.

A. ETIOLOGY

1. General environment

Table 1 shows the sex and race distribution of our sample. These 123 infants stayed in the nursery from their fourteenth day to the end of their first year and in a few cases up to their eighteenth month. No selection was made in the infants observed. We invariably tested and followed each child admitted to the nursery up to the day when it left. The observations took place at weekly intervals, and totalled approximately 400 hours for each child. All these infants shared the same environment, the same care, food, and hygiene.

An apparently milder form of the syndrome presented in our three case histories, with a similar drop in developmental quotient, was observed in 26 cases.

We shall now proceed to investigate the factors in the background and in

TABLE 1.

	White	Colored	Totals
Male	37	24	61
Female	40	22	62
Total	77	46	123

the environment of these cases in order to isolate those that are etiologically significant.

2. Factors without demonstrable influence on the causation of the syndrome

a. Race and Sex. Tables 2 and 3 show the distribution of the different degrees of depression according to color and sex.   The factors of color and of sex do not appear to exert demonstrable influence on the incidence of the syndrome.

TABLE 2. DISTRIBUTION ACCORDING TO RACE

	White	Colored	Totals
Severe depression	7	12	19
Mild depression	17	9	26
No depression	32	18	50
No diagnosis[a]	21	7	28
Total	77	46	123

TABLE 3. DISTRIBUTION ACCORDING TO SEX

	Male	Female	Totals
Severe depression	9	10	19
Mild depression	13	13	26
No depression	26	24	50
No diagnosis	13	15	28
Total	61	62	123

b. Chronological age. The youngest age at which the syndrome was manifested in our series was around the turn of the sixth month; the oldest was

[a] As in any psychiatric study, no exact diagnosis could be made in a certain number of cases. We include them in our tables for the purpose of showing the proportion of such undiagnosed cases within unselected total of observed children.

the eleventh month. The syndrome therefore seems to be independent of chronological age, within certain limits.

c. *Developmental and intellectual level*. It might be objected that in early childhood the developmental age is more significant than the chronological age. A hypothesis might state that a certain level of intelligence is prerequisite for any psychiatric syndrome. However, we have found the syndrome in question in children whose development was advanced by two months beyond their chronological age, just as well as in children whose development was one month retarded, as compared to their chronological age; the developmental quotients of the children affected would vary from 91 to 133; nor did the syndrome appear earlier in the children with the higher developmental quotient. So it would seem that within reasonable limits these factors play no significant role in the formation of the syndrome. Table 4 shows the average of the developmental quotients of the children with no disturbance, with mild disturbance, and with severe disturbance.

TABLE 4.

	Average developmental quotient
Severe depression	110
Mild depression	109
Others	109

3. *An etiologically significant factor*

There is one factor which all cases that developed the syndrome had in common. In all of them the mother was removed from the child somewhere between the sixth and eighth month for a practically unbroken period of three months, during which the child either did not see its mother at all, or at best once a week. This removal took place for unavoidable external reasons. Before the separation the mother had the full care of the infant, and as a result of special circumstances spent more time with the child than is usual in a private home. In each case a striking change in the child's behavior could be observed in the course of the four to six weeks following the mother's removal. The syndrome described above would then develop. *No* child developed the syndrome in question whose mother was *not* removed. Our proposition is that the syndrome observed developed only in children who were deprived of their love object for an appreciable period of time during their first year of life.

On the other hand, not all children whose mothers were removed developed the same syndrome. Hence, mother separation is a necessary, but not a sufficient cause for the development of the syndrome. The additional etiological factors which are required to make it effective in producing a depression will be touched upon in a later part of this paper, and discussed at length in a paper in preparation.

4. Reactions to the loss of the love object

The syndrome in question is extremely similar to that which is familiar to us from Abraham's (1912) and Freud's (1917b) classical descriptions of mourning, pathological mourning, and melancholia. The factor which appears to be of decisive etiological significance in our cases is the loss of the love object; this brings the syndrome closer to the consequences of the loss of the love object, as described by these authors. In melancholia there is added the feeling of being unloved, along with an incapacity to love, self-reproach, and suicidal tendencies. The absence of these symptoms in the child can be attributed to two reasons: (1) the child's fewer resources; (2) the difference in psychic structure between adult and infant.

As regards the greater resources of the adult: an adult suffering from melancholia is capable of expressing verbally that he feels unloved and that he is incapable of feeling love for anybody. We suspect that a child who up to a certain point was outgoing and friendly, but who now withdraws from every friendly approach, is expressing the same thing with the equipment at his disposal. We have of course no way of verifying this suspicion, just as we have no way of knowing whether anything like self-reproach can exist in a ten-month-old baby, even though it deprives itself of its usual enjoyment of toys or food. Nor can the infant enact a suicide; but it is striking that these cases one and all show a great susceptibility to intercurrent sickness.[1]

The difference in psychic structure between child and adult is far-reaching in its consequences. In the adult we have a well-established organization consisting of id, ego, and superego. Particularly the manifestations of the superego are conspicuous in melancholia.

In the infant, during the first year, only an id and a still weak—one might nearly say nascent—ego are available. The weakness of the ego makes it especially vulnerable to such a trauma as the loss of the love object is to the adult. On the other hand, we may expect that just because the infantile ego is not yet well-knit nor firmly established, it may be more amenable than that of the adult in accepting a substitute love object. Severe traumata in the case of the adult impinge on a solid, complete ego organization, and force it into

---

[1] This is strongly borne out in another series of cases observed in another institution. These were of a more severe nature—the resulting mortality among the children involved took on the aspect of a major catastrophe. See "Hospitalism," this volume.

a regression to an earlier fixation point. Not so in the case of the infant. Here the injury will be manifested in the form of a disturbance of the ego development. This can take the form of a retardation, or a deformation, or even of a destructive paralysis of ego development, dependent on the severity and the duration of the trauma.

Accordingly, clinical pictures vary in severity from temporary developmental arrest to loss or inhibition of already acquired functions (one of the children observed by us was already able to stand alone when he lost his mother; for the following three months he stayed supine or at best stayed in his cot), and in extreme cases result in irreversible progressive personality distortion. On the other hand, since the infant's ego organization is in the process of development, recovery from damage that is not irreparable is swifter, more dramatic than in the case of the adult.

The clinical picture of the consequences of the loss of the love object will be as varied in the infant as in the adult. In the adult we encounter mourning, pathological mourning, depression, melancholia. We cannot yet distinguish the phenomena observed in infants in such detail. For the time being and for the purposes of the present paper, we discuss that form of the clinical picture which in our belief comes closest to what Fenichel described as "simple depression," in his elaboration of the earlier findings on preoedipal infantile depression, called by Abraham (1912) "primal parathymia." In view of the etiological factors which appeared in our findings, we prefer to follow a suggestion of R. M. Kaufman and to call the picture observed by us "anaclitic depression."

B. THE CONCEPT OF EARLY DEPRESSION IN THE LITERATURE

The psychoanalytic significance of the clinical symptomatology of melancholia was described by Abraham (1912, 1916, 1924), and Freud (1917b). Both emphasized its similarity to cases of mourning, a psychic manifestation belonging to the field of normalcy. In all publications on the subject it was stressed that both melancholia and normal mourning originate from the same kind of trauma, i.e., a loss of the love object, the difference between normal mourning and pathological mourning being in the existence in the latter of fixation points on the oral-sadistic level. The primal parathymia observed by Abraham is placed in the years immediately preceding the oedipal conflict, and the examples given are typical of precursors of oedipal experiences.

These suggestions of Abraham of course do not exclude the existence of a depression in the first year of life. Accordingly, Fenichel (1945) states:

> The formulation can now be made that the disposition for the development of

depressions consists in oral fixations which determine the reaction to narcissistic shocks. The experiences that cause the oral fixations may occur long before the decisive narcissistic shocks; or the narcissistic injury may create a depressive disposition because it occurs early enough to still be met by an orally oriented ego. It may also occur that certain narcissistic shocks, because they are connected with death (and the reaction to death is always oral introjection of the dead person), create the decisive oral fixation.

Regarding the factors that create oral fixations in the first place, the same holds true as for other fixations; the determinants are extraordinary satisfactions, extraordinary frustrations, or combinations of both, especially combinations of oral satisfaction with some reassuring guarantee of security; actually traumatic experiences in the nursing period can be found more often in subsequent manic-depressive patients than in schizophrenics [p. 405].

On the basis of our findings on 19 severe and 26 mild cases we believe that we are now in the position to offer clinical evidence for Fenichel's assumption that the equivalent of the primal parathymias described by Abraham can be observed during the first year of life.

In order to avoid the assumption that we are here speaking of what Melanie Klein (1944) calls "the depressive position" in infancy we now discuss her theoretical views.

In psychoanalytic theory, depression is an abnormal psychic manifestation, expressly considered the result of a specific environmental constellation. In the Kleinian system, depression is not only different in principle, but is also of primary significance as the cornerstone of the whole system. Melanie Klein (1932, 1940, 1944, 1945) considers depression the *fons et origo* of all human psychic development. She and her school (Heimann, Isaacs, Rickman, Riviere [1936], Rosenfeld, Scott, Winnicott) postulate the presence of a so-called "depressive position" in infancy. This, in their opinions, is the fundamental mechanism of the infant's psyche, disposing of powerfully operating instruments of introjection and projection, upon which all further psychic development is based.

Our findings do not represent a confirmation of the view of Melanie Klein and her school. She states (1944):

> The infantile depressive position arises when the infant perceives and introjects the mother as a whole person (between three and five months) . . . the assumption seems justified that the seeds of depressive feelings, in so far as the experience of birth gives rise to a feeling of loss, are there from the beginning of life. I suggest that the "depressive position" in infancy is a universal phenomenon.
>
> The coordination of functions and movements is bound with a defense mechanism which I take to be one of the fundamental processes in early development, namely the manic defense. This defense is closely linked with the "depressive position."

In other words: Melanie Klein posits a "depressive position" as an immutable stage in infantile psychic development, appearing between three and five months, irrespective of the child's individual history, experience, and environmental circumstances. She views the "depressive position" as part of the congenital equipment of every human being.

We are accustomed to consider our anatomical and physiological equipment as congenital. Of recent years, the tendency has been to restrict which psychic functions are to be considered inherited or congenital. Nonetheless, such endowments as neural patterns based on anatomic and physiological premises, as well as on developmental sequences; perceptive modes as expressed in the principles of Gestalt; perhaps even certain basic reactions as described in the Watsonian triad of love, fear, and rage are generally accepted as congenital and universal.

But the psychic element posited by Melanie Klein is of a very different nature from all of these. It is hard to conceive of the "depressive position" as a universal keystone of personality. We have become familiar with depression from the study of mental disease (of melancholia) in grown-ups. Psychoanalytic research, specifically that of Freud and of Abraham, demonstrated that it is a result of a regression to the oral-sadistic level of ego development. It would seem as if this finding had provoked a misinterpretation on the part of Melanie Klein. She appears to have concluded that since melancholia was a regression to the oral-sadistic level of the libido, the infant on progressing to this oral-sadistic level would have to develop melancholia. This of course is circular reasoning. Melancholia is the consequence of several factors, *one* of which is a fixation point at the oral-sadistic level of development. That fact in itself, however, is insufficient for the emergence of melancholia. Without the concurrence of certain experiential events dependent on environmental constellations, no melancholia will occur. The experiential events in question are of a severely frustrating nature and they presuppose the existence of some part of the ego organization which is to be frustrated. If these specific experiential events do not take place, or if they take place in a modified form, a completely different mental disease or perhaps even only a special character formation will emerge.

Melanie Klein, on the other hand, assumes that human beings are born with a finished and complete psychic structure. Here she falls into the same category as do other modifiers of psychoanalytic theory, like Adler, Jung, Rank, and Reich. Mostly they had an axe to grind, whether that was for the purpose of eliminating the problems of infantile sexuality from psychoanalytic theory, or of satisfying the postulates of an ideological allegiance. Thus, with the help of the trauma of birth, Rank (1924) saddled heredity plus the experience of birth with the responsibility for the etiology of neurosis, and reduced the role of infantile sexuality, oedipal experience, and environmental influence to insignificance.

In contrast to Melanie Klein and her group, when we speak of anaclitic depression in infants, we do not consider depression as *the* typical or as *a* typical mechanism of infantile psychic development. We do not consider depression as an integral element of the infantile psyche. To state that all human psychic development is determined by a "depressive position" in infancy makes as little sense as to state that erect human locomotion is determined by fracture or luxation in infancy—though some infants' gait at the outset may be vaguely reminiscent of a fractured or luxated limb. We speak of depression as a specific disease in infants arising under specific environmental conditions.

III. Diagnosis and Prognosis of the Syndrome

A. DIAGNOSIS.

The problem of diagnosis of psychiatric disturbance in early infancy, during the preverbal stage, is difficult. In the first place, the question arises whether in this stage anything in the nature of psychosis can exist. Psychosis is by definition a disturbance in the relations between the different spheres of the personality. It would therefore look as if the formation of a superego or, at the very least, those abstractive functions of the unconscious parts of the ego that ensure conceptual thinking, would have to be present to enable us to speak of psychosis in the infant. For if anything is certain, it is that the infant is not ruled by a superego, nor does it dispose of abstractive functions in any way demonstrable before the age of approximately 18 months. Therefore that part of the psychotic destruction in the personality that involves the higher functions of the ego will not be manifested.

However, psychosis is characterized not only by delusion, disturbance of thought processes, abnormal thought production and mental confusion (memory defect, confabulation, impairment of apperception and attention, disorientation, ideational disorders, suspicion, etc.). It also involves modification of motility, grossly expressed by hypermotility, specific motor phenomena, or by hypomotility (catatonia, cataplexia, etc.); and it is more subtly manifested in the form of postural changes and pathognomonic expression. And finally, the most outstanding changes in the psychotic personality are those manifested in the affects. The changes in motility and the affective disorders are manifestations that do not require the presence of a fully organized ego capable of conceptual thinking, let alone the presence of a superego. Disturbance in these two fields presupposes an elementary organization of the ego, enabling it to perform the function of a coordinating center for elementary perception and apperception, for elementary volitional coordination of motility, as well as a capacity for such elementary differentiation of affect as is involved in the capacity to produce distinctly discernible positive or negative affective reactions on appropriate stimulation. This stage is reached when the child arrives at the second half of the first year of life (Hetzer and Wolf, 1928; Spitz, 1945a).

At this stage the child is capable, as we have stated above, of reacting to environmental experience by demonstrable affective disorders. We will show further on that gross disorders of motility are also manifested. The more subtle disorders can be detected in the dejected pathognomonic expression and posture of these infants. They show an obvious distaste for assuming an erect position or performing locomotion. It is in such behavioral changes that we have to seek the evidence of the pathological process.

Manifest evidence of this process is unmistakable to the practiced eye. The poverty of the symptomatology reflects the exiguousness of the modes of expression and the number of activities available to children of this age. As a consequence of the pathological process even this small number of expressions and actions is reduced—or expressions and activities achieved in the normal course of development by the one-year-old do not materialize. Such a reduction in the performance, emotional and otherwise, of the infant are apt to impress the psychiatrist as an arrest in development rather than as a personality disorder. We believe—and we will bring proof of this in the further development of our case histories—that to consider the phenomena in question as an arrest in development only is to take a superficial view. The inadequacy of our means of communication with the infant is of course a severe handicap for diagnostic recognition of possible psychiatric disorders at this age. We are limited to the observation of behavior and its deviations; to the interpretation of visible manifestations of emotions; to the taking of a detailed anamnesis with the help of our own observation and that of the persons living with the child; and finally, to the quantifiable results of testing procedure. Thus the diagnostic signs and symptoms fall into the groups of static ones, genetic ones, and quantitative ones.

1. The static signs and symptoms

The static signs and symptoms are those observable phenomena that we are able to ascertain in the course of one or several observations of the infant in question. We have mentioned them in Part II of this study. One of the outstanding signs is the physiognomic expression of such patients. The observer at once notices an apprehensive or sad or depressed expression on the child's face, which often impels him to ask whether the child is sick. It is characteristic, at this stage, that the child makes an active attempt to catch the observer's attention and to involve him in a game. However, this outgoing introduction usually is not followed by particularly active play on the part of the child. In the main it is acted out in the form of clinging to the observer and in sorrowful disappointment at the observer's withdrawal.

In the next stage the apprehensiveness deepens. The observer's approach provokes crying or screaming, and the observer's departure does not evoke as universal a disappointment as previously. Many of the cases observed by us fall into the period of what has been described as "eight months anxiety" (C. Bühler, 1931; Hetzer and Wolf, 1928; Shirley, 1933; Jersild and Holmes, 1935).

The so-called "eight months anxiety" begins somewhere between the sixth and eighth month and is a product of the infant's increasing capacity for diacritic discrimination (Spitz, 1946d) between friend and stranger. As a result of this the approaching stranger is received either by what has been described as "coy" or "bashful" behavior, or by the child's turning away, hanging its head, crying, and even screaming in the presence of a stranger, and refusing to play with him or to accept toys. The difference between this behavior and the behavior in anaclitic depression is a quantitative one. While in anaclitic depression, notwithstanding every effort, it takes upwards of an hour to achieve contact with the child and to get it to play, in the eight months anxiety this contact can be achieved with the help of appropriate behavior in a span of time ranging from one to ten minutes. The appropriate behavior is very simple: it consists in sitting down next to the cot of the child with one's back turned to him and without paying any attention to him. After the above mentioned period of one to ten minutes the child will take the initiative, grab the observer's gown or hand—and with this the contact is established, and any experienced child psychologist can lead from this into playing with the child's active and happy participation. In the anaclitic depression nothing of the sort occurs. The child does not touch the observer, the approach has to be moderately active on the observer's part, and consists mostly in patient waiting, untiringly repeated attempts at cuddling or petting the child, and incessant offers of constantly varied toys. The latter must be offered with a capacity to understand the nature of the child's refusal. Some toys create anxiety in some children and have an opposite effect on others; for example, some children are attracted by bright colors but are immediately made panicky if a noise such as drumming is provoked in connection with this brightly colored toy. Others may be attracted by the rhythmic noise. Some are delighted by dolls, others go into a panic and can be reassured by no method at the sight of a doll. Some who are delighted by a spinning top will break into tears when it stops spinning and falls over, and every further attempt to spin it will evoke renewed protest.

When finally contact is made the pathognomonic expression does not brighten; after having accepted the observer the child plays without any expression of happiness. He does not play actively and is severely retarded in all his behavior manifestations. The only signs of his having achieved contact is, on the one hand, his acceptance of toys; and on the other, his expression of grief and his crying when left by the observer. That this qualitative distinction is not an arbitrary one, can be seen from the fact that in a certain number of the cases in which the anaclitic depression was manifested late, we could observe the eight months anxiety as well as the anaclitic depression at periods distinct from each other. In one case, for instance, the eight months anxiety actually appeared at 0;7 + 14 and had already completely subsided and disappeared when the anaclitic depression was manifested at 0;11 + 2.

In the next stage the outward appearance of the child is that of complete withdrawal, dejection, and turning away from the environment. In the case of these children, even the lay person with good empathy for children has no difficulty in making the diagnosis, and will tell the observer that the child is grieving for his mother.

2. The genetic signs

The genetic signs can be disclosed with the help of a longitudinal investigation of the infant's development. A careful anamnesis reveals that before the above described attitude set in, the child was a pleasant, smiling, friendly baby. If the observer is lucky he may ascertain whether the child is already past the eight months anxiety, that it has come and gone. If the nursing staff reports a sudden development of changed behavior in the child without demonstrable organic disease and if this can be correlated to a separation from the child's mother or mother substitute, our suspicion as to the presence of anaclitic depression will be confirmed. It should not be overlooked that when we speak of the mother we are using a term which should really cover a wider field. "Love object" would be the more correct expression and we should say that these children suffer a loss of their love object.

3. Quantitative signs

Quantitative signs can be detected by consecutive developmental tests which, if compared to each other, will at the beginning of the anaclitic depression show a gradual drop of the developmental quotient; this drop progresses with the progression of the disorder.

B. PROGNOSIS: WITH INTERVENTION

In the three case histories given by us in the beginning we ended by stating that a certain measure was taken in each case, whereupon the syndrome disappeared. The measure taken was in the nature of environmental manipulation. It consisted in returning the mother to the child. The change in the children's observable behavior was dramatic. They suddenly were friendly, gay, approachable. The withdrawal, the disinterest, the rejection of the outside world, the sadness, disappeared as if by magic. But over and beyond these changes most striking was the jump in the developmental quotient, within a period of twelve hours after the mother's return; in some cases, as much as 36.6 percent higher than the previous measurement.

Thus one would assume that if adequate therapeutic measures are taken, the process is curable with extreme rapidity and the prognosis is good. The last statement requires some qualification. To our regret we have not been and are not in a position to follow the children in question beyond a maximum of 18 months. It is therefore open to question whether the psychic trauma sustained by them as a consequence of being separated from their mothers will leave traces which will become visible only later in life. We are inclined to suspect something of the sort. For the sudden astonishing jump in the developmental quotient on the return of the love object is not maintained in all cases. We have observed cases in which, after a period of two weeks, the developmental quotient dropped again. It did not drop to the previous low levels reached during the depression. However, compared to these children's predepression performance, the level on which they were functioning after their recovery was not adequate.

The spectacular recovery achieved by the children we observed again places before us the question whether we are justified in calling the syndrome a depression and, if so, whether it should be considered as a phenomenon of more than transitory importance, whether it should not be equated to the transitory depression observable in adults—whether indeed it should not be equated to mourning rather than to depression. (See Appendix, A1., paragraph 2.)

C. PROGNOSIS: WITHOUT INTERVENTION

The main reason why, apart from all physiognomic, behavioral, and other traits, we feel justified in speaking of an anaclitic depression going far beyond mourning and even beyond pathological mourning is that we have observed a number of cases in which no intervention occurred and where it became only too evident that the process was in no way self-limiting. These cases were the ones observed in Foundling Home.[2] In that institution, where medical, hygienic, and nutritional standards were comparable to those obtaining

[2] Described in an earlier paper ("Hospitalism," this volume). As there, to facilitate distinction between the two institutions, we call the one in which cases described up to now were cared for. "Nursery," and the one we are about to describe, "Foundling Home."

in Nursery, the separation from the mother took place beginning after the third month, but prevalently in the sixth month. However, whereas in Nursery the separation was temporary and the love object was restored after approximately three months of absence, in Foundling Home the love object was not restored. The picture of depression was as clear-cut as in Nursery, with some additional developments: for the picture of children in advanced extreme cases varied from stuporous deteriorated catatonia to agitated idiocy.

If we compare the pictures of the two institutions we are confronted with a syndrome of a progressive nature which after having reached a critical point of development appears to become irreversible. It is this characteristic which causes us to call the picture depression and not mourning. And beyond this, in Foundling Home we encounter a phenomenon more grave than melancholia. Notwithstanding the satisfactory hygiene and asepsis, the rate of mortality of the infants reared there was inordinately high. In the course of two years, 34 of the 91 children observed died of diseases varying from respiratory and intestinal infections to measles and otitis media. In some cases the cause of death was in the nature of cachexia. This phenomenon savors of psychosomatic involvement.

No intervention was effective in the case of the longer lasting separation in Foundling Home. This finding is one of the reasons why we spoke of three months as a critical period. The second reason is that in Nursery we observed towards the end of the three months the appearance of that kind of frozen, affect-impoverished expression which had strongly impressed us in Foundling Home. Furthermore, a curious reluctance to touch objects was manifested, combined with certain unusual postures of hands and fingers which seemed to us the precursors of the extremely bizarre hand and finger movements composing the total activity in those infants of Foundling Home whom we described as presenting a picture of stuporous catatonia.

After their recovery in the course of their further development, which to our regret could not be followed beyond 1½ years, the children in Nursery did not show any spectacular changes. As indicated above it, is therefore impossible at this point to state whether this early depression left any visible traces. One would be inclined to expect it. One would be inclined to expect some fixation.

IV. The Therapy: Dynamic and Structural Considerations

A. THE RUDIMENTARY EGO

1. As in melancholia (Fenichel, 1945, p. 402; Harnik, 1932) there occur in anaclitic depression more or less successful attempts to regain the lost objective world. The term "attempts at restitution" has been reserved by

Freud for certain phenomena in schizophrenia. The attempts to regain the lost objective world in melancholia and also in anaclitic depression take the form of finding a substitute object (Abraham, 1924; Jacobson, 1943; Fenichel, 1945, p. 404). We will therefore call this trend "attempts at substitution." These attempts form part of recuperative trends which become visible in anaclitic depression as they do in any other disease. We will encounter them in the course of our further discussion.

During the depressive stage of melancholia when the superego intolerably oppresses the ego, the outcome can only be a complete destruction of the individual, as in suicide. Against these demands of the superego we have the reaction of the id drives. This reaction, however, is unsuccessful because the superego produces anxiety, forcing the id drives along the path dictated by the pleasure-pain principle; thus one part of the id drives is put into the service of the destructive superego demands. This part is represented by the desexualized id drive.

In case of a favorable outcome, however, the aggressive id drive is not completely desexualized. The sex-fused portion of the aggressive drive then may remain available to the ego. If such is the case it may be used in the interest of those self-curative tendencies which every living organization will manifest both in organic and psychic sickness. In its attempts to comply with the superego's demands the sex-fused id drive is used in the establishment of a compulsive system. Through the compulsive neurotic behavior and its rigid adherence to arbitrarily established rules, the superego can be at least temporarily satisfied that, with great sacrifices, its demands are being complied with. With this a remission (in the picture of an obsessional neurosis with compulsive ritual) begins, and thus interrupts the progress of melancholia.

2. Another outcome is possible if the ego does not succeed in putting the sex-fused id drives in the service of the appeasement of the superego, but the superego on the other hand does not succeed either in putting the defused drives into the service of its own destructive tendencies. In this case the id drives, aggressive and sexual, are shunted into an ego reinforcement. This then enables the ego to overpower, as it were, the superego, and to incorporate it into itself. As in the depressive phase, the imago of the love object is introjected, whereupon the fury of the superego is unleashed against it; so in the manic phase, the superego, which in itself is the recipient of the archaic imagines of the original love objects, is now incorporated in the ego. The result is that the limits between the systems are abolished, and the manic picture develops.

Both outcomes of the manic-depressive process center around the ego and can be considered as representing attempts of the ego to escape annihilation;

and it is in view of this that we consider them recuperative trends even when they are unsuccessful.

Such trends presuppose, however, the presence of the three systems, id, ego, and superego. In the infant the superego is absent, so that it is impossible to assume destructive hostility of the superego. However, the loss of the love object in itself is equivalent to a hostile deprivation for the infant. The organization with which the infant can react to this deprivation is its ego, inadequate as it is at this period. As Freud established, the ego at this early age is mainly a body ego. The organizations of which the ego disposes are (1) a very rudimentary ideational organization, barely adequate for diffuse hallucinatory processes, and (2) a rapidly developing locomotor system.

B. RECUPERATIVE TRENDS VERSUS INSTITUTIONAL CARE

At this same period the id drive in regard to the object is patterned on the anaclitic model. All locomotion will therefore be put in the service of an attempt to get gratification of the drive for anaclitic social relations.

The demand for social relations is subject to development in the course of the first year of life. Up to the sixth month these demands can be and are expressed only in a passive manner, since the infant has not achieved locomotion yet. Therefore the social demands of the infant are initiated not so much by the infant's activities as by the adult's activity.

From 6 to 12 months, however, its social demands are expressed actively, as shown in the results of the Hetzer-Wolf tests. At the age level of 7 months, one of the test items consists of observing whether the infant already creates contact actively. At the level of 9 months, the test consists in observing whether without intervention of the examiner the infant will grasp the hand or the coat of the averted adult.

One might also formulate this by saying that before the sixth month, the passivity of the social demand is expressed in the fact that it is only manifested in the pathognomonic reaction of the infant to the adult. Before the sixth month, the social contact manifestation is initiated by the adult and the child follows him; whereas after 6 months, the infant takes the initiative and seeks for the adult.

In a certain percentage of our cases of anaclitic depression we have found that the infants did not show the anxious attitude immediately after being deprived of their love object. We were informed by the staff that these children were disturbed by the absence of their mothers. Nevertheless they seemed to turn with eagerness to the observer. We might interpret this behavior as an attempt at substitution of the lost object along the anaclitic mode.

However, if active attempts at substitution are to be initiated through social contact, locomotion is a necessary prerequisite for such an attempt. In institutionalized children both the opportunity to reestablish anaclitic object relations through social contact, and the opportunity for locomotion, are severely handicapped.

From the dynamic point of view, locomotion and motility in general fulfill the important task of offering a necessary channel of release for the aggressive drive. When motor activity is inhibited in infancy, all normal outlets of the aggressive drive are blocked. In this case only one alternative remains for dealing with the aggressive drive: that is, to direct it against the self. The resulting dynamic picture is identical to the one we have previously described for melancholia. The only difference is that whereas in melancholia it was the superego which made use of the aggressive drive against the ego, in the case of inhibited motor activity in infancy the intervention of the superego is unnecessary.

Actually the difference between the dynamics in melancholia and those in anaclitic depression are not as great as might appear from a theoretical point of view. The hostile ego-oppressive authority in melancholia is the superego. In anaclitic depression the restriction of motility and the deprivation of the love object is imposed by the surrounding grown-up world. This world of grown-ups which forms the immediate environment of the infant is the identical one from which in the oedipal stage the imagines will be taken for the purpose of forming the superego. In other words, both in melancholia and in anaclitic depression the sadism which threatens the patient with extinction originates from the same source, except that in melancholia the source is an intrapsychic representation, while in anaclitic depression the source is the living original of the later intrapsychic representation.

An objection might be raised at this point: If anaclitic depression is provoked by inhibiting the locomotion of infants separated from their love object, why is it that a significant number of the infants observed by us in Nursery, the majority in fact, remained unharmed? And what is the reason for the severe nature of one group of infantile depression, for the milder course of the others?

The answer is that in both cases the outcome depends on the measure of success achieved in this institution in providing the infant with a substitute love object. The separation of the infants from their mothers takes place in Nursery between the sixth and the ninth month. Another of the inmates is then assigned to the care of the motherless child. The substitute mother thus cares for her own child and for a stranger. Though the enlightened management of Nursery exerts the greatest care, their selection is limited by the available number of inmates. Also it is hardly to be expected that a group of delinquent girls, as these were, will furnish very high grade mother substitutes.

We suggest that when the mother substitute is a good one, depression does not develop. Where the mother substitute turns out to be an aggressive, unloving personality, the parallel to adult melancholia is enacted in real life. Just as in melancholia the ego is oppressed by a sadistic superego, here the body ego of the infant is oppressed by a sadistic love object substitute.

Inhibited in its motor release, the pent-up aggressive drive is turned against the ego. The ego then is caught between a hostile love object substitute and its own aggressive drive. Bereft of locomotion, it cannot actively seek replacement for the lost love object among the other grown-ups in the institution.

An indirect confirmation of this view is contained in Table 5, which refers to the original mother-child relationship. In it we tabulate the number of children and the nature of their depression, on the one hand, the nature of the relations between the child and its mother, on the other. The mother-child relation was established by our observation of the way the mother behaved to her child. For the purpose of corroboration these observations then were compared with the information gathered for this purpose from the unusually able headmatron of Nursery. This somewhat complicated procedure made it impossible to procure reliable data on all the 95 children in question; but we did get them on 64, appearing in Table 5.

TABLE 5. MOTHER-CHILD RELATION

	Good			Bad		
	Intense	Moderate	Weak	Intense	Moderate	Weak
Severe depression	6	11	—	—	—	—
Mild depression	4	—	3	7	—	4
No depression	—	—	2	11	2	14

The figures speak for themselves. Evidently it is more difficult to replace a satisfactory love object than an unsatisfactory one. Accordingly depression is much more frequent and much more severe in the cases of good mother-child relationship. In bad mother-child relationship not a single severe depression occurs. It seems that any substitute is at least as good as the real mother in these cases.

In institutions, motor activity is inhibited for organizational reasons: lack of adequate nursing staff requires that the children be mostly confined to their cots, and move freely on the floor only for very restricted periods, if at all. The ego therefore is impoverished by being deprived of the release of motor activity. The aggressive drive is pent up and directed against the ego.

This restriction, however, also precludes the children's actively seeking replacement for the lost object among the grown-ups present in the institution or through contact with other children. Thus institutional routine will jeopardize the chances of substitutive attempts of the ego both in the motor and in the emotional sector.

C. FACILITATION OF RECUPERATIVE TRENDS IN INSTITUTIONS

The theoretical considerations elaborated above on the parallelity of the roles played by the superego in melancholia on the one hand, and on the other by the originals of the later imagines in an anaclitic depression, hold promise of a much more successful and effective therapy in the latter. Changing the superego in melancholia or assuaging it is a laborious, time-consuming, and all in all not very hopeful task. Providing a mother substitute (if restoring the mother is precluded) for a child suffering from a not too advanced anaclitic depression, refraining from inhibiting its motility, should be matters for an efficient and adequate environmental manipulation. The correctness of the latter statement is borne out by our observations on the prompt results after restoration of the love object to the deprived infants. It is also borne out by the favorable results of liberating motility and providing an adequate mother substitute for those infants for whom the original love object could not be restored.

It is easy to visualize that these elements in the picture of infantile depression will be subject to a wide scale of variations, depending on the rapidly developing changes in personality that take place during the first year of infancy; and on the wide gamut of environmental facilitations offered by the different types of institutions.

As regards the first, the changes in personality, it is self-evident that no imaginable motor activity exists in the first six months of life which could conceivably be used for attempts at substitution of the lost object. During this period, routine care of the infant, at least during the first three months, covers a large part of its social requirements. This picture changes completely in the second half of the first year of life. Locomotion develops rapidly and the demand for love switches from previous passivity to activity.

Institutional confinement of infants to their cots after the sixth month thwarts their use of locomotion in attempts at substitution. The infant's active attempts to make contact with other infants or adults in the environment are blocked. The infant is at the mercy of the compliance of its environment, and of the ability of the institution to provide an adequate substitute object.

Hence we will find clinical pictures of increasing severity according to the capacity of the institution in question to afford children deprived of their love objects an outlet in the form of free locomotion and substitute love objects. This is the reason why the results of child care in the worst foster homes surpass (with a few exceptions) those of the best institutions.

In the case of the infants observed by us in Nursery, we found that in so far as the object was not restored, or an adequate substitute object not supplied, the depression progressed rapidly. Beginning with sadness and weeping, it continued into withdrawal, loss of appetite, loss of interest in the outside world, dejection, retardation, and finally, a condition which could only be described as stuporous.

D. THE ACTUAL THERAPEUTIC MEASURE

Our dynamic and structural model of the anaclitic depression suggests the obvious therapeutic measures. It is gratifying to find that for once in psychiatry they appear to be really effective where they can be applied. They fall into three classes: (1) prophylaxis, (2) restitution, (3) substitution.

1. Prophylaxis: deprivation of infants, during the first year, of love objects for a prolonged period, should be strenuously avoided. Under no circumstances should they be deprived for over three months of love objects, during the second half of their first year.

2. Restitution: if infants have been deprived of their love objects during their first year for a prolonged period, restitution of the love objects within a period of maximally three months will enable them to recover, at least partially, from the damage inflicted.

3. Substitution: where neither prophylaxis nor restitution is possible, the substitution of the love object by another one is advisable. Particular attention should be given to the facilitation of the infant's locomotor drives in the largest measure possible, and to the supporting of its tendencies to choose actively its own substitutes for the love object of which it has been deprived.

V. SUMMARY

A. A psychiatric syndrome of a depressive nature is observed in a series of infants and classified as anaclitic depression.

B. Its etiology is related to a loss of the love object, combined with a total inhibition of attempts at restitution through the help of the body ego acting on anaclitic lines.

C. Prophylaxis and treatment is suggested on the basis of these structural and dynamic findings.

D. Some of the results of such treatment are reported.

E. Theoretical assumptions concerning melancholia are discussed.

A. VARIOUS OBSERVATIONS WITH THEORETICAL IMPLICATIONS

In the course of this study a number of observations were made which we have not cared to include in our general conclusions for several reasons. Some of these observations appear to us to lead to conclusions which are still of too speculative a nature for the purposes of the present study. Others again are too scattered and irregular to represent satisfactory findings for the purpose of establishing or confirming any theory. We therefore bring them here in order to call the attention of other investigators to these phenomena, in the hope that they may be utilized in later work.

1. The variations of the developmental quotient in the course of anaclitic depression

In all our cases without exception a gradual decline of the developmental quotient began when the infant was deprived of its love object. This decline paralleled the increasing severity of the developing symptoms. This is a welcome confirmation of our observations; an unexpectedly surprising and dramatic change in the developmental quotient occurs when the love object is returned. We had the opportunity to test such cases immediately after the return of the love object, i.e., within 12 hours. Developmental quotients would jump as much as 36.6 percent in this brief period. The developmental age of the children would take a jump from $0;11+0$ to $1;4+0$; or from $0;9+0$ to $1;1+0$. This in itself is surprising enough, but it is still more surprising that in the case of a child whose developmental age had jumped within three days from $0;11+0$ to $1;3+28$, it receded again, and for the following two months moved between $1;1+21$ and $1;1+24$.

It is an extremely striking finding that faculties already acquired should be lost in the course of the anaclitic depression, that when the love object returns they should be regained suddenly in a manner far surpassing the actual age of the child, but that after a short while the level of achievement should settle back again more closely to the performances to be expected according to the child's actual age. In view of our discussion of the fact that the ego at this period is mainly a body ego, that on the other hand the tests applied to establish the developmental quotient require a good deal of body activity, one gets the impression of a sudden ego expansion having taken place on the return of the love object. This ego expansion is out of proportion to the age-adequate capacities of the child, and sinks back to a more normal proportion if no further disturbances intervene. The curious phenomenon of this sudden ego expansion which on the return of the love object replaces the depression makes us inclined to speculate whether there may be any analogy between this manifestation and the replacement of a depression by a manic episode.

2. Some considerations in regard to assumptions of psychoanalytic theory and their verification

The predominant role of oral eroticism in melancholia has always been stressed in psychoanalytic literature (Abraham, 1924). It is assumed that a regression to the oral biting phase takes place, with fantasies of introjection. Anal-sadistic trends appear enormously increased. Therefore we would expect to find striking oral biting and anal-sadistic phenomena in our depressed infants. Such was not the case, at least not in that measure which one would expect in view of the comparatively simple, elementary structure of early infantile psychic patterns.

a. Oral biting manifestations. The one oral symptom common to all of the children was loss of appetite; on the other hand, we observed a greater tendency of the depressed children to stuff everything—hands, clothes, toys—into their mouths, and to keep them there. Prior to the depression these children were not noticeably prone to finger-sucking. During the depression finger-sucking increased conspicuously. We encountered biting phenomena in some of the depressed children, but not in all. In those cases in which we could observe them, they had not been present prior to the depression. It is an outstanding fact that the biting activities *never* were in evidence *during* the depression; they appeared after the depression had lifted. Interesting manifestations will be found in the following quotation from the protocol of one of our cases.

Aethelberta. White female. "From the beginning far advanced in her development, friendly, well liked. At 0;7 + 16 slightly depressive expression in the face noted, simultaneously with a decrease of the developmental quotient. Inquiry elicits that she had been separated from her mother ten days before. In the following weeks she becomes weepy; by the time she is nine months old, the nursing staff observes that the child is getting thinner and suffering from insomnia; she seems to be watching everything and allegedly cannot go to sleep for this reason. She finally is isolated for the purpose of overcoming her insomnia. Approaching her becomes difficult; she is mostly sitting in her bed, her dress in her mouth, or sucking her hand. In the following weeks she refuses to touch toys and lies dejected on her bed, face averted from the experimenter. Films taken by us during these weeks show a pathetic picture of sorrow, helplessness, and demand for assistance. The developmental quotient drops further. The child, up to this point vigorously healthy, develops a stubbornly persisting cold. At 0;10 + 22 a mother substitute is delegated with instructions to be particularly loving to the child. The effect of this measure becomes immediately visible, though the child is by no means cured. She now accepts contact with other children in an aggressive form. At 0;10.29 she is biting, scratching, and pinching other children to the point of drawing blood. By 0;11 + 5 she tries for a prolonged period to bite the observer's nose, chin, neck, and hand. During these attacks she reaches out with her hands and vocalizes different incoherent sounds, among which the word "ma-ma" returns several times. At

0;11 + 19 the mother is returned. Simultaneously she has become friendly and positive, and her developmental quotient has suddenly risen 29.28 percent.''

There are many traits in this picture which could be used to confirm psychoanalytic theory and we have quoted it for this reason. We do not at this point feel justified, however, in drawing conclusions because similar phenomena are manifested only by a minority of our cases.

b. Anal-sadistic manifestations. Anal activities showed a somewhat different pattern. Like oral biting phenomena they were very striking in some cases and absent in others. However, in those cases where they were present they could be observed both during the depression and after the depression had lifted. The phenomena observed in these children were playing with feces, with or without accompanying genital masturbation, and in some cases, coprophagia. Fecal games and oral biting manifestations appeared frequently, although not necessarily, in the same children. In the case of Aethelberta, for instance, as well as in that of another child, the games consisted in rolling fecal pellets, which seemed to be the only toy these children enjoyed. Aethelberta continued the fecal games after the depression had lifted, in the form of social games, trying to feed her play partner with the pellets. In another case in which biting and fecal games were simultaneously present, the pellets were used for covering the bed with a layer of feces and for throwing out through the bars of the cot, so that the surroundings of the bed were also completely covered with feces. Genital masturbation, which at this age is not particularly frequent in infants, was observed in nearly all of the children in whom fecal games were observed.

Autoerotism:
Some Empirical Findings and Hypotheses on Three of Its Manifestations in the First Year of Life

with the collaboration of KATHERINE M. WOLF, Ph.D.

I. INTRODUCTION

A behavioristic investigation of autoerotism in the first year of life is confronted by various obstacles.[1] The first of these is the definition of our term. We shall use it in the sense in which it was used by Freud (1913):[2]

> These manifestations of sexual impulses can be recognized from the beginning, but at first they are not yet directed at any outer object. Each individual component of the sexual impulse works for a gain in pleasure and finds its gratification in its own body.

On the basis of this definition of autoerotism we propose to investigate some autoerotic activities that occur during the first year of life.

One of the difficulties in such an investigation is that of observing a relevant number of cases over sufficiently long periods. A really unimpeachable study would have to offer continuous 24-hour observation of the infant during the whole of the first year of life. For obvious reasons this is hardly feasible.

Reprinted from *The Psychoanalytic Study of the Child*, Vol. 3/4. New York: International Universities Press, 1949, pp. 85–118.

[1] Extensive bibliographical research has been undertaken in connection with this article and the whole literature on autoerotism during the first years of life published in psychiatric, psychoanalytic, pediatric and pedagogic fields has been investigated. [This survey was published. See Spitz, 1953. Ed.]

[2] See also Freud, 1905b. [The *Standard Edition* translation of this passage, which is cited in the references, appears on p. 88. Spitz is quoting here from "Totem and Taboo," *Basic Works of Sigmund Freud*, New York: Modern Library, 1938, p. 865, a slightly different translation. Ed.]

Another difficulty lies in the abundance of phenomena to be studied. Activities of the oral zone in infancy would require a whole monograph; one sector of these activities, thumb-sucking, has formed the base of the well-known monograph of Lindner (1934) and of numerous later publications.

The detailed investigation of the oral autoerotic activities would indubitably yield some interesting facts. We have however, for practical reasons,[3] excluded them from the present study, limiting ourselves to a detailed investigation of the following three autoerotic activities: (1) The well-known "rocking" of infants during their first year; (2) genital play; (3) fecal games.[4]

Like sucking, these three activities are characterized by their rhythmicity, their character of self-stimulation, and the fact that the child appears to derive some sort of pleasure while performing them (Freud, 1905b).

Thus what we have set out to do in our present paper will be more in the nature of a description than in the nature of classification; it will be an attempt at illustration, and our interpretations will be tentative. If certain regularities do appear in the course of this procedure we will consider them in the nature of approximations; an orientation, as it were, within the map of the ontogenesis of sexuality.

II. Sample and Method

The main body of our investigation was conducted in an institution on a total of 196 infants. Of these, 26 have not yet reached the age at which according to our observations autoerotic activities usually begin nor did they show any tendency toward such activities at the time. We have therefore excluded them and bring the results of our observations on the remaining 170, as shown in Table 1.

---

[3] The objection may be raised that it is not possible to discuss autoerotism in infancy intelligently without using oral autoerotism as the basis of our observations and discussions, as a frame of reference, so to say. For by definition infancy is the oral phase. The reasons why we have not done this are mainly of a practical nature. While the three autoerotic activities observed by us are amenable to direct observation, much of the oral activity is not. That oral activity takes place in the first year of life is a statement of the obvious. It is not so with the other autoerotic activities we have observed. We would therefore have to use a completely different approach to be able to make any statements about oral activity, namely an experimental approach in which the oral activity would be modified either in the sense of its being artificially increased or in the sense of its being artificially decreased. Either would present great difficulties in regard to the policies of the institutions involved, as well as to the attitudes of the parents and nursing personnel. Sucking frustration experiments can be performed on dogs, as D. Levy has done. One is loath to perform them on infants. Furthermore, 24-hour observation would become necessary, and this, with our observational setup, is unfeasible. There is also a problem, even with a 24-hour observational program, of how much of the oral activity should be considered as autoerotic—how to differentiate between oral activity which is gratified during the feeding procedure and therefore does not require autoerotic gratification, and how much is not.

We have therefore, very much against our wishes, been forced to neglect the oral autoerotic activities, though we possess extensive observations on the oral behavior of the infants discussed

TABLE 1. CHILDREN OF NURSERY OBSERVED FOR AUTOEROTISM

	Male	Female	Total
White	50	56	106
Colored	35	29	64
Total	85	85	170

The institution in question is a penal institution[5] in which the infants observed by us were raised from birth to the end of their first year by their own mothers under the supervision of personnel experienced in child care. The hygienic and environmental conditions of the institution were satisfactory, as witnessed by the fact that no child died during the four years in which we made observations in the institution and that serious diseases did not occur during this time (Spitz, 1946b). This is a finding which is quite exceptional for any institution housing children during their first year of life; it is actually much more favorable than the mortality rate during the first year of life for the United States as a whole, where during the same years it was 40.7 per thousand in 1943 and 39.4 per thousand in 1944. This represents an average for the country as a whole. In the state where the institution is located the death rate is somewhat below the average of the U.S., namely 32.8 per thousand (Wolff, 1944).

As in all our investigations, the unselected total sample of the children

by us. We have limited ourselves to three autoerotic activities and consider our approach justified for the following reasons:

a. We have observed the incidence of each of these activities. The comparison of these incidences has given us certain information on their relative frequency, information which we consider instructive independent of whether other autoerotic activities, even those as important as the oral ones, are present or not.

b. In comparing this incidence with the one environmental variable established by us, namely the mother-child relation, certain regularities have become apparent. These regularities have a significance of their own. This significance is independent of the answer to the question whether oral autoerotism is covariant with, or varies independently of the regularities found by us.

The final verification or modification of the theoretical assumptions made on the strength of the regularities observed by us will depend on future findings on oral activities made under similar conditions.

[4] It should perhaps be stressed that we do not use the term anal play because we have not been able to observe any instance of active tactile approach to the anal region at this period of life, whereas we have been able to observe a significant number of cases in which feces of the children became their favorite and preferred play object. We also use the term "genital play" instead of "masturbation." As will become evident below, we consider masturbation too specific a term for the activities observed at this age level.

[5] For a detailed description of this institution, under the name of "Nursery," see "Hospitalism," this volume.

present in the institution was observed by us and used for our study. Each child was observed at weekly intervals for 4 hours per week, over a period of one year or more, averaging over 200 hours of observation per child. This method of observation will surely miss many instances of autoerotic activities of these children. Therefore our figures on the absence of such activities cannot be regarded as conclusive. We, nevertheless, believe that the method will yield a sufficiently informative cross-section of the more striking items of behavior. We believe that with this method we have been able to achieve some insight into the incidence of the three above-named autoerotic activities, into their frequency, and into their phenomenology. Actually the observation of the latter gave us the possibility to distinguish the three classes we mentioned, the rocking, the genital play, and the fecal play.

We conducted regular weekly interviews with the nursing personnel as well as with the mothers of the children. Rorschach tests were administered to approximately 30 percent of the mothers.

Simultaneously we investigated the emotional climate of each child studied and we attempted to correlate the children's emotional background to their observable autoerotic behavior.

The total study up to the present day has been running for close to four years.

III. RESULTS

We wish to stress that the results obtained in the present study are limited to the age group represented by our sample, i. e., from birth to 15 months. Our conclusions therefore apply to the first year of life and to the first year *only*. Any comparisons with phenomena observed at a more advanced age can only be misleading.

We found that from the point of view of autoerotic activities these infants could be divided into four groups (if we neglect oral activity):

1. Those children whose autoerotic activity consisted predominantly of rocking,

2. those whose autoerotic activity consisted predominantly of genital play,

3. those whose autoerotic activity consisted predominantly of fecal play,

4. and finally those in whom none of these activities was ever observed by us.

A. INCIDENCE

Out of 170 children, autoerotic activities of at least one of the above three types were observed in 104 up to the time of this writing. Rocking was observed in 87 children. Genital play was observed in 21 children. Fecal play was observed in 16 children. These figures overlap to a certain extent because more than one autoerotic activity was observed in certain children.

These figures in themselves do not tell us very much if we accept the finding that *in this environment* both genital play and fecal play appear to be rarer during the first year of life than we had been led to expect by scattered remarks in the literature.

The sex distribution and the race distribution of autoerotic activities can be seen from Table 2.[6]

TABLE 2. RACE AND SEX DISTRIBUTION OF AUTOEROTIC ACTIVITIES IN NURSERY

	Male	Female
White	76%	45%
Colored	63%	62%

A sex difference in autoerotic activities with a predominance in the males appears in the white group. No such differences were observed in the colored group.

Differences between the races appear ambiguous. We do not believe that the numbers involved are large enough to justify any conclusions from these results.

B. DISTRIBUTION

The distribution of the autoerotic activities is shown in Table 3, in which genital play and rocking are illustrated. We did not include fecal play because of the comparatively small numbers involved.

It appears that it is infrequent that both genital play and rocking should be

TABLE 3. RELATION BETWEEN GENITAL PLAY AND ROCKING

	Rocking	No rocking	Total
Genital play	7	14	21
No genital play	80	69	149
Total	87	83	170

[6] Our sample was not evenly matched in regard to either race or sex. Instead of the number of subjects involved we have therefore given the percentage of these subjects in relation to the population of our sample.

present in the same child. We shall discuss later the conclusions that we believe can be drawn from this incompatibility.

The age distribution also presents some points of interest. First, that of genital play: (See Figure 1).

From this chart it appears that a certain level of general development is a prerequisite for the appearance of genital play. That is not unexpected. After all, directed activity and a certain capacity for adequate handling of objects as well as a certain discriminatory perception, are prerequisites for such play.[7]

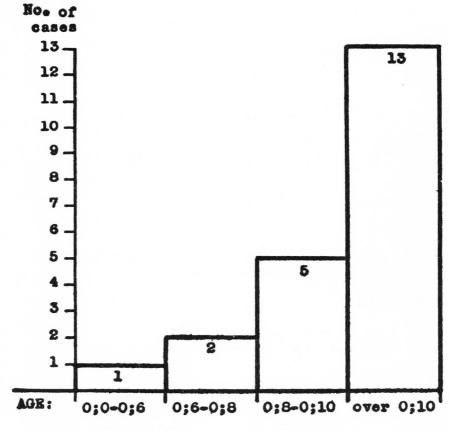

FIGURE 1. GENITAL PLAY: AGE DISTRIBUTION

[7] In the literature on infantile autoerotic activities collected by us references to exact age of the inception of genital play are almost absent. The only exact reference which coincides with our observations is that of Lauretta Bender (1939) who states that genital play starts between the eighth and ninth month with normal children.

The more significant distribution, however, is seen in Figure 2, in which we compare the age distribution of rocking and genital activity.

Figure 2 shows that the rocking activities reach their maximum at an age at which genital activity is the rare exception and that from there on they successively decrease until the end of the first year. In both charts it is not the incidence of the activity itself that is shown, but its inception, that is, the age at which the activity was first observed in a given child. We have no factual data for the explanation of the inverse course of these two activities. It suggests, however, the assumption that genital play is a more mature activity of the infant than rocking and that in this capacity genital play will progres-

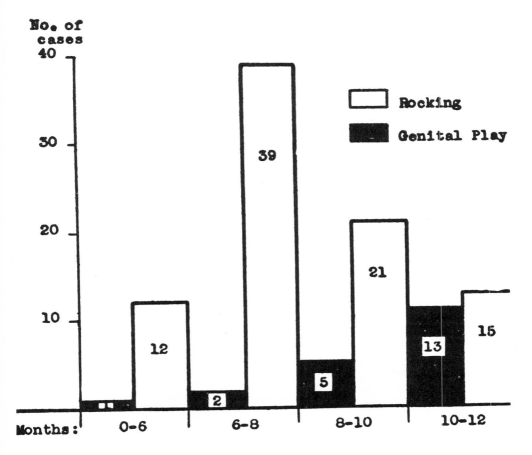

FIGURE 2. AGE DISTRIBUTION OF ROCKING AND GENITAL PLAY

sively increase with the progressing age, whereas the more archaic rocking will decrease with maturation.

This assumption suggests somme further questions. They are of an etiological nature and therefore cannot be answered by a mere behavioristic observation of the phenomenon itself.

C. ETIOLOGY

1. Methodological Consideration

Our observations up to this point have yielded figures on the incidence and age distribution of three groups of autoerotic behavior in the first year (excluding oral activities), namely: rocking, genital play, and fecal play. Our figures have further shown that some of these activities appear to inhibit the manifestations of the others in one and the same child. We will therefore ask ourselves:

1. Why do certain children indulge in rocking games during the first year, others in genital play, others in fecal play, and others finally in none of these?

2. Why does the presence of certain of these activities seem to exclude indulgence in the remaining ones?

In attempting to find the answer to these questions we shall first have to investigate the etiological factors operative in determining the selection of one autoerotic activity rather than another.

The etiological factors which can be distinguished in this group can be divided into hereditary, congenital, and environmental ones. As regards heredity, at present no reliable criteria are available. Actually we have the impression that in the case of such gross phenomena as those with which we are dealing here hereditary differences may not be very significant. That at least has been our conclusion in an investigation directed at the differentiation of the developmental quotients in our group according to white and colored race, where the results during the first year show such minimal differences between the developmental quotients, such small fluctuations between the two developmental curves, as to lack any kind of significance. We were able to demonstrate that such differences at best can only represent a fraction of the difference provoked by the environment, as demonstrated by a second curve in the same investigation (Spitz and Wolf, 1947).

This finding regarding racial differences applies also to the congenital factor. It may be added that in our population there were no gross findings of congenital disfunctions demonstrated either by the medical examination at birth, nor by results of the test examinations beginning with the second week after birth.

This leaves us with the environmental factor as the decisive one. In infancy and particularly in a nursery setting, environment is restricted and elements easily analyzable. In our case certain factors were uniform for all the subjects involved. They were food, housing, clothing, hygiene, cots, toys, and the daily routine.

There remains one possible environmental variable: the human element. This variable, however, is also that which represents, at this age at least, the highest emotional valence, one might nearly say, the only emotional valence. The variable "human element" will at the same time provide us with information about the role and significance of emotions as a factor in autoerotic activity—as could be expected by anybody familiar with psychoanalytic propositions.

The human element and its emotional corollary is provided in the first year of life by the mother, a term by which we mean both the child's actual mother and/or any other person of either sex who may take the place of the child's physical mother during a significant period of time. Our variable therefore will consist in the difference of the attitudes of the mothers of the children in question, in the differences in their behavior toward their children. These differences will be predicated upon the varying personalities of these mothers.

This analysis suggests our next step, namely that of correlating the variable we have found, the mother-child relationship, with our other findings in regard to autoerotism. But, while our findings in regard to all other elements of the child's environment were lacking in variety, we discovered that the variable which we are investigating now presents us with a diversity which appears to offer well-nigh insurmountable obstacles to classification. The mothers of these children vary widely in their personality, in their intellect, in their emotional attitude toward sex, toward each other, toward authority, and toward their children. Some of them are of low intelligence and good-natured, many of them have an infantile personality, others again are more on the psychopathic side with manifest aggressions. There are a few borderline cases, some are even definitely psychotic, though not disturbed. There are a number of prostitutes on one hand and quite a few small town girls who had the bad luck to be caught.

As heterogeneous material as the above does not lend itself readily to the establishment of a leading hypothesis. For the purpose of establishing a leading hypothesis one would normally choose the performing of a series of controlled experiments in which certain variables would be held constant and only one permitted to vary. Such experiments are unfeasible in our case; but it is at least possible for us to choose groups in which within the group itself most of the factors are relatively homogeneous and their variations not too significant; and to isolate one factor as a variable in which quantitative variations of a rough and ready kind can be ascertained. The factor in question is the intensity of the mother-child relationship. For this purpose it appears advisable to approach our problem from two opposite poles and to try to find one environment in which the mother-child relationship is at its lowest, and to oppose to it a second environment where the mother-child relationship can be expected to be at its optimum. The diversity presented in the picture of "Nursery" would thus be reduced to a minimum—since it cannot be completely eliminated. It is of course not easy to find a group of children whose environmental background on one hand, and whose relationship to their mothers on the other, is sufficiently homogeneous. Certain environmental situations, however, make a rough approximation of such a desideratum feasible.

Once such environments can be found we will be in the position to compare the autoerotic activities of the groups with each other.

For our first environment we have chosen a group of 17 children raised in white-collar-worker private homes where close personal exploration of the child and the parents convinced us that the mother-child relationship was either an exceptionally good one, or that at least efforts were being made to achieve this. This environment we have considered as offering optimal relations from the point of view of maximal intensity.

It was easier to find the second environment, the one in which mother-child relations were nonexistent. For this purpose we chose Institution 2, a foundling home[8] situated in another country in which the children were raised without their mothers, and by an insufficient number of nurses; officially one nurse cared for 8 children; in practice one nurse took care of 10 to 12, thus providing the child with one-tenth of the attention a mother normally gives her offspring and with even less love. As regards food, housing, clothing, hygiene, the conditions were comparable to those encountered in Nursery.

2. The Etiological Factor Responsible for the Incidence

The findings made in these two environments are distinctly startling. In the case of the children reared in private families, we found that of 17 children, 16 manifested genital play within the first year, at ages which were on the average two months earlier than those observed in Nursery. Only in one child was rocking observed exclusively.

In Foundling Home, where emotional relations were completely absent, we observed 61 children in their first 18 months. Of these, only one (CC 62, age 1; $1 + 10$)[9] manifested any genital play. As far as rocking is concerned, it was observed in 2 of the children *after* the first year (CC 41, age 1;3 + 10, and CC 45, age 1;1 + 12) and in 2 children before the first year (CC 11, age

---

[8] For detailed description of the institution under the name of "Foundling Home," see "Hospitalism," this volume.

[9] The designations CC, P, N, etc., refer to individual cases in the several environments.

0; 10 + 1, and CC 58, age 0; 11 + 3). There was very little thumb-sucking. The only other activity which—by any stretch of imagination—can be called ''autoerotic'' were shaking movements of the nature of spasmus nutans as described by Moro (1918).

Our findings in these three different environments can be summarized as follows:

Environment 1. 17 children (private families, excellent mother-child relations):

Autoerotic activities were observed in all,

rocking in 1 case,

genital play in 16 cases.

Environment 2. 170 children (nursery, mother-child relations varying from emotionally very good to emotionally very bad):

No autoerotic activity was observed in 65 cases,

rocking in 87 cases,

genital play in 21 cases,

fecal play in 16 cases.

Environment 3. 61 children (foundling Home, complete absence of emotional relations):

Practically no autoerotic activities (rocking in 4 cases, genital play in 1 case).

We are forced to conclude that:

1. Autoerotic activity appears to be covariant with the pattern of emotional relations between mother and child, since when these emotional relations are absent, no autoerotic activities are observable. Where mother-child relations are at their maximum all subjects produce autoerotic activities.

2. The closer the mother-child relation of the particular given environment, the more infants we find manifesting genital play in the first year of life. This finding is confirmed by a case published by Emmy Sylvester (1947).

3. Etiological Factors in Different Types of Autoerotic Activity

a. Genital play. Our leading hypothesis thus appears established: the presence of mother-child interrelation is a necessary prerequisite for the appearance of autoerotism in the first year of life. A further qualification of the leading hypothesis from the same table follows: it appears that the amount of genital play varies with varying mother-child relations, a statement which will not surprise psychoanalysts. It is therefore incumbent upon us to examine more closely the elements constituting what we up to here have called mother-child relation, as well as its variations in the different environments studied by us.

Deprivation of Mothering

In investigating the mother-child relationship we have to realize that in this relation, barring severe sickness of the child, there is only one partner who can take the initiative or be active in any way: the mother. It is she therefore who determines the nature of the relationship. Consequently we will have to visualize the relationship from the angle of the mother. Before doing this, however, we will again consider our three environments:

Foundling Home: no mother-child relation, no genital play; developmental quotient progressively dropping down to level of imbecility.[10]

Nursery: mother-child relation shifting from extreme closeness to extreme rejection. Moderate percentage (13 percent) of genital play, fairly good average of developmental quotient (107) of the second half of the first year.

Private families: extreme closeness of mother-child relation, genital activity 94 percent, average developmental quotient 135.

The covariance between closeness of mother-child relation, genital activity, and developmental level is striking.

At this point an examination of the term "closeness" imposes itself. For physical closeness of the mothers to their children in Nursery is at least as great as that of the mothers in private homes.[11] The problem arises: since it is the mother's personality which determines the mother-child relationship, how does the emotional personality of the mothers in Nursery differ from that of the mothers in private homes?

There appear to be two main differences, the one based on social background and social adaptation, the other on problems of emotional balance.

The mothers in Nursery came there because of a failure in social adaptation. In a large percentage of the cases this maladaptation is not severe, consisting mainly in sexual indiscretion at the wrong age. (Compared to the figures of the Kinsey report on present day morality in private families, extramarital intercourse of females of the average age of 20 does not impress us as differing fundamentally from the general attitude toward sex.) Thus the background of the mothers of children in private homes contains emotional factors which are potentially similar to those of the mothers in Nursery. We suspect that the difference between the mothers in this institution and other mothers of an urban background is one based on cultural attitudes of their immediate environment and on the diversities of their economic status. Such differences

---

[10] For exact comparison of the developmental quotient figures see Figure 3.

[11] It is this physical closeness, this luxuriation of a great variation of emotional interchange between the mothers and the children which we stressed in a previous study (Spitz, 1945b). There we contrasted the overprotection in Nursery with the complete libidinal impoverishment and lack of contact observed in Foundling Home. A differentiated analysis of the mothers' personalities was not significant for the purpose of that study. We pointed at the probable role of these factors, though at the time we were not yet in the position to be more specific in our statements, as we had not yet collected sufficient data on the personalities of the mothers.

in themselves seem insufficient to warrant the assumption of basic dissimilarities in the emotional attitude of the two groups of mothers to their children. However, in Nursery, motherhood has been penalized by social disapproval going to the point of internment (which inevitably will elicit feelings of resentment and guilt) and involving a separation of the mother from the father of her child.

This brings us to the other main difference between the mothers of private children and the mothers in Nursery: the mothers of private children have a sexual partner, their husband; the mothers in Nursery have none.[12]

This difference has far-reaching psychological consequences from the dynamic and economic point of view. In the private homes the mother is able to discharge a goodly part of her instinctual drives, both libidinal and aggressive, on the marriage partner and does so not only in a particularly effective manner in the course of normal sexual activity, but, as we know, through the exchanges of everyday life. Apart from this it will be comparatively easy for a woman with a husband, particularly during the lying-in period, to direct any additional hostile tendencies which her baby might provoke to a concerned and, in this situation, generally particularly considerate partner.

Not so in the institution. In Nursery the mothers have no adequate and accepted outlet for their libidinal or their aggressive drives; they are separated from their husbands and therefore the only possible outlet for the libidinal drive are relations of a homosexual nature with the other inmates. Such relations are discouraged and as far as possible frustrated. In a large percentage of the cases the mothers in question would not even be capable of indulging in such relations because of their personality structure. In those cases where homosexual contacts were possible we found the libidinal balance of the mothers in question so seriously upset in consequence as to make their relations with their children abnormal, to say the least. As for the aggressive drives, they have to be repressed when directed to the authorities of Nursery and they find their outlet partly in quarrels with other mothers, partly in modified relations with the children.

It can be seen from these considerations that the role of the father for normal relations between mother and child is an extremely significant and important one. This is an assumption which had been made frequently in psychoanalytic literature regarding disturbances of the preschool child, school

---

[12] We may disregard the frequently observed condition in private families, that when a mother was unresponsive to her child, the father would often manifest a strikingly loving, one might say "motherly," attitude and thus offer compensation. That probably is a factor of chance which in the institution might also be manifested through the interest taken by somebody besides the mother.

child, and adolescent. To my knowledge it was not made yet regarding infants in the first year of life.

We must argue from this that the concept of "close" mother-child relationship should be qualified. It appears that in this relationship "closeness" alone is not the determining criterion, but that balance, a modicum of instinctual equilibrium, is a further prerequisite. It is imperative for the mother to be able to discharge her instinctual drives, particularly the aggressive ones, without involving her child.

Where those drives do not find an adequate discharge, where they are dammed up and finally are discharged on the child, overprotection or hostility to the child results. Mostly, however, the two alternate in violent ups and downs.

The modification in autoerotic activity to which such violent extremes lead is the subject of a later section of this study. As we have shown above, violent unchecked emotions in respect to the child are absent in those cases in which genital play develops already during the first year of life. In these cases we have therefore a "close" mother-child relationship in which a relatively consistent attitude prevails which does not show the extremes of libidinal neediness or of aggressive hostility.

It follows from this statement that we consider a "close *and* balanced" mother-child relationship an important prerequisite for the development of genital play during the first year of life. This statement should not be confused with the assumption frequently made in the literature[13] that genital play is induced by a maternal approach equivalent to a genital seduction. Hygiene and the washing of the genital parts, cleanliness in connection with evacuation, inappropriate caresses on the part of the mother, are again and again mentioned as probable cause of genital play in early infancy. We do not share this opinion, we definitely believe that the factor responsible is not only a local physical one but an emotional one. After all, not only do we have a large number of children in Nursery who never were observed to indulge in any kind of autoerotic activity, but we also observed *rocking only* in 80 cases; all of these children, who did not indulge in any genital play, were also exposed to the same kind of "genital seduction" in matters of hygiene—the washing of genitalia, cleanliness in regard to evacuation, etc.—as were those children who did indulge in the genital play.

Striking evidence that the physical and local seduction by the mother in the close mother-child relationship need not lead to genital play, was provided by our observation of actual cases of genital stimulation which did not lead to genital play at all, let alone to excessive masturbation, but to psychiatric

---

[13] Already in 1912 this assumption was rejected by Federn who in his theoretical point of view anticipates a number of our empirical findings.

conditions of a quite different nature. We will present two unequivocal cases from our material: one that of a medical treatment of the female genital at an early age, the other that of deliberate genital seduction during a large part of the first year of life.

Case N 18. This child was infected with gonorrhea and subjected to local treatment during her first 2 months. Nevertheless during the whole subsequent year in which we observed this child she was never seen to indulge in genital play. On the other hand she was probably the most persistent rocker in our experience, she rocked with such violence that one would hear her from several wards and corridors away.

Case N 3. Beginning at 4 months and up to 11 months the mother (latent manic depressive) regularly performed cunilingus on the child: she was repeatedly observed doing so by reliable witnesses. In this child also no genital play developed. Instead the child developed excessive thumb-sucking, from the fourth month on. At 9 months thumb-sucking was replaced by excessive fecal play which reached its climax at 1 year and 1 month. Every time the child was observed she was found sitting in her cot with a dreamy absent-minded expression, collecting feces from her diaper and alternatingly putting the excrement in her mouth or throwing it out of her cot, frequently vomiting the eaten excrement.

The two cases in question lead us to assume that genital seduction in the first year of life is not responded to by genital activity. The response appears to be rather one which is appropriate to the phase of the sexual organization in which the child happens to be at the time of the genital stimulation. In the case of the first child we have extremely early genital stimulation through the local therapy for gonorrhea. The resulting response is of the nature of diffuse muscle activity corresponding to the early level of the organization of this child's personality, namely the level of primary narcissism.

In the case of the second child the response to consistent genital stimulation up to the eleventh month again is one that is manifested in the age adequate sector of sexual development, namely in the oral sector from the fourth to the ninth month and in the anal sector at the end of the first year. In other terms, we believe that the early genital stimulation of Case N 18 resulted in rocking, whereas the genital seduction of Case N 3, taking place in the transition from the oral to the anal stage, resulted first in excessive thumb-sucking and later in coprophagia.

Of course we are aware that beyond this gross difference in the age level at which the local genital stimulation took place there also were significant differences in the personalities of the mothers of the two children. The role which the personality of the mother plays in the development of rocking and fecal play will be the subject of a later section.

There is further evidence that genital stimulation in itself is not sufficient to provoke genital play. It so happens that at certain periods in the institution in which these children were observed, eczema was rampant. In addition to the children suffering from eczema we also observed a small number of children (five in all) suffering from various other itching skin conditions like impetigo, rash, etc. As the skin irritation would cover many of these children from head to foot, including the region around the genitals, the theory of genital masturbation in infants being provoked by local stimulation like ox-iuris, eczema, etc., would lead one to assume that all the children suffering from eczema would have also manifested genital play. Obviously the number of our cases is not large enough to establish significant correlations. Nevertheless, as far as it goes, our material shows that eczema and genital play are independent of each other. (See Table 4.)

TABLE 4. RELATIONSHIP BETWEEN ECZEMA AND GENITAL PLAY IN NURSERY

	Eczema	No eczema	Total
Genital play	3	18	21
No genital play	21	128	149
Total	24	146	170

The stimulation itself, be it of a general nature like eczema, or of a local circumscribed nature directed at the sexual organ itself, as in the two cases mentioned by us, does not appear to be that factor which elicits genital play in the first year of life.

Thus we have at present no adequate explanation of why a "close" mother-child relation, without particular genital stimulation, should result in genital play when local stimulation does not. We have only tentative observations to offer to guide us if we want to formulate a hypothesis.

The observations in question are of a physiognomical and behavioristic nature. We have recorded them with the help of motion pictures made from the subjects during their autoerotic activities. From the beginning it has struck us that there was a wide difference in the physiognomical expression which accompanies the three autoerotic activities investigated.

While in the case of rocking, whether supine, knee-elbow, or standing, the children's expression was one which could go to the point of orgiastic delight, while in fecal play and coprophagia the expression was one of dreamy withdrawal, of a turning inward, going to the point of depressive daze and psychotic suspicion—we saw nothing of the kind in any of the children we observed during their genital play. Here we saw regularly a facial expression which might go from indifference to alert attention or to friendly sociability.

In other words, the children in question did not seem to be emotionally more involved when playing with their genitals than when playing with any other part of their body, their feet, ears, etc. In some of these children it is quite instructive to compare the facial expression during genital play with the infinitely more absorbed and orgiastic expression manifested during ingestion of food, be that at the breast or with a spoon from a plate.

We suspect that genital play in the first year of life has the significance of one of the many normal bodily activities and games of the infant. However, normal activities develop equally in all sectors only when the emotional climate is adequate, when the relations between the child and its mother are satisfactory. As soon as they become unsatisfactory an imbalance is manifested in some of the sectors of bodily and mental development, some activities being retarded or arrested, others unduly facilitated. It would seem that genital play, possibly because it has relatively little specificity in this phase of infantile sexuality, is one of the earliest victims of unsatisfactory mother-child relations.

The third covariant mentioned, the developmental quotient achieved in the three environments, supports this hypothesis. It is vividly illustrated by Figure 3 showing the variations of the average developmental quotients of the three environments throughout the first year of life.

It might be concluded from this that the genital play is nothing but a part of the whole developmental pattern during the first year of life; that therefore a high developmental quotient will involve the early appearance of genital play just as it involves the early appearance of other motor and play activities also.

We prefer to assume that both autoerotic activity and the developmental quotient itself are but the manifestations of a more basic factor, namely of the mother-child interrelation. Where this interrelation is at its best, genital play will be general in the first year of life and general development will surpass the average. Where this interrelation is absent, genital play will be missing and general development will drop far below the average and deteriorate progressively.

The next sections will deal with those cases which fall between the two extremes, complete absence and optimal presence of mother-child interrelations.

b. Rocking. The mother's personality. As indicated above, rocking is one of the autoerotic activities found in those children where the mother-child relation is neither completely absent nor of the really well balanced, close type. However, the mother-child interrelation which obtains in these intermediate cases no longer lends itself to such large generalizations as were possible in the case of complete absence of autoerotic activity or even in the case of genital play. We are therefore compelled to narrow down our field

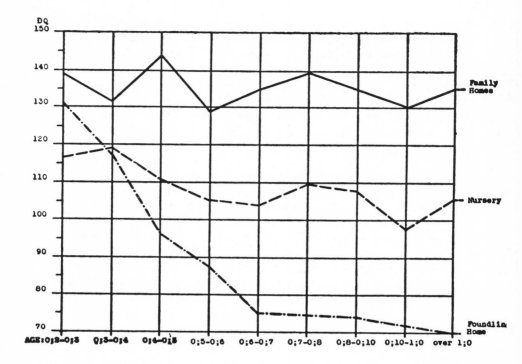

FIGURE 3. DEVELOPMENT QUOTIENTS IN FAMILY HOMES, NURSERY,
FOUNDLING HOME ACCORDING TO AGE IN THE COURSE OF THE FIRST YEAR
OF LIFE

of investigation. We can no longer make a simple sweeping generalization, all-inclusive for the whole group but will have to inspect every single individual within the group. Regrettably enough this was not evident at the beginning of our study and we therefore have only been able to get detailed data on one-quarter of the individuals involved. As shown in Table 3, we have a total of 80 children in our group who manifested rocking exclusively. The mothers of 20 of these were given a battery of psychological tests: the Rorschach, the Szondi, the modified Stanford Binet, the Pass-A-long, the Minkus, etc., and a personal interview. Obviously, the findings cannot be considered conclusive for the whole group. They are, however, consistent with our personal impressions of the mothers: and since the findings within the 25 percent closely investigated by us have been unusually consistent, we consider them fairly indicative of what to expect in the rest of the group.

Of the 20 mothers so tested we have found that 17 have a psychological structure which shows striking similarities, as follows:

1. The general level of maturity of the mothers residing in Nursery is definitely below average. However, the 17 in question are unusually infantile even for this environment. This is expressed not so much in their intellectual level; it is more closely expressed in the incapacity to plan, as evidenced in a number of tests. It is further manifested in the Rorschach, by something which gives the appearance of a defectiveness in the elaboration of defense mechanisms, particularly sublimation.

2. The 17 mothers in question are definitely extrovert personalities with a readiness to intensive positive contact. They show definitely alloplastic tendencies; this agrees well not only with their extrovert attitude, but also with their infantilism, which is in definite contrast to the autoplastic tendencies found in neurotics.

3. All 17 lack the faculty to control their aggression and present both in the tests and in our observations frequent outbursts of negative emotion, of violent hostility.

Accordingly these mothers who are subject to the emotions governing them at any given moment and who do not have the foresight (lack of planning, infantilism) to measure the consequences of their behavior, are unusually inconsistent in their approach to their environment. As already mentioned, their babies are of necessity the main outlets for their labile emotions. Consequently their babies will be exposed alternately to intense outbursts of love and equally intense outbursts of hostility and rage. This is the parental relationship described by Wilhelm Reich (1925) in his study of the impulsive character. We shall discuss why in our opinion the children of such mothers develop rocking as their only autoerotic activity in the first year of life.

The rocking child's personality. The similarity of the rocking children's personalities is perhaps even more impressive than that of their mothers. In contrast to the mothers, where as yet we have detailed personality evaluations and test protocols in only 25 percent of the cases, we are thoroughly informed on the large majority of the children observed by us; each of these children was tested at regular intervals and closely observed once a week during one year. It is by the objective data of the testing procedure, quite apart from any personal impression gained through observation, that the conviction was forced upon us that rocking children show a characteristic personality structure all of their own. No such uniformity is demonstrable in the children who do not rock.

To explain this statement it becomes necessary to give a brief summary of the developmental profile method used in the Hetzer-Wolf Tests (1928). These tests investigate with the help of standardized items (10 per month of age) six sectors of the personality: Body Mastery, Social Adaptation, Memory plus Imitation, Manipulative Ability, and Intelligence. In the profile the ordinate represents the developmental age achieved in the different sectors.

The points reached at a given age level in the different sectors are connected. To the expert the structure of the resulting profile reveals, beyond individual personality constellations, typical developmental and characterological patterns.

The striking finding is that rocking children regardless of their general level of development show two characteristic low points of the profile in two-thirds of the cases. These low points may represent absolute retardation in respect to the chronological age of the infant, or relative retardation in regard to performances in the other sectors of the personality. The two sectors in which the overwhelming majority of rocking children are retarded are their social adaptation and their manipulative ability.

On checking this finding with the total of our sample we find a significant relationship between the above-described —S —M Profile[14] and rocking behavior in infants. This is shown in Table 5.

The two personality sectors in which retardation is evident have to do with activities that measure the child's methods of dealing with his environment, that is, with interrelations between child and environment in which the initiative of the child himself becomes increasingly manifest with advancing age. The sector of manipulative activities has to do with the way the child handles and masters toys, tools, inanimate objects in general. It purports to

TABLE 5. RELATIONSHIP BETWEEN —S —M PROFILE AND ROCKING BEHAVIOR

	Profile		
	—S —M	No —S —M	Total
Rocking	49	28	77
No rocking	4	60	64
Total	53	88	141
Insufficient records indicating tendency to —S —M Profile			29
Total number of children			170

[14] The "—S —M Profile" refers to the pattern of low points in developmental testing which occur in the social adaptation and manipulative ability sectors. Ed.]

measure the child's relation to "things," or, as we have preferred to call this category of the environment, to "objects" which are identical and constant with themselves in time and space.

The sector of social relations, on the other hand, is that in which relations to the human environment are evidenced. These relations include the one which in psychoanalysis is called the relation to the libidinal object. We also speak of constancy of the libidinal object. This constancy is described in analysis as a historical one. Obviously this is a rough differentiation; for a large part of the human environment will never attain the dignity of a libidinal object for a given individual; and in the individual's history a number of his contemporaries will run their course as "things." On the other hand, it is altogether possible (and it regularly occurs at one time or another in the development of the individual) that an inanimate object is by a particular constellation of events enabled to fulfill needs which correspond to the drive structure directed toward the libidinal object.

The consistent retardation of the majority of rocking infants in the sectors of "things" and libidinal objects is a measurable proof of these infants' disturbance in the field of object relations in general. For we find it permissible to assume from unpublished observations of K. M. Wolf that libidinal object relations have to be firmly established to enable infants to form relations with inanimate objects.

Our attention is aroused by the fact that in both sectors it is the relation to environmental objects that is disturbed. Of course, from the point of view of dynamic psychology, we usually consider the relation to libidinal objects as the only one worthy of attention. We are apt to take the relations to things as granted and as of subordinate importance—and so they are. But our finding in the case of infants is a reminder that the world of the psyche is one and indivisible; so that we cannot encounter a disturbance in one sector of the objectal relations without its involving a disturbance of the relations to all other objects, be they even as insignificant as a toy. The disturbance with which we are confronted in the case of the children whose main autoerotic activity consists in rocking is one of complete incapacity to form object relations.

We will ask ourselves now whether this finding sheds any light on the form of autoerotic activity selected among the many possible ones by these children. We believe that a tentative proposition is justified. If we pass in review the different forms of autoerotic activity available to the infant during its first year, such as thumb-sucking, playing with the lips, playing with the ears, nose, hair, or certain privileged limbs, playing with the genitals, or playing with feces, we realize that each of these forms involves an "object" and necessitates cathecting an object representation. The cathexis is of a secondary narcissistic nature, but nevertheless distinguishes the particular "object" of autoerotic activity from the rest of the body.

The only autoerotic activity which does not require such a privileged "object" is rocking. For in rocking the whole body of the infant is subjected to the autoerotic stimulation. The activity is an objectless one—or rather the object activated is the object of the primary narcissistic drive.

With this proposition we have postulated a parallel to the "impulsive personality" described by Reich (1925). In Reich's "impulsive personality" the alternation of extreme permissiveness and extreme hostility on the part of the parents resulted in a personality which is incapable of introjecting a consistent parental imago and as a result of this incapacity cannot develop a normally functioning superego. As a result of this the relations of such impulsive personalities to their environment are as variable and unpredictable as were the original imagines and no object relation is possible, only the acting out of impulses preponderant at any given time, regardless of consequences.

In the case of our infants it is not a question of introjecting parental imagines[15] for the purpose of forming a superego. It is the question of forming the memory traces of an object constant in time and space and consistent with itself. In our proposition the primal object is the libidinal object which forms the pattern for all later object relations. As this object, the mother, is so contradictory that it does not lend itself to the formation of an object which can remain identical with itself in space and time—nor is it sufficiently consistent to remain genetically identical with itself because of the vagaries, ups and downs, in its emotional temperature,—the formation of the primal object relation pattern becomes impossible. Consequently the formation of all later object relations, even with the nonlibidinal objects, with things, will be impaired through the inadequacy of the original experience. It is the original experience with the libidinal object which creates an expectancy pattern. Where that is lacking each single object will have to be approached as an experiment, as an adventure, and as a peril.

Rocking as a dominant autoerotic activity in the first year thus appears as the symptom of the arrest of object relations of every kind, resulting from the inconsistency of the environment's emotional interchange with the child. As such it is to be considered as a pathological sign when it is the exclusive autoerotic activity of the infant and not replaced by more normal ones. Nevertheless it does imply the presence of emotional interchange, be it ever so unsatisfactory, and it is a manifestation of the original drive. This places it in stark contrast to the complete absence of all autoerotic manifestations we have observed in cases of extreme emotional starvation in Foundling Home.

Another aspect of rocking which corroborates our assumptions is that this

---

[15] [Spitz uses the secondary plural of "imago"; the more common plural is "imagoes." Ed.]

is one of the few autoerotic activities at this age in which the child frequently manifests a wild delight, an orgiastic pleasure. The fractioning of the libidinal drives in the different subordinate modes of discharge which one witnesses in genital play, and play activity of all kinds, does not take place in rocking. Here the drive in its totality is directed toward the narcissistic object, the role of which thus becomes comparable to the role of the genital at a much later stage, when the primacy of the genital concentrates upon itself the energy obtained from the partial drives. In the same manner the energy from the different sectors of the infantile personality is concentrated in rocking upon the narcissistic object—of course the concentration in the case of the genital is a genuine one, whereas the concentration in the case of rocking is simply due to the fact that a division of the drive components has not taken place (i. e., that the drive components have not been allocated to their appropriate sectors).

To summarize: Inconsistent, contradictory behavior of the mother makes the establishment of the adequate object relations impossible and arrests the child at the level of primary narcissistic discharge of its libidinal drive in the form of rocking.

c. Fecal Play. In discussing this, the last of the three autoerotic activities observed, we are obliged to change somewhat our presentation. While in the case of genital play and in that of rocking a few words were sufficient to describe the activities in question which are familiar to all observers in the field, such is not the case with fecal play. We shall therefore begin by defining and describing it.

Fecal play in the course of the first year of life is not frequently seen. In the comparatively large number of children (384) observed by us we have not found it in more than 16 cases, all of them in the institution we have called Nursery. As regards onset, the earliest age for which we have it recorded is 8 months and 3 days. The vast majority of our cases fall between 10 and 14 months. In 11 out of these 16 cases the fecal play culminated in coprophagia. We will therefore speak interchangeably of coprophagia or of fecal play. Though the fecal play itself was prolonged and contained many varieties, we had the impression that all this playing was but a preliminary to the final aim of putting the feces in the mouth and, in a number of cases, swallowing it. In those cases in which coprophagia was not observed it may well have occurred during our absence. Therefore we came to the conclusion that fecal play during the first year of life is intimately connected with oral ingestion.

It is a handicap of this presentation that the behavior cannot be shown in the form of the motion pictures we have made of our observations. We must perforce give as close a description as we can from the protocol of one of our cases:

Case N 117 (1; 1 + 26). Female, white. "In standing position when approached by observer offers her hands filled with feces which she tries to put into observer's mouth. She is not unfriendly, reciprocates play and smiles.

When observer withdraws to a distance she sits down, an abstracted expression on her face. The expression is not really depressive. She takes a pellet of feces, rolls it between her thumb and index, then smears it over the sheet and over her legs. She takes another one, manipulates it, passes it from one hand to the other. She uses large walnut size gobs for manipulation. From these she forms pea-size pellets which she puts into her mouth at rare intervals, chewing them. As she does not spit them out they are probably swallowed. The abstracted expression of her face deepens and she passes an audible fecal movement. She lifts her skirt, looks at the full diaper, her face lightens with pleasure while she listens to the flatus she is passing. Except when listening to the flatus she vocalizes a lot.

When the fecal provisions in her hand are exhausted, she begins to manipulate the full diaper with one hand, lifting her skirt with the other and looking at her manipulations. Now she bends forward, seizes the full wet diaper between her teeth and alternately chews and sucks the urine soaked fecal mass through the diaper. From time to time she sticks two fingers sideways into the diaper, picks out some feces, forms a pellet and slips it into her mouth.

This play was observed for 1 hour and 20 minutes. The observer's presence did not disturb her, on the contrary: she related her play to him in a flirtatious, smiling, laughing, vocalizing, contact creating manner, without any apprehension, from time to time offering feces to the observer."

This protocol is presented because of its completeness; it contains approximately all the behavior patterns of the coprophagic child.

However, not all coprophagic children show each of these behavior patterns; neither the offering of feces to the observer which we have observed in three instances, nor the contact seeking, the smile and the laughter, can be seen in all the cases. On the other hand the forming of pellets and eating them is a characteristic of the typical coprophagic child. Only one child (Case N 60), though he smeared feces just like the others, did not form pellets but stuck large pieces of feces into his mouth. This child was mentally deficient.

Our previous findings in the case of complete absence of all autoerotic activities, our findings on children showing genital play, and on those showing rocking, have led us to expect that a specific form of autoerotic activity implies a concomitant specific form of mother-child relation. We found this expectation fully justified when we investigated the mother-child relationship of the coprophagic children.

The mother's personality. We have already previously stressed the variability of the personalities of the mothers in Nursery, but also the fact that psychoses and psychotic trends are relatively rare. It came as a surprise to find that the bulk of the psychoses which came to our attention in this environment was concentrated in the group of those mothers whose children manifested fecal play. Eleven out of the 16 mothers showed the clinical symptoms of depression, reactive or otherwise; 2 of them were paranoiac. Of the remaining 3, 1 was very severely disturbed, but no diagnosis was made; on 2 we have no information. The picture is still more striking when we compare the incidence of depression in the mothers of the group showing fecal play with that of the mothers of the other children, as shown in Table 6.

TABLE 6. RELATION BETWEEN THE MOTHER'S DEPRESSION AND THE CHILD'S FECAL PLAY

Child	Mothers		
	Depression	No depression	Total
Fecal play	11	5	16
No fecal play	5	132	137
Total	16	137	153

The correlation between depressive mothers and children with fecal play is significantly positive in spite of the small sample.

A closer study of these depressive mothers reveals further meaningful details. In the first place we have found that 11 of our 16 cases (70 percent), in accordance with their diagnosis, showed definite intermittent changes of the mothers' behavior toward their children. The duration of these changes varied from a minimum of two to a maximum of six months. In the cases where shorter periods occurred we could observe such swings up to four times in the course of one year. As for their character, the swings varied from extreme hostility with rejection to extreme compensation of this hostility in the form of "oversolicitousness."

We have put the term "oversolicitousness" in quotation marks for a good reason. In a high number of our coprophagic cases, our protocols reveal that remarks to the effect that the mother is tender or loving to her baby are qualified by the statement that this love has some exaggerated traits. We find, for instance, a hungry, fascinated incapacity of the mother to tear herself away from the child. Or we find a statement of a mother that she "cannot look at other children, only at her own." Or such a mother may dislike the other children to the point where she not only neglects them, but does them actual harm. The rejecting or hostile behavior is, in its way, just as peculiar. Overt rejection usually takes the form of a mother declaring that she does not want her child, and offering it for adoption. However, these overt rejections are in the minority; equally infrequent are overt hostile statements of mothers about their children, like that of a mother who "hates her child to be called 'darling.'"

Whatever the overt manifestation of feeling, we found unconscious hostile behavior in all our cases. A surprisingly large number of the coprophagic children (Freud, 1917b) have suffered injury at the hands of their mothers. They suffer burns; they are scalded; one swallows an open safety pin; one is dropped on his head; one is nearly drowned during bathing—we got the impression that without the attentive supervision of the staff few of these children would survive. It is worth mentioning in this connection that the only two cases of actual genital seduction of children by their own mothers which have come to our notice are to be found in this particular group of depressive mothers.

The "love" period is mostly manifested (seven cases) in the beginning of the baby's life and the hostility comes later. But in five cases the obverse holds good. In four cases our records are incomplete in this respect.

The child's personality. The children who manifest coprophagia show also a definite character structure. Of the 16 coprophagic children, 10 are depressive.[16] Table 7 shows the relations of these figures to each other.

Coprophagia is not limited, however, to the depressive episode of the child. We observed also after the depressive episode the following phenomenological differences: These children tried to feed their feces to any person available, be that another child or be that the observer. We could observe this behavior in 3 of our 16 coprophagic children. These subjects showed a smiling expression during their fecal play and took up smiling contact with the observer.

The dynamic effect of the mother-child relationship. The picture presented by the mothers of these coprophagic children is that of a personality with a deep-seated ambivalence. Periodically the superego has the upper hand, the

---

[16] For the criteria of depression in the first year of life we refer to our previous publication (Spitz, 1946a). For the sake of simplification we shall in the following speak of depressive children. The concept of psychiatric disturbance in infancy is so recent that adequate differentiation of syndromes has hardly begun. We have been able to differentiate such syndromes as hospitalism, marasmus, and depression. In the above quoted article we have already hinted that the anaclitic depression syndrome probably shows certain subdivisions, one of which we have qualified as "mild depression." We believe that in the coprophagic cases another of these syndromes will in due time become discernible, for, though these children may present many of the signs and symptoms of the anaclitic depression, a certain percentage of them show striking physiognomical differences. While the facial expression of children suffering from anaclitic depression is actually comparatable to that of a grown-up suffering from severe reactive depression, more than half of the coprophagic children showed a facial expression which resembled far more that of paranoiac suspicion or that of catatonic daze. Furthermore the basic phenomenological difference between the anaclitic depressive and the present category lies in the coprophagia, for children with anaclitic depression present oral symptoms, if any, mostly *after* they have come out of their depression. Coprohagic children on the other hand, though frequently depressive, manifest their oral symptoms *during* this depressive state.

TABLE 7. RELATION BETWEEN THE CHILD'S DEPRESSION AND THE CHILD'S FECAL PLAY

Child			
	Severe depression	No depression	Total
Fecal play	10	6	16
No fecal play	24	115	139
Total	34	121	155

hostile components are repressed, the presenting picture is that of a self-sacrificing, self-debasing mother, who envelops her child with her love. Such a mother may for instance pester the observer consistently during this period with her worries about her child, particularly during the first months, when they frequently assume that the child is deaf or blind. Or in another case the mother said: "My baby is so little [at the time it was one year old] I am afraid to hurt it." Or again in another case a naive observer, a nurse, remarked about a mother: "She is defiant, like a lioness with her cub."

In the case of the 11 mothers with periodical changes these "love" periods lasted for an appreciable time, never less than two months. After that they would be replaced by a swing to the opposite attitude, to overt hostility or to overt manifestation of unconscious hostility. In all cases such hostile periods again lasted for an appreciable time, again not less than two months.

Thus the child is confronted with a libidinal object which presents one consistently maintained attitude during a period which appears to be sufficiently long to permit the forming of object relations. When this period is at its end the object of these object relations becomes the opposite of what it was before. But then again it remains consistently the same for a sufficiently long time to permit on the one hand the formation of new object relations, on the other the formation of a compensation reaction to the loss of the previously established object. It is of this compensatory reaction that we will speak further on.[17]

Prior to that, however, we wish to compare the dynamic picture of the mothers of the rocking children to that of the mothers of the coprophagic children. In the case of the rocking children we had stressed the inconsistency of the love object, of the mother. We mentioned that they expose their children

---

[17] Such a picture has been assumed by Rado (1927). He extrapolated from adult analysis and postulated the presence of a "bad mother" as distinct from a "good mother," at the age of early ego-ideal formation.

alternately to intense outbursts of love and equally intense outbursts of rage. But it would be an error to confound this picture with the periodicity observed in the mothers of the coprophagic children. The infantile personality of the mothers of the rocking children does not permit a consistent attitude lasting for days, let alone months. Their tantrums alternate with kissing jags within the hour and at no time is their behavior predictable from the point of view of the child. Its libidinal object alternates so rapidly between the opposite poles and passes so rapidly through every point of the compass of emotions that all attempts at forming an object relation must fail.

It is interesting to note that the correlations between genital play and rocking on one hand, and genital play and coprophagia on the other, offer support to our proposition. We have called rocking the most archaic of our three activities, with only thumb-sucking going back possibly to an earlier level. Rocking is preobjectal. Its object is a primary narcissistic one and therefore it is observed in a number of cases before the appearance of genital play as a simple infantile form of autoerotic behavior without any pathology attached to it. It becomes pathological only when it persists throughout the whole of the first year. When it does that it excludes in the large majority of cases the coexistence of genital play, understandably so, as genital play presupposes a certain level of object relation. This mutual exclusiveness is evident in Table 3.

Fecal play on the other hand consists in the actual manipulation of an object. Therefore it presupposes object relations of a sort, even though they may be pathological ones. It is noteworthy that in 5 out of our 16 cases of fecal play, genital play was also observed. Furthermore, in most of these cases genital play appeared before coprophagia, thus implying the presence of object relations, which later were disturbed. One might say that in these cases the subsequent fecal play appears as a distortion of the original object relations.

However, this does not provide us as yet with an explanation of why fecal play and particularly coprophagia is chosen by these children. We believe that such an explanation involves speculative assumptions, a step we are hesitant to take. We offer a hypothesis on the question therefore with diffidence, as a working hypothesis, and feel ready to renounce it if a better one can be found.

Our hypothesis is in the first place based on the assumption of the oral introjection postulated for depression by Freud (1917b) and Abraham (1924). This oral introjection in the depressed person is of course unconscious. But its manifestations are perceptible enough to the observer. The devouring oral attitude of the mothers in question was evident, going to the point of cunilingus. Our proposition therefore is that the children identified with the unconscious tendencies manifested by their mothers. This identification led the children to the oral introjection of their object. It took place as a result of the change in the personality of the original love object, which was thus lost to the children. As this loss, or one of these losses, coincides with the end of the first year—in our opinion the transition to the anal phase—the object which becomes available at this point is the fecal object. Of course the fecal object becomes an object only at the moment when it is discovered in the diaper. Whether the deep absorption of the infant's face during the expulsion of its feces at this age denotes its perception of the excrement as an object or only its perception of the anal stimulation; and whether the following expression of gratification, when expulsion has been completed, is amenable to an interpretation; whether this interpretation can be expressed in the terms of the fecal mass becoming an object already during the expulsion and whether therefore the expulsion is experienced as a repetition of the loss of the libidinal object—that we are not prepared to say. However, when the expulsion has been completed and the visibly pleasurable sensations of the child have been savored and come to their end (that is, half a minute later), a new act begins. The child turns again to the outside world. In many cases he sits up, looks around, discovers the diaper and visibly interested, reaches for the fecal mass. At this point the fecal mass in the diaper has become an object, and a libidinally cathected one. Witness the way these children handle the feces-filled diaper and how they rapidly proceed either to put the whole diaper with the fecal mass in their mouth and chew it, notwithstanding the acrobatic contortions necessary for this; or, in the other case, take out a piece of the mass and go through the procedure already described in our case history. At this point the object has become one which is introjected. It is an open question whether we should think of this introjection in terms of a part-object.

This hypothesis is not quite as speculative as it would appear. The question of the child's identifying itself with the mother's unconscious wishes is not at all problematic at this age. As published elsewhere (Spitz, 1946a), the ego of the infant in the first year is rudimentary and is only able to subsist thanks to the circumstance that it is supplemented by the mother's personality. As a result of this circumstance which we have described as the "mother-child dual"[18] most of the infant's functions take place in closest concomitance and interaction with the mother's actions and attitudes, either as their prolongation, or as their origin, or paralleling them all along the way. Such a function will of course amount to something which (if we wish at this early age to avoid the term of identification which implies a specific mechanism) could be called a practical identity, a lack of differentiation between ego and environment.

[18] A similar concept of the unity between mother and child, object and the precursor of the ego, was described by Ernst Paul Hoffman (1935) and called "Zweieinigkeit" (p. 367).

If we add to this that at this period, conscious and unconscious, ego and id are not yet delimited in the infant, it is easy to imagine the infant enacting unconscious attitudes of the mother.

There is some support for this assumption in our figures also. Not only do 11 of the 16 mothers of the coprophagic children suffer from depression, but 2 of the 5 remaining mothers show similar periodic changes in their attitudes to their children, bringing this relationship up to the impressive total of 13 out of 16. Furthermore we find that out of a total of 11 of these mothers who were depressive, 8 have children who had also manifest depressions. This should not be taken as an indication of heredity.

Thus our assumption would be that coprophagia as autoerotic activity in the first year of life is covariant with depression in the mother. The effective factors in the mother's depression are two: its periodical nature and its unconscious oral introjective tendencies. In the child we find three factors: (1) the compliance of the child's structural level for the purpose of identification with the mother's trends; (2) the child's reaction to the loss of its libidinal object, a dynamic compliance; (3) the phase compliance or genetic compliance of the child's being situated at the transitional period from the oral to the anal phase.

IV. THEORETICAL CONCLUSIONS

If we consider now the three autoerotic activities we have observed and discussed, we find that they represent stages of object relations. The nature of the objectal relations is the determinant of the particular autoerotic activity chosen. The nature of the object relation also is expressed by the form the autoerotic activity takes.

From this point of view our presentation should in reality have started with rocking. Here the nature of the object relation was the most primitive one, a primary narcissistic relation, or to be more exact, a regression to the primary narcissistic stage. It is caused by a maternal personality which does not permit the formation of any object relation whatsoever. The form it takes is a non-objectal activity of the libidinal drive.

The coprophagic activity is on another level. Here we have a real object relation, though a distorted one, to a part-object. The formation of the object relation is made possible by a consistent attitude of the mother lasting for an appreciable time. The distortion of the object relation is caused by a change in the mother's personality, which change in its turn is maintained for an appreciable period. The object centers upon itself the aggressive and the libidinal drives.

In genital play the object relations are satisfactory and remain attached to the libidinal object, thanks to its consistent facilitation of such object relations. Here the autoerotic activity remains within the framework of the whole of the objectal activities of the child and is a subordinate activity of minor importance.

V. SUMMARY

A group of 170 children was observed during their first year of life for the incidence of three autoerotic activities: genital play, rocking, and fecal play. The mother-child relations were established as the variable among the environmental factors which could affect this group. Two control groups were used in which the variable was kept as constant as possible: one group of family children with optimal mother-child relations and one group of institutionalized children where mother-child relations were so to say absent.

It was found that autoerotic activities are a function of the object relations prevailing during the first year of life. They are absent when object relations are absent; when object relations are so constantly contradictory that object formation is made impossible, rocking results. When object relations change in an intermittent manner fecal play results. When object relations are "normal," genital play results.

The dynamics of these different object relations were investigated and discussed.

Editor's Commentary: The Pinneau-Spitz Controversy

By 1955, the preceding four papers had become enormously influential in clinical and social welfare circles. In that year Spitz was stunned by an extensive criticism of these papers published in *Psychological Bulletin,* which many considered devastating. Pinneau (1955) found little in Spitz's work that was convincing from a research standpoint and stated that considering the data presented, Spitz's conclusions were unwarranted. As succeeding issues of the *Bulletin* document, Spitz replied to Pinneau and Pinneau then to Spitz. This controversy is significant not only for its historical interest, but also for the light it casts on the contrasting approaches of the experimental psychologist and the clinician-researcher. Paradoxically, Pinneau's criticism, while valid in many respects, serves to emphasize the strengths as well as the weaknesses in Spitz's approach. Consideration of these issues may instruct both the clinician and developmental researcher of today.

The major brunt of Pinneau's criticism concerned Spitz's inadequate descriptions of ecological background, of samples, and of observational methods. The studies had no description of interobserver reliability or of the conditions under which observations were made. Data were presented in such a way that one could not determine how many cases were observed longitudinally and how many cross-sectionally. Further, Spitz did not specify the initial health conditions of infants. How many were abnormal at birth? How many were assessed during illness—perhaps having succumbed to the notoriously lethal measles epidemic of the Hospitalism study? Because of the manner in which data were presented, one could not determine accurate relationships between the decline of infants and the times of separation from mothers. Certainly by today's editorial standards these papers would probably be accepted for publication only after these matters were clarified. Pinneau then attacked the validity of the developmental test instrument, the Hetzer-

Wolf test. He pointed out that this instrument was inadequately standardized on a poor Viennese population, that the test contained an overestimation of the developmental quotient in the early months, and that the test's predictive validity had not been established.

Subsequent studies have provided evidence that Spitz's inferences were correct regarding the links between maternal separation and depression and regarding the differential effects of acute separation before and after six months of age. Given this evidence, and acknowledging Pinneau's valid criticisms about data presentations and the developmental instrument, we might ask what Pinneau missed in not appreciating the meaningfulness of Spitz's work. Perhaps there was something about the nature of the clinician's perspective that was not accounted for in Pinneau's criticism. Spitz followed a number of infants longitudinally and noticed that after separation from their mothers, they became weepy, had sad facial expressions, and were immobile; their faces often had dazed looks; and they sometimes engaged in autoerotic activities. Spitz felt saddened and was reminded of the adult state of depression. Even though infants could not tell him how they felt, *he* felt they were depressed, and he related their plight to the loss of a loved one. Spitz felt something inside himself that was communicated by these infants, and he made use of that feeling to facilitate a widened perception. After this, he was able to see a clinical syndrome that included a pattern of behavior, affective communication, and events occurring over time. Spitz used the developmental tests, not so much as a predictor of retardation, but as a way of assessing the infant's level of functioning in the context of current interactive circumstances.

In his published reply to Pinneau, Spitz (1955d) chose not to address many of Pinneau's criticisms directly. Nor did he delineate the clinician's perspective. Instead, he restated what he considered to be his conclusions. In their emphasis on the process of mothering, on affective interchange, and on reciprocity, these conclusions sound quite modern:

1. That affective interchange is paramount, not only for the development of emotion itself in infants, but also for the maturation and the development of the child, both physical and behavioral.
2. That this affective interchange is provided by the reciprocity between the mother (or her substitute) and the child.
3. That depriving the child of this interchange is a serious, and in extreme cases, a dangerous handicap for its development in every sector of the personality [p. 454].

Much of the recent scientific literature has emphasized the effects of the early caretaking experience on subsequent development. We now appreciate that such effects are complex and bidirectional, with influences going from infant to parent as well as from parent to infant (Bell and Harper, 1977). The typical caregiving experience is certainly not limited to one caregiver (Clarke-Stewart, 1977; Lamb, 1978). Further, the young child who has experienced early deprivation is remarkably "resilient"; given a major salutary and enduring change in the caretaking environment, major cognitive deficits can be made up and psychopathology need not result (see Clarke and Clarke, 1977; Kagan, Kearsley and Zelazo, 1978; for a critical review, from the psychoanalytic point of view, see Emde, 1980).

As his response to Pinneau illustrates, Spitz became less concerned with loss of the mother and more concerned with affective reciprocity as the key ingredient missing in those deprived infants who so bothered him. The following paper, "Anaclitic Depression in an Infant Raised in an Institution," shows the continued growth of his thoughts as he discarded two of his initial ideas about anaclitic depression. At first, Spitz thought that anaclitic depression was irreversible after three months and that it was linked to the loss of a primary mothering figure. This later paper describes a prolonged anaclitic depression syndrome in an institutionalized infant who then recovered. Although Spitz is not the senior author, the paper is included to show the extension of his thinking in the face of new clinical and research data.

Anaclitic Depression in an Infant Raised in an Institution

with Robert N. Emde, M.D. and Paul R. Polak, M.D.

Anaclitic depression was originally described as a psychiatric disturbance in infancy which results from maternal deprivation in the second half of the first year of life (Spitz, 1946a). The original description states: "If the nursing staff reports a sudden development of changed behavior in the child without demonstrable organic disease and if this can be correlated to a separation from the child's mother or mother substitute, our suspicion as to the presence of anaclitic depression will be confirmed."

Since the original description, other authors have questioned whether such a syndrome could develop in the absence of a preceding bond with a mother or mother substitute. Orlansky (1949) has stated: "It should be noted that in the cases of anaclitic depression reported by Spitz the children affected had been accustomed since birth to the care and attention of their mothers. One wonders if the same reaction would have taken place had they not been accustomed to such personal attention during their first year of life." Casler (1961), in a later extensive review of the maternal deprivation literature, continued this line of thought by stressing the importance of differentiating between cases in which there is a rupture of an existing maternal-infant bond and cases in which no such bond developed.

In the course of our research in a residential nursery for infants, we had the opportunity to observe the development of one of the maternal deprivation syndromes. The syndrome of anaclitic depression was noted to develop without the rupture of an existing mother-infant bond and to resolve without a mother-child reunion.

The residential nursery has been described in a previous publication (Polak, Emde, and Spitz, 1964a). Prior to his developing anaclitic depression, the infant of this study was among many followed in a longitudinal study of the smiling response. Because of this, a large amount of background data and movie films were obtained before the syndrome developed. Historical and

Reprinted from *Journal of the American Academy of Child Psychiatry*, 4: 545–553, 1965.

chart information from the professional staff of the nursery supplemented our direct observations and movie analysis.

CASE HISTORY

George, a 6 lb., 8 oz. male infant, came to the residential nursery at eight days of age. Of Spanish-American parentage, he had been born at a local hospital. No abnormalities were noted in his delivery or in his physical examination at birth. During his first month at the nursery he was noted by a nurse to exhibit a good deal of "fussy crying"; he seemed to be very demanding and wanting more attention than other babies his age. However, at other times, he was described as being "shy," preferring to remain in bed rather than being held. As was the usual nursery procedure, he was moved at age 1 month from the room where he had been since his arrival to an adjacent room with infants from 1 to 2 months of age. At age 2 months he was again moved, this time to a large crib dormitory housing infants from approximately 2 to 6 months of age. Each of these moves was accomplished easily and without any noted change in behavior on the part of George.

During his first month in the crib dormitory, it was noted that, unlike other infants his age, George objected to sitting in the teeter chair. During this time, Mrs. L., one of the staff members who most often took care of George, went away on a 10-day vacation without any noticeable effect on him. At 2 months and 20 days, George began to smile regularly to the nodding human face and was included in weekly observations for our smiling study (Polak, Emde, and Spitz, 1964a). He was observed by the authors regularly throughout the duration of his smiling response.

At age 3 months, Mrs. L. noted that George began to demand attention more actively. Prior to this time, it was felt that he needed more attention because of his fussiness, but now he would actively seek attention; when he was not picked up at such times, he would evidence what was described by Mrs. L. as an "angry cry." George's sensorimotor development, as observed by the authors, progressed well within the range of normal from 3 to 5 months. In our discrimination study comparing the moving human face and the moving photograph of the face (Polak, Emde, and Spitz, 1964b), George evidenced clear discrimination by smiling preferentially to the human face at 3 months and 7 days. Preferential vocalization to the human face (as compared to the photograph of it) occurred at 4 months and 4 days. Both discriminations took place at typical ages for our nursery population. From 3½ months through 5 months of age, George continued to smile strongly to the nodding human face, but he did not smile at all to a similarly nodding photograph of the same face. Within single experimental sessions, George's smiling, by our measures, appeared more regularly than that of other infants with little variation in magnitude on successive stimulus presentations. He almost invariably responded to the nodding human face with a quick, broad, long-lasting smile. As was typical of our sample, George's smiling response to the nodding human face began to diminish a few weeks before he reached 6 months of age. At 4 months, George was tested using the Bühler developmental tests (Bühler and Hetzer, 1932). His developmental quotient was 114, again within the normal range for our population.

At 6 months of age George was again transferred; this time, the transfer was to a room at the other end of the nursery which contained older children, usually from 6 months up to 2½ years of age. One week after the transfer, Bühler testing was repeated. The developmental quotient was 90. Not only was this considered below the norm for this age of our nursery population, but it represented a decrease of 21 percent compared to his developmental quotient of 2 months earlier. Three-and-one-half weeks after the transfer, the smiling response to the human face disappeared. At the age of 8 months and 10 days, stranger anxiety was noted during a routine visit to the nursery. That is, George cried and turned his head away when approached by one of the experimenters. As in the original description of stranger anxiety (Spitz, 1946a), when the experimenter offered his back to George, making sure that his face was out of George's line of vision, George established contact by exploring the back of the experimenter. After establishing contact, it was possible to interact with George face to face without the dramatic crying which resulted from an initial face to face approach. A few days later, Mrs. L. took note on George's chart of his display of crying in response to strangers, which she found unusual for nursery babies. In our observations of George during the next 2 weeks, marked stranger anxiety persisted. Approximately 3½ weeks after the onset of stranger anxiety, at the age of 9 months, George was found in the pathognomonic posture of anaclitic depression. He refused contact by any of the authors, *even when the gradual back approach was used*. During the following weeks our visits to the nursery would invariably result in finding George in the same posture—lying in his crib in the knee-chest prone position with the pathetic facial expression of anaclitic depression. Three months after George's anaclitic depression began, a small experiment was performed. The purpose of this experiment was to see if George responded to "friend" (i.e., nursery staff) in the same way as he did to "stranger" (i.e., one of the experimenters). George was found in his usual position, lying on the crib mattress in the pathognomonic position. One of us approached and George screamed and turned away as anticipated. Some time after the intruder withdrew, George once again ceased crying and assumed his original posture. At this point one of the two nursery staff members who was largely responsible for caring for George approached him. Not only did George not cry, but he seemed somewhat easily comforted as N. picked him up in her arms.

In total, we estimated the period of anaclitic depression to last approximately 7½ months. A slight change in George's anaclitic depression began to appear when he was almost 14 months old, 5 months after the onset of the anaclitic depression. At that time a chart notation indicated that he was beginning to crawl again; he had ceased to crawl after the onset of anaclitic depression, spending much of his time in the pathognomonic position described above. His crawling behavior occurred at the same time he began to accept a neighbor infant of the same age, Lynne, as his playmate. Lynne had been in the nursery since birth but was not depressed as she was walking and interested in adult contact. Although we could not approach George directly at this time, we observed that he would play with Lynne, engaging in such activities as give and take of soft toys. We also noted that if we engaged Lynne in play, George's interest could be attracted. At these times he did not actively avoid looking into our faces, although he still resisted any advances by us. At the age of 16½ months, George began to make increasingly successful attempts at walking. Coincident with this, his anaclitic depression resolved. George once again appeared to enjoy human adult contact.

Subsequently, George progressively increased his mobility, walking through the nursery whenever he was allowed. He made more friends among the other children his age in the nursery and we would frequently find him actively playing with them when we arrived. He continued to welcome adult contact and began to seek it actively by giggling and jumping up and down in his crib when we entered the crib room. Incidental observations, however, revealed that he showed some abnormal distress at times, by crying, when one's approach to him was sudden and when it involved physical contact. He made some successful trial weekend visits to the homes of some volunteer workers, and at the age of 20 months was adopted. Our initial reports from his adoptive home indicate that he is doing well.

At first we were quite puzzled by the development of this case of anaclitic depression. A biological mother seemed not to be involved, as George had been separated from her since birth. George was taken care of by many different people, but two of them, L. and N., were most consistently involved with him. Both women were employed full time by the nursery and were responsible for 20 or more children at any given time. As a first step we checked the vacation schedules of these two mother surrogates in order to ascertain the time correlation with George's anaclitic depression.

Although the actual anaclitic depression did not begin until age nine months, we began to observe behavioral changes in George shortly after his transfer to the crib room at age six months. Approximately one week after this transfer the developmental quotient of 90 was obtained, and two months later stranger anxiety was noted. It was found that shortly after the event of transfer, N. went on vacation for one week and, following this, L. went on vacation for ten days. While some relationship between their temporary absence from the nursery and George's state seemed possible, it was not a satisfactory explanation of George's behavior. The anaclitic depression had its onset after their return, and was not resolved by their presence. Further investigation of changes at the time of transfer was therefore undertaken.

Before transfer, George resided in a dormitory with 16 other infants, under the care of four regular nursery staff members. After transfer, he was in another room containing 17 infants, but with only two regular staff members in attendance. Thus the transfer resulted in a 50 percent decrease in regular staff members taking care of the infants. In addition, it was discovered that teenage summer volunteers visited the infants of the two- to six-month age group much more frequently than they visited the older infants. In the former room, there were many regular volunteers who came on specific days to play with, cuddle, and feed the babies. According to L., George seemed to get to "know" some of the teenage volunteers who came regularly. He sought their attention, and his "fussy crying" often subsided when one of them picked him up. When he was moved to the room with older infants, George found far fewer volunteers coming to see him, and they came less regularly. To add to his loss, when school resumed four weeks after George's transfer, teenage volunteers' visits decreased further.

Another change occurred in the way feeding took place before and after transfer. In the two- to six-month nursery, infants were routinely held by a staff person or volunteer during feeding, and meals were given four times a day. In the six-month-and-over nursery, the infants were suddenly graduated to high chairs and meals of junior foods three times a day. This clearly involved a good deal less physical contact with the feeder. The importance of skin contacts in the feeding and mothering of infants has been emphasized (Spitz, 1950d).

A detailed consideration of the time during which George's anaclitic depression resolved was equally revealing. When he was 16 months old, two weeks before we considered the depression to have resolved, the end of the school year brought another influx of enthusiastic teenage volunteers. Initially, according to L., George sat in his crib and cried on approach of the volunteers, but they persisted, frequently picking him up and giving him much attention. Their persistence bore fruit, and L. stated that eventually George no longer cried at their approach and began to show that he enjoyed them.

DISCUSSION

The case of George appears to extend the clinical picture of anaclitic depression. This syndrome is known to occur after separation interferes with an existing mother-infant bond. However, it does not occur after each such instance. The original description (Spitz, 1946a) emphasized that maternal separation should be considered a necessary but not a sufficient cause of the syndrome, because not all infants with maternal separation develop anaclitic depression. The case of George reveals a classical clinical picture of this syndrome developing in an infant who had never established a relationship with a mother, or a single mother surrogate. George was cared for by a large number of people, and it was apparently a sudden decrease in the amount and quality of this mothering from many people that was associated with the onset of anaclitic depression, and an increase in this mothering from many sources that was followed by his restoration to health.

The role of a peer infant in the recovery from anaclitic depression may have been more important than we at first thought. There is a correspondence of George's beginning to crawl again and of his beginning to play with Lynne, an infant placed next to him. More recent experiments by H. and M. Harlow (1964) have shown that the mother-infant relationship in the rhesus monkey could, to a large extent, be substituted by permitting the infant monkeys to play with other age-matched infant peers. These peer monkeys could be equally deprived or nondeprived infants. However, caution must be used in applying these findings to the human infant. In terms of maturation the rhesus monkey is born with a physical and mental development which corresponds to the human infant of 1 to 1½ years. It would seem the human infant is much more vulnerable. If an analogy from Harlow's work is useful, it may be that in humans peer interaction can substitute for mothering only when such play is possible—i.e., after the first year of life (see Spitz's discussion of Harlow and Harlow, 1964).

The importance of locomotion in the treatment of anaclitic depression has been pointed out (Spitz, 1946a), and in this case there is a correlation between increasing locomotion and George's improvement. It is uncertain whether this was an added factor in his improvement or a natural concomitant of it, but it is likely that both were involved. During the time of his initial improvement, George was often placed on the floor and allowed more opportunity for crawling and, later, walking.

George's anaclitic depression followed what we diagnosed as a classical case of eight months anxiety. With time, one syndrome fused into the other. This was recorded dramatically on film and serves again to underscore Spitz's original statement that the difference between eight months anxiety and anaclitic depression is basically a quantitative rather than a qualitative one.

An unexpected finding was the duration of George's anaclitic depression. Originally, a period of 3 months was considered critical, after which the process of depression appeared to be irreversible (Spitz, 1950d). George does provide an exception to this, as his anaclitic depression lasted 7½ months.

There remains an intriguing question. Why should George develop anaclitic depression in a situation of a relative decrease in mothering when most of the infants in the institution experienced the same relative decrease with no visible problems? A partial answer may lie in George's personality before the age of six months. He was described as shy, withdrawn, fussy, and at the same time demanding. Another consideration arises from the finding that all of the cases of severe depression occurred in situations where there was an estimate of a "good mothering" relationship (Spitz, 1946a). In this study, the majority of infants with no depression, and maternal separation, were found to have an estimate of "bad mothering." This led Spitz to comment: "Evidently it is more difficult to replace a satisfactory love object than an unsatisfactory one." Was it because of the "good mothering" George had at the nursery that he became susceptible where others did not? Or is it possible that by some combination of heredity and environmental factors, he was more vulnerable to decreases in mothering than other infants? Unfortunately, at our present state of knowledge we feel it is not possible to answer these questions.

Part 2

THE EMERGENCE OF DIALOGUE

Editor's Introduction

As the preceding section illustrates, Spitz's thought became increasingly concerned with the mothering process. Having started with what was missing in those infants who so poignantly represented tragic "experiments in nature," Spitz turned his attention toward discovering what promoted growth in healthy infants. As he considered the ways normal infant development took place under conditions of affective reciprocity, he came to his concept of the "dialogue." Although this concept does not appear until 1963, its origins may date from his extensive study of the infant's "Smiling Response." The major portion of a brief but delightful 1946 monograph on this topic begins this section. "Autoerotism Reexamined" presents another preface to this concept, whose full development is offered in "Life and the Dialogue," "The Derailment of Dialogue," and "The Evolution of Dialogue."

The concept of dialogue refers to the socially dynamic situation that is required for caregiving. Although the word "dialogue" may at first seem paradoxical when applied to infancy—a period of development named for its characteristic of being without speech (from Latin, *in* + *fans:* unable to speak, *Oxford English Dictionary*)—Spitz chose this word to emphasize that a basic communication process does exist in infancy. Although communications are not verbal, they are complex, emotional, and two way, providing adaptive information for both parent and infant. Writing in the early 1960s, Spitz thus not only extended the psychoanalytic concept of "object relations" in the social sphere, but also gave a legitimate focus to the study of the ways in which the infant sends and receives signals and the ways in which the infant influences his or her own experience of being cared for. Approaches hinted at by Spitz are now in the forefront of research (see Brazelton, Koslowski, and Main, 1974; Bell and Harper, 1977; Stern, 1977; Osofsky, 1979).

Excerpts from "The Smiling Response: A Contribution to the Ontogenesis of Social Relations"

with the assistance of Katherine M. Wolf, Ph.D.

I. THE PROBLEM

A. INTRODUCTION AND SURVEY OF THE LITERATURE

One of the first manifestations of positive emotional experience in the infant is the smile. We realize that we lay ourselves open to criticism when we speak of the baby's smile as a manifestation of positive emotion, or as we will call it from now on, of pleasure. We have no way of knowing whether the infant really experiences pleasure when it smiles. An old wife's adage states that, on the contrary, when the baby smiles it has a bellyache. As a general statement the adage is certainly false, but the slight amount of truth it contains makes it necessary to discuss it and to elucidate the question as to what the smile of the baby really is.

Whenever we speak here and in the following of "smiling" we will refer to the facial configuration of lips and face known as "smile" in grown-ups. We shall also include those pathognomic[1] activities such as grinning and laughing which in grown-ups, or in the older child, are considered as even more pronounced manifestations of the emotions which evoke a smile.

Smiling in the form of the pathognomic activity of widening and curling of lips appears quite early in the baby—according to Bühler (1933) as soon as the tenth day of life. We have observed and filmed an infant smiling on the eighth day of life. A few earlier observations are reported in the literature (Moore, 1896; Dearborn, 1897, 1900; Ament, 1899; Blanton, 1917; Watson, 1924). There seems no reason to question the possibility of smiling imme-

---

Reprinted from *Genetic Psychology Monographs*, 34:57–125, 1946.

[1] Pathognomic (from the Greek *pathos*—suffering, passion, and *gnome*—judgment)—the recognition of emotions and passions through their outward signs and expression. (*Webster's International Dictionary*, 1943.) Modern scientific tradition has limited the usage of this term more or less to facial expression.

diately after birth, since at this early age smiling does not appear to be correlated with any specific stimulus or situation. It is one of the numerous expressive movements of the face observed in the baby, such as frowning, opening and closing of the mouth, protruding of the tongue, and facial distortion which we consider to be in the nature of the overflow phenomena. It does not differ in this from the squirming, writhing movements of arms, legs, and trunk, which appear indiscriminately at this age whenever a stimulus strong enough to overcome the very high perceptive threshold of the first week of life is offered. Under these circumstances it is obvious that any of these manifestations, including smiling, can occur in response to any stimulus; thus the old wife's adage, according to which the baby smiles when it has a bellyache, is justified in a way. The baby may smile when it has abdominal pain, to be sure. But it may also squirm or frown or do any number of other things for the same reason. This period of indiscriminate manifestation of pathognomic activity, however, is outgrown very soon in the course of the baby's development. By the third month his smile has become a reaction distinctly linked to certain stimuli. The nature of these stimuli differentiates them definitely from any experience which could be called painful or disagreeable in the grown-up. From this point on it will not be possible to say that when the baby has a bellyache it smiles. From this age level on (more accurately from this developmental level on, since the chronological age varies) smiling will not be manifested in any psychological situation in which pain, rage, anger, boredom, or neglect is experienced. These are the situational configurations in which neither the infant, the toddler, the school child, the adolescent, nor the grown-up will smile except in one of those conventional elaborations of the smiling gesture which are developed into a semantic system of facial expression in the process of growing up. It appears therefore that there is an unbroken genetic line for a large number of situational configurations which do *not* act as a stimulus for smiling.

On the other hand, from this developmental level on the infant does produce the smiling response in a certain well-defined situational configuration. As Gesell and various other authors have stated, this situational configuration can be described in psychological terms as the anticipation of the gratification of a specific need. We will discuss in the last part of this paper the characteristics and factors involved in this "need gratification." Suffice it to say here that it takes place on the social level and that the infant's behavior in response to it manifests physiognomic characteristics of *striving toward* the stimulus configuration; two months later it gives the impression of striving for, and of pleasure in, reciprocity. Since pleasure is an emotional shading which can only be ascertained with the help of introspection, the physiognomic characteristics of the infant's behavior alone would be insufficient to justify our assertion that the infant smiles because it experiences pleasure.

We find, however, that the specific situations of need gratification in which the infant smiles are the same as those in which the toddler, the school child, the adolescent, and the grown-up smile. Furthermore, introspection among older children and adults reveals that the emotion they experience in these situations is pleasure. Inasmuch as the older child and adult introspectively reveal as pleasurable those situations which bring forth a smile, and inasmuch as the infant's smile is evoked in the same kind of situations, it is clear that there is an unbroken genetic line connecting the pleasurable experiences of the infant and the adult.

Three statements can be made about the infant:

1. A wide range of emotions exists in which the smile never occurs from the third month on.

2. The situation in which smiling is produced from the third month on is always *one of a specific need gratification.*

3. The physiognomic characteristics of the infant's behavior in the smiling response remains the same from the third month on, and can be defined by the behavioristic term of *Zuwendung,* turning towards.

As soon as verbal communication becomes possible, these three elements as well as smiling are connected with the introspectively recognized emotional shading of pleasure. We feel therefore that the evidence is overwhelmingly in favor of assuming that the infant also experiences the emotion of pleasure when it smiles.

In the baby, however, at least during the second quarter of the first year, it is not *every* satisfactory or pleasurable experience which evokes the smile. Thus the infant does not smile consistently at its food or at its toys. The stimulus by which its smiling can be consistently evoked must be a stimulus coming from a human partner (C. Bühler, 1937a; Murphy and Murphy, 1931). Various manifestations of the human partner can evoke the baby's smile. Referring to what we have said about psychology being the science of human interrelations, it is of interest that smiling develops at a very early age into an essentially social manifestation, the manifestation of pleasure experienced when beholding the presence of a human partner.[2]

This in itself is quite unexpected. However, it is put into still more striking relief by the fact that it stands out as by far the most advanced among the child's reactions at this period. For if we study closely the behavior inventory

---

[2] That the human face is the most potent visual stimulus during early infancy has attracted the attention of investigators in fields so far removed from our present study as that of ophthalmology. It has been put to use there in studying eye movements (Kestenbaum, 1930).

of the third month of life—or even that of the fourth—we find that no other behavior pattern shows as much perceptive discrimination or of specificity as does the smiling response on beholding a human being. It is as if the infant had suddenly developed a behavior pattern far in advance of the rest of its behavior. This phenomenon of the early appearance of the smile as a fully differentiated diacritic manifestation, at a period when no such manifestations exist in any other sector of development is a further support of our assumptions on affects. We assume affects to be the prerequisite for perception as well as for all other mental activity. We find in studying the behavior of the child that affective discrimination is the earliest of all and breaks the trail for all the rest of the development.

I do not believe that most psychologists have visualized the phenomenon in these terms and it is tempting to speculate why they have overlooked this fact. Probably since the newborn is unconsciously considered a human being right from the beginning, the fact that at times its social behavior resembles that of a human being, does not surprise them. We are all inclined to overrate the intellectual performances of the infant, we are prone to what I call an "adultomorph" approach. In its earlier stages the whole theory of the infant's mental life was impregnated with this error. Later workers in the field of infant psychology on the other hand became conscious of this source of error and sought to compensate for it. They did so by treating the infant as a machine to be observed only in stimulus-response terms. This resulted in an atomization of the infant's whole personality into a multitude of small sectors. It is hardly surprising that in this process *total* personality reactions and emotions were lost and that this procedure erred as much in its way as the "adultomorph" method.

Nevertheless, there are some indications in the writings of these psychologists that they do have an inkling of the momentousness of this period. For instance it is hinted at, though by indirection, when Sigismund (1856) calls the first three months of life *Das dumme Vierteljahr* (the dumb trimester). But it is only in the last 20 years that the attention of even a few psychologists has been directed toward the smile of the baby as a psychological phenomenon which might perhaps warrant at least as much consideration, say, as whether the infant is able to support its own weight by its hands. But even their writings are meager on the subject. In Murchison's *Handbook of Child Psychology* (1933), for instance, there are only two references to smiling as a form of infant behavior, and two to smiling as a social behavior. The three first references are in the article of Charlotte Bühler, the last one in the article by Mary Cover Jones. Truly an impressive poverty in a collection of articles on child psychology by the best known authors in the field, allegedly covering every phase of the subject in a volume of 956 pages! In Gesell and Thompson's book, *Infant Behavior* (1934), the index contains no reference to smiling, while laughing is only cursorily touched upon in the frame of reference of language behavior.

Nevertheless even at that time there existed a detailed study of smiling in infants by R. W. Washburn (1929). The phenomenology of the infant's smiling behavior is described in Chapter 1 of this monograph in utmost detail. In another chapter methods of stimulating smiling and laughing in infants are investigated in similarly great detail. This analysis shows that social stimulation is far and away the most effective method for provoking smiling. The results are then correlated with age, frequency of smiling or laughing responses, developmental level, developmental quotient, age level, weight-height indices, and age of mother. The detail and exactitude with which measurements seem to have been conducted would make this monograph appear a very valuable one.

There are, however, two major objections to this study: (1) Exiguity of the material. The study has been conducted on a total of only 15 subjects, of which 4 were observed eight times. Half of the subjects were observed five times or less. This is the material on which the author bases all her conclusions, including a typology which comprises four groups: the serene, the emotionally labile, the cheerful, and the sober. (2) Neglect of certain indispensable methodological safeguards, to wit: (a) The subjects are removed from their habitual environment to a special examining room in another part of the city, an interference which is disturbing to any small child. The intensity of this disturbance, what is more, varies not only with the child's personality and background, but also with the child's age. Thus a new variable is introduced into the experiments which cannot be expressed in terms of the variables investigated by the author. (b) The author does not take into account that making these experiments in the mother's presence, in many cases with the child sitting on the mother's lap, in many others provoking the child's laughing response through the mother's intervention, falsifies her results.

Nonetheless the author has revealed a number of facts which are of value for the understanding of the smiling response. One of these is that inanimate objects alone do not elicit smiling or laughing. Another is that the constantly smiling face of the observer was the most effective stimulus for eliciting the child's response. A third is that the period in which the smiling response can be provoked extends from 12 to 40 weeks and that after that time it becomes difficult to elicit it. These are statements which conform with the observations of later investigators (Washburn, 1929; Murphy and Murphy, 1931; Kaila, 1932; C. Bühler, 1937b) who observed and were interested in the phenomenon in various ways. The interpretations range from the assumption that the child is imitating (here again the problem arises as to what imitation is, why it occurs and how it is provoked), to the assumption that he is behaving spontaneously.

Other investigators have discovered that the infant reacts by smiling to three classes of sensory perceptions of the human being, namely the visual, the auditory, and the tactile. Of the three, visual perception elicits the infant's smile by far the most frequently and regularly, which explains why the current interpretations of smiling behavior refer quite exclusively to its appearance in response to the visual stimulus offered by the human face.

Arnold Gesell (Gesell & Ilg, 1937) believes that in the course of development the human face is connected with a large number of "expectancies" associated with satisfactions and that the infant finally reacts by smiling to the element most frequently seen in connection with these expectancies—a sort of conditioned reflex, as it were. Charlotte Bühler (1927) believes that the smile of the baby is a social phenomenon from the outset, that the smile is *the* specific reaction to social contact, to the voice and the glance of the human being. She states explicitly that of all visual stimuli which can be expected to elicit the newborn's interest, the human face is the only one which provokes a smile by the end of the second month (Bühler, Hetzer, & Mabel, 1928).

Hetzer (Hetzer & Ripin, 1930) states that even in the fourth month the presentation of the bottle does not elicit a smile.

The finding that children between the age of two and six months reciprocate the smile of grown-ups who approach them, was interpreted by Charlotte Bühler (1927) to mean that the child reflects the expression, smiling or serious, of the grown-up. She obviously chose the term "reflects" to avoid an interpretation of the reasons underlying this behavior of the child. It is, however, hardly possible to avoid the assumption that this imitative behavior must take place by means of some sort of rudimentary identification.

On the strength of a series of cleverly devised experiments Eino Kaila (1932) has stated that between the child's third and fifth month the smiling reaction occurs in response to certain Gestalt configurations in the human face.

Kaila's experiments were made to determine whether the infant imitates the adult's smile and whether this imitation is indicative of a process of identification with the adult's attitude. His experiments showed that the smile between the third and the fifth month has nothing of the nature of imitation in it, but is a reaction to a stimulus configuration. The configuration fulfills certain, though not all, of the conditions of a visual Gestalt. He continued his experiments beyond the fifth month and could show that imitation starts much later than the smile and that it starts with much more elementary movements of the facial muscles than the complicated action of smiling. He assumed that the imitative activity is, at its beginning at least, not directed toward pathognomic expression of emotions, but toward the reproduction of perceptions which have the qualities of a visual Gestalt.

Kaila showed experimentally that it is not a specific person (the mother, as it was generally believed) whom the infant recognizes and greets with a smile between its third and sixth month. Having shown this, his problem was then to isolate those factors in the human face in general which become effective as a stimulus for the child's smiling response.

Kaila further found that the child stops smiling if the experimenter turns sideways (in profile) or if he covers his eyes. He also found that it is not necessary for the experimenter to smile to induce the child's smiling response; it is sufficient if he shows his head *en face,* making any kind of movements, nodding, for example. Not only is it unnecessary for the experimenter to smile under these circumstances, but he can even cover his mouth and the child will continue smiling.

To summarize Kaila's experiments and conclusions, he found that from the third to the sixth month babies respond with a smile to the stimulus of the adult's face under specific, well-defined conditions. These conditions consist of a stimulus configuration composed of two factors:

1. The stimulus offered has to consist of two eyes plus nose and forehead (the forehead must be smooth, not frowning). If this stimulus configuration is modified, if for instance the experimenter turns his head in profile or frowns, the child stops smiling and loses contact with the experimenter.

2. The stimulus must be accompanied by motion in the rest of the face. If the smiling infant is confronted with an unsmiling, motionless face, it stops smiling, loses contact, and often appears upset. The nature of the motion of the experimenter's face may be smiling, or talking, or head-nodding, etc.

Our summary of Kaila's findings and of the way he formulated them makes it evident that he eliminated the problem of emotion from his approach. Charlotte Bühler, on the other hand, emphasized the factor of emotion by formulating the hypothesis that the child "reflects" the grown-up's friendly or serious expression. Kaila succeeded in disproving the assumption of the child "reflecting" anything at this early age (simultaneously he disproved the assumption of Guernsey (1928) who assumes that infants imitate the facial gestures of adults from the second month on). Having disproved imitation, he had to use another explanatory framework, and for this purpose he employed Gestalt concepts. The question as to the role played by emotion thus vanished as by an act of sleight of hand and the problem was returned again to the old mechanistic terms of the nineteenth century. To disprove that the child imitates the emotional expression of the grown-up, however, does not at the same time disprove the emotional nature of the child's manifestation, nor does it disprove its social character.

Kaila's experiments are both brilliant in their originality and precise in their method. We are indebted to him for some of the most stimulating findings on early infancy. It is with this debt in mind that we shall examine those points in which his findings fall short of our own aims.

For the purpose of a first orientation to the problem of the smiling response his material was adequate. But if we wish to understand and evaluate the phenomenon, we must admit that this material is insufficient, for it comprises a total of 71 infants from one single institution, all of the same racial, national, and cultural background. This is a very one-sided sample, further restricted by the fact that he selected only those infants who smiled readily.

Of these infants, 37 were observed only for one week and the rest for longer periods, the maximum being a group of six infants, for nearly two months.

The briefness of the observation period may be attributed to circumstances beyond the investigator's control. Nevertheless, it also fits into Kaila's scientific bias as Gestalt psychologist for whom the structure of a psychic phenomenon at a given moment is important but who is not concerned with the genetic viewpoint. Accordingly, the development of the phenomenon is hardly touched upon and the fact that modifications of developmental factors may lead to completely different manifestations is overlooked.

This brief survey of the literature suffices to show that the greatest part of the significance of the infant's smile is still unexplored and unexplained. But the fact remains that the smile is, after all, one of the two possible pathways for the understanding of emotions during the early stages of preverbal development. It was this insight which started us on our present investigation, the objectives of which may be enumerated as follows.

B. GENERAL PURPOSE OF PRESENT STUDY

1. To revise the findings of Kaila's study of the smiling response on the basis of an extensive sample diversified according to race, cultural background, and environment.

2. To establish the developmental pattern of the smiling reaction and the age range within which it is manifested, by investigating it on comparable numbers of infants at several age levels within the first year of life.

3. To investigate the necessary and sufficient conditions for provoking the infant's smiling response.

4. To establish whether the smiling response is an individual peculiarity, a cultural acquisition, a racial trait, or a universal pattern.

5. If the latter is the case, to investigate the exceptions in the smiling pattern and to attempt to find the conditions under which such exceptions occur.

6. To investigate the significance of the smiling response as an emotional manifestation as well as its significance from the point of view of the child's emotional development.

II. IS THE SMILING RESPONSE UNIVERSAL?

With these points in mind, I devised a new series of experiments with the aim of clarifying the issue and following it up to its logical conclusion. We shall now describe our experimental sample and methods.

A. THE SAMPLE

A total of 251 children, 139 males and 112 females, was investigated. In any such experiment the problem of nature versus nurture arises, i.e., the question of congenital and that of environmental influences on individual response. With the intention of throwing some light on this question in regard to our problem we diversified our material according to two leading principles. (a) *According to heredity.* For this purpose we investigated children belonging to three races, distributed as follows: 105 white, 39 colored, 107 Indian. (b) *According to environment.* For the purpose of elucidating the possible effectiveness of environmental influence we investigated five different environments: private homes (upper-class professionals), a baby nursery, a foundlings' home, a delivery clinic, and an Indian village.

Table 1 shows the total distribution of the children according to environment and race. Other than diversification as to race and environment no further selection was attempted. In each environment the *unselected total* of the available infants was examined. Within this unselected total four age groups

TABLE 1. ENVIRONMENT

Race	Nursery	Private home	Foundlings home	Delivery clinic	Village	Total
White	57	15	21	12	—	105
Colored	39	—	—	—	—	39
Indian	—	—	48	33	26	107
Total	96	15	69	45	26	251

were distinguished as the result of the average appearance and disappearance of the smiling reaction. They are:

1. A group of 54 children observed from birth to their twentieth day.

2. One hundred and forty-four children observed from the age of 20 days to 60 days.

3. A group of 132 children (this group covers the previously mentioned 144, less 12 who for varying reasons could not be followed) tested during their third, fourth, fifth, and sixth month. To this has to be added a group of 13 children who came under observation only after their third month, bringing the total of this group to 145.

4. A total of 147 children were followed from their sixth month to the completion of their first year. Of these 108 had already been followed from their third to their sixth month.

An additional group of 39 children came under observation for the first time only after their sixth month.

In all our experiments (both those mentioned up to now and those to be discussed subsequently) we introduced certain basic safeguards. As far as possible each experiment was performed on each child by a male experimenter and by a female experimenter separately, at different times to determine whether there were differences in reaction to one or the other sex. Talking to the child (or in its presence) or touching it either before or during the experiment was avoided. Where it was necessary to move the arm of the child for photographic purposes we were careful to take hold of the clothing only. Thus the exclusively visual quality of the stimulus offered to the children was preserved.

Finally we narrowed down the visual stimulus to that offered by the experimenter's face. To avoid falling into the error committed by Washburn (1929), we were careful to perform our experiments in the absence of the mother or at least to exclude her from the visual field of the child during the experiment. We were investigating the nature of the stimulus of the child's smiling response and the presence of the mother would have introduced an unpredictable variable into the test situation, because the emotional relations of infants with their mothers vary from one emotional extreme to the other. Furthermore, a smile of the child in the presence of the mother would have to be interpreted in the light of the fact that a preexisting emotional relation was coloring the child's attitude, whereas a smiling response to the experimenter is a response to a stimulus seen for the first time. Finally the difference between the mother as instigator (Dollard, 1939) and the experimenter as stimulus of the baby's response varies greatly at different developmental levels of the infant, as we hope to show in subsequent publications.

With the exception of the 26 children in the Indian village, each child was submitted to the smiling stimulus from 5 to 30 times during the critical period of the third, fourth, fifth, and sixth months. Since each experiment was performed both by the male and the female experimenter, whenever both were available, the number of reactions is nearly double the above figures. Furthermore, as will be explained in the experiments described below, the smiling reaction of the babies was provoked 8 to 10 times in each experiment, as a consequence of the modifications which were added to the experiment. The very large number of experiments thus performed on each child excludes the possibility of accidental results. These repetitions bore valuable fruit in other directions too. They provided us, for example, with data which contribute to an understanding of the deviations in the usual pattern. Of these deviations, more later.

B. METHOD

In our first set of experiments we presented a smiling or nodding face as a stimulus fully *en face* so that the children could see both eyes simultaneously. When the child responded with a smile we slowly turned our face into profile, continuing either to smile or to nod. If the child now stopped smiling, we turned the face back *en face* and tried to provoke the smile again.

C. RESULTS AND DISCUSSION

The first important result to emerge from our investigation is the age distribution of the smiling response, the rise and fall of which is vividly illustrated in Table 2.

The age limits indicated in this table should be considered as zones merging imperceptibly into each other. For instance, the smiling response does not

TABLE 2.

Response	Age			
	Birth to 0;0+20	0;0+21 to 0;2+0	0;2+1 to 0;6+0	0;6+1 to 1;0+0
Smile	—	3	142	5
No smile	54	141	3	142
Total	54	144	145	147

disappear suddenly after the sixth month. This disappearance is a gradual one and becomes complete by the end of the eighth month. It should also be stressed that the significant contrast between the first and the second half year of life lies in the fact that in the first six months the infant smiles *indiscriminately* at *every* adult offering the appropriate stimulation, whereas in the second half it *may* smile at one person or another, if so inclined, but will not smile indiscriminately at everybody.

Perhaps it should also be mentioned that even during the peak of the smiling response infants will only respond if the experimenter has the ability to focus their attention, and if there are no gross interfering circumstances such as sickness, sleepiness, disturbances with screaming and crying, to inhibit the reaction of the child.

As expected, children of less than 20 days do not respond to the smiling stimulation. After all, it is generally conceded that during the first few weeks the infant's reactions are diffuse and uncoordinated, their perception inadequate, their attention unfocused. The minimal necessary conditions for a stimulus to evoke a reaction are: (1) that the stimulus be perceived; (2) that the attention be focused on it sufficiently to permit a reaction to take place; (3) that the neuromuscular reaction patterns be sufficiently coordinated to make reaction possible.

None of these conditions is fulfilled at this age and accordingly none of the infants examined by us showed any of these reactions. Of course, smiling as a spontaneous movement could sometimes be observed just as any other facial contortion.

We also expected to find the largest number of reactions in the group covered by the third, fourth, fifth, and sixth months. All previous investigators spoke of these age levels as being the ones characterized by smiling; smiling has, therefore, been incorporated as a test for infant development in the testing procedures of Hetzer and Wolf (1928), Gesell (Gesell & Amatruda, 1941), and others. Again our expectation was fulfilled, though in a measure far surpassing anything we had imagined. The unfailing presence of the smiling reaction at these age levels makes the few exceptions, which comprise only 2.07 percent, all the more significant and worthy of investigation.

The concentration of the smiling response on the age group between the third and sixth month induced us to limit the main body of our investigation to this period. The distribution of this age group according to environment, race, and presence of smiling response is shown in Table 3.

Table 3 shows that neither in regard to race nor in regard to the sociological structure of the environment was any gross difference in the reaction to the smiling stimulus discernible. We can, therefore, conclude that the smiling

TABLE 3. ENVIRONMENT AND RACE

Response	Institution			Private home		Total
	White	Colored	Indian	White	Indian	
Smile	53	26	23	14	26	142
No smile	1	1	—	1	—	3
Total	54	27	23	15	26	145

response is a universal human pattern, which is not influenced either by race or by environment.

As we shall see, there is good reason to believe that certain environmental factors can have a very marked effect indeed on the development of the smiling response. These particular environmental factors, however, were not operative in the environments which we studied, for age groups up to the point where the smiling response is at its peak.

These uniform results over a widely diversified range of subjects are strikingly consistent and contribute to our conviction of the universality of the smiling pattern; we are also impressed by the hardiness of this pattern, a finding which makes deviations all the more interesting for us.

As we have stressed above, these results were more or less to be expected, except for the extraordinary reliability of the presence of the smiling response during the second trimester of life.

We have, on the other hand, found some rather unexpected phenomena. One is the appearance of the smiling response in a few rare cases as early as the twenty-fifth day of life. In our material, the cases in which the smiling response occurs before the end of the second month total 2 percent. (The rarity of the phenomenon no doubt explains why it was not noticed by previous observers.) The scattered nature of its inception during this period places it into marked contrast with the uniformity of the reaction in the second trimester of life. We shall attempt to find an explanation for these exceptions later on.

Another unexpected result is the extinction of the smiling pattern after the sixth month. The proportion of children in the last third of the first year who smile indiscriminately at the approach of a smiling stranger is less than 5 percent. In our later discussion we shall analyze these exceptions and try to find out whether factors within the individual history of these children offer any explanation of their divergent behavior.

All in all, we can say that this part of our investigation has shown us a phenomenon in infant behavior which is narrowly circumscribed as to the age levels at which it appears, but which within these age levels seems to be as unshakably consistent as the patellar reflex. For this reason we shall be able to make use of it in the same manner as we make use of a tendon reflex: its absence, or its atypical manifestation, will call our attention to a dysfunction within a certain area of the personality. We have said in the introduction to our problem that the psychological area to which we are referring is that of the infant's emotions. If, after the manner of physiological concepts, we can speak of a homeostasis of individual emotional life, disturbances in the infant's smiling reaction in the period covering the third to sixth month will indicate an imbalance of emotional homeostasis. On the other hand the presence of the smile during the second trimester is *not* a sufficient indicator of emotional homeostasis. Like any tendon reaction, when positive, the smile is *one* of the signs of normal functioning, a necessary, but not a sufficient index. The same holds true of the patellar reaction: when absent it shows a disturbance in some part of the reflex arc, including the posterior spinal tract. But this statement cannot be reversed: even if the patellar reflex is present there may be a disturbance in the lower part of the posterior spinal tract.

By claiming that the presence of the smile in the second trimester of life is a necessary (though not sufficient) indicator of emotional homeostasis we have implicitly voiced our skepticism in regard to the explanations offered by previous investigators, be they introspective ones (like that of the child "reflecting" the grown-up's expression) or stimulus-response explanations (like that of the child reacting to the stimulus of a Gestalt configuration). It now becomes incumbent upon us to investigate two sets of problems. The first is that of what are the conditions, physical and otherwise, which provoke the child's smiling response; in other words, we will have to undertake a detailed analysis of the stimulus which becomes operative in provoking the infant to smile, and this analysis must proceed both from the point of view of the stimulus-phenomenon's physical appearance and from the point of view of its possible psychological significance. Our second problem will be to investigate the emotions expressed by the infant when it responds to the smile. We shall deal with these two sets of problems separately and shall now proceed to investigate the first, the conditions which provoke the smiling response. In order to do so, we have applied to the relevant sectors of our sample, the 145 children between the age of two months and six months, a new series of experiments which will be described below. These experiments were also conducted with the 144 children between the ages of 20 days and two months and with the 147 children between the ages of six months and one year. These two last groups, however, were investigated only for purposes of completeness as well as to find out whether they showed any striking response. The main body of data for the discussion of this problem is based on the two- to six-month age group.

III. WHAT ARE THE NECESSARY AND SUFFICIENT ATTRIBUTES OF A SMILE-PROVOKING STIMULUS?

A. PURPOSE OF INVESTIGATION

Our aim in these experiments was a twofold one. In the first place, we wished to ascertain whether at this early age the child is capable of perceiving, understanding, and evaluating the emotional expression of the human face. The second problem which I tried to elucidate was whether the human face in its human quality is the stimulus for the child's reaction, or whether the stimulus is a configuration *within* the human face.

B. METHOD

With these problems in mind three series of experiments were developed. In the first series the emotional quality of the stimulus was removed while conserving the configurational elements. In the second series of experiments the human attributes of the stimulus were removed, again retaining its configurational factors. The third series of experiments is merely an elaboration of the second under more stringent conditions.

1. Experiment 1

The emotional quality characterizing a smiling, nodding grown-up's face is that of friendliness, at least for other grown-ups. The configurational factors of a smiling face, on the other hand, are the forehead, the two eyes, the nose and the mouth, with a widening movement of the mouth-lips-cheeks region. In this experiment we exaggerated this movement in the extreme and achieved an effect similar to that of certain Japanese theatrical masks used in the No-plays, a species of *rictus* or *risus sardonicus*. A similar mimic expression is to be found in the headpieces of Japanese armor and also in certain ancient Greco-Roman theatrical masks. The purpose of all these masks was to inspire terror; the expression is perhaps best described as that of a savage animal baring its fangs. No grown-up would be inclined, even for a moment, to mistake this expression for one of friendliness, or of pleasure. Its savagery is unmistakable.

a. Results. This stimulus was offered to 142 children between the third and sixth month. Films were made in 33 cases, on 16 mm. film, with 24 exposures per second. In 141 of the cases in which the smiling reaction was positive the rictus experiment was equally positive. In one case where the smiling experiment was positive, the rictus experiment was negative. This child was approaching the upper age limit of six months (0;5 + 10).

Between the third and fifth month of life it was never negative when the smile was positive. It was, however, positive in one case before the second month in which the smile was negative.

We then proceeded to investigate whether the response to the rictus stimulus obeyed the same laws as did the smile, namely disappearance on turning in profile and reappearance when turning back *en face* again. We offered the infant our full face while rhythmically widening and narrowing our mouth. When the infant's smiling reaction reached its maximum, we slowly turned our head into profile, continuing at the same time the alternate widening and narrowing movements of the mouth. The infant immediately became serious, lost contact with the experimenter and often became upset. In some experiments head-nodding was added to the mouth-widening movement, thus increasing the movement factor of the stimulus. Both movements were continued when we turned our head into profile. All the infant's reactions remained the same as above.

b. Discussion of Experiment 1. These results show that the *emotion* expressed in the human face has no significance for the smiling reaction of the child between its third and sixth month. The child's reaction is no sign of its understanding of the partner's emotional attitude. Whether smiling, speaking, nodding in a friendly manner, or baring its fangs in a terrifying expression of savage rage, the human face is seen *en face* and in motion remained for the child the signal of a human partner and was reacted to with a smile.

Though it has nothing to do with the question of recognition of emotions, such as love or friendliness in the human face, we introduced at this point another experiment for the purpose of clearing up a very widespread superstition.

Many profundities have been uttered about the magic power of the human eye. People have argued that the special quality inherent in the human eye manifests itself in the fact that even the smallest children are attracted to the eye more than to any other human feature. The objection, therefore, might be raised that the smile of the baby was provoked in our experiments by this mysterious power of the human eye.

We reasoned that if it were the human eye which has such power, one eye should be as good as two. So during the experiment, while the child was smiling at our smiling face, we covered up one of our eyes, continuing to smile or nod as we had done before. The child's face immediately lost its smile, became serious, even bewildered, and the child quickly lost contact. A film of this experiment was taken.

2. Experiment 2

The second series of experiments was designed to remove the human attribute of the stimulus while conserving its configurational factors, in order to investigate the validity of the statement that the smile of the three-month-old infant is a reaction to a Gestalt perception. In these experiments we pursued this idea to its logical conclusions. If the three-month-old smiles in response to a Gestalt-perception, and to a Gestalt-perception *only,* then there is no reason why this Gestalt-perception should be linked with the human being itself.

We, therefore, introduced a new experiment which consisted in covering our heads with a black skull cap and in putting one of the current Halloween masks over our faces. The mask, of course, could not smile. But, knowing from the previous experiment that smiling movements of the mouth can be effectively replaced by any other facial movements, the experimenter presented his face, covered with mask and skull cap, to the children, sticking his tongue rhythmically through the mouth-slit of the mask. When this experiment had proved completely successful in provoking the smile of the babies, the experimenter, still retaining the mask, replaced the tongue movements with a nodding movement of his mask-covered head. The children's reactions were the same as before: they smiled, laughed, or crowed, according to the individual child's inclination.

a. Results. The stimulus was presented to 142 infants between two and six months. Of these 140 reacted with a smile to the mask. Two (one aged 0;4 + 15, the other aged 0;5 + 12) who had reacted positively to the smile did not react to the mask. These two cases will be discussed further on.

b. Discussion of Experiment 2. Just as the previous experiment indicates that it is not the emotional quality of the mimic movements offered, but the Gestalt-quality which acts as stimulus for the child's smile, the mask experiment seems to show that this Gestalt-quality is not restricted to the human being's face or person. The reaction can be provoked just as well by a few colored pigments on a piece of cambric, as long as three essential conditions are provided: (1) the presentation must take place completely *en face;* (2) two eyes must be shown; (3) the configuration must include the factor of motion.

We consider condition No. 1 as one of the most essential in the whole series of experiments. Both in the experiment of the mouth-widening and in that of the mask we included the additional variation of turning the head in profile. In both cases, as shown by all the films we have taken of those experiments, the effect is instantaneous; the child stops smiling, takes on a bewildered look, then either becomes serious or loses contact and looks away. It is obvious that whether it be a smiling human face, or a human face baring its fangs, or the face of a cardboard mask, the essential Gestalt-quality which serves for recognition of a pleasurable stimulus for the child is that these shapes be seen *en face,* and that the Gestalt consists of the *two* eyes, forehead and nose—plus motion.

The mask experiment should have been conclusive. But one school of psychologists in the past, in particular that of C. D. Broad (1925), has in all seriousness tried to explain imitation and contact by "telepathy" between the child and its partner. Even if one did not take this argument seriously, however, the objection might be raised that the human being hidden behind the mask is betrayed by the human, nonmechanical movement of the nodding.

3. Experiment 3

To remove this objection I constructed a primitive life-size puppet by stuffing a bag roughly into the shape of a head, attaching the mask to it and covering the top with the skull cap. A "body" was provided by hanging a dark shirt on a clothes hanger and fixing the artificial "head" into the collar of the shirt, so that it could be nodded.

This scarecrow, which really had nothing human in it, was presented to the child by the experimenter, who carefully hid himself behind the furniture at the foot of the cot. To our surprise we found that the very first time we applied this stimulus its effect seemed to be identical with the effect of the experimenter himself bending and smiling over the baby. The child greeted the nodding scarecrow by smiling, laughing, gurgling, or crowing in the same way as it had responded to the experimenter's smiling face in previous experiments.[3]

C. SUMMARY OF RESULTS OF THE TWO EXPERIMENTAL SETUPS

Table 4 shows the results of our experiments. As will be seen from this tabulation we are again faced with an impressive total of positive reactions. It follows that during this age period discrimination between the recognition of the human face and the recognition of a mask has not yet developed except in a few rare cases.

D. CONTROL SERIES

[3] This article was about to go into print when Dr. K. Wolf kindly called my attention to the fact that Gardner and Lois Murphy (1931, p. 251) had suggested experiments with a mask for provoking the smiling response. To our knowledge this suggestion has not been acted upon.

TABLE 4.

Response	Stimulus		
	Rictus	Mask on experimenter	Mask on stuffed head
Smile	141	140	140
No smile	4	5	5
Total	145	145	145

The extremely positive results achieved with the help of a stuffed, lifeless mask made it tempting to investigate whether there are any other lifeless objects to which the infant reacts with a smile. For the purpose of finding an answer to this question we made a systematic selection of material to be offered to the children.

The attributes of a perceptual stimulus which could elicit the smile of an infant can be roughly divided into the following categories:

1. *Intensity*. It could be that the child smiles to perceptual stimuli which are neither too strong nor too weak. We, therefore, offered: (a.) A strong, a medium, a weak flashlight; (b.) a loud, a medium, a soft bell.

2. *Specific sensory quality*. There are several possible perceptual stimuli of a definite qualitative nature to which a child might respond. Warm colors and light colors and high-pitched sounds or euphonic sounds may be more likely to induce smiling than cold colors or dark colors and low-pitched sounds or noises. Color might be preferred to white, black, or grey; color combinations to uniform color. We, therefore, presented the child with a series of stimuli each of which offered one of these variations or a combination of several of them. To give only a few examples: (a) a musical rhythmical sound versus an unrhythmical and "disagreeable" noise; (b) red cardboard versus white cardboard; (c) rattles of different color combinations versus plain rattles.

3. *Surface structure*. It might be that the child prefers either a plain surface or a surface with a complicated structure. We, therefore, contrasted the stimulation of a shock of red knitting yarn with the stimulation of a smooth square of red cardboard of approximately equal size.

4. *Shape*. Conceivably, the child might prefer round objects to square ones, or pointed objects to objects without a point and that these preferred objects would be more likely to provoke the smile of the infant. We, therefore, presented the infants with objects of various shapes, such as: (a) a ball; (b) hollow blocks; (c) a bath thermometer.

5. *Size*. Finally, the effectiveness of a stimulus might be dependent on its size. Variations in size might modify its emotional appeal. We, therefore, offered the child objects of different size: (a) various sizes of paper; (b) colored blocks of different size; (c) red blocks of different size; (d) balls of different size, etc.

These stimuli were presented to each child by the male and by the female experimenter alternately. They were offered in such a manner that the experimenter could not be seen by the children; when no smile was elicited the stimuli were moved before the child by the hand of the hidden experimenter, so that the human element was present in the child's perceptive radius, although the experimenter's face was hidden. The hiding of the face, incidentally, is imperative at the three- to six-month level, because at this age the child's fascinated gaze often cannot be distracted from a human face by any toy whatsoever.

These experiments, which were made with all the 145 children in question, gave completely negative results. None of the children smiled on perceiving the toys. When their attention was captured by any one of them, their expression became concentrated and intent, but they never smiled.

These findings confirm prior statements of Washburn, Murphy and Murphy, and C. Bühler to the effect that infants do not smile at their toys.

Since none of these perceptual variations led to a smiling response, we investigated whether it might be a subjective rather than an objective factor which transforms a stimulus into a smile instigator. We, therefore, investigated the frequency of smiling response in relation to degree of familiarity with an object. We first offered the child a completely new object, then we offered an object to which he was used to for many weeks, endeavoring to eliminate any possible spurious factors by selecting two objects as similar as possible. For instance, we offered the child its own rattle with which it had played almost throughout his whole life and contrasted this with an offering of an unfamiliar rattle. Neither the new nor the familiar object elicited any smile.

Even when we exaggerated the strangeness of the object by using one which the child had never seen before, a toy which did not resemble any of its own toys, a child under six months showed interest or attention at best, but never a smile.

We then proceeded to present the children with an object which we considered as having emotional significance for the infant. For this purpose, taking account of the importance of food in the infant's life, we used the nursing bottle (the great majority of the infants in question had been bottle fed or had received supplemental feedings from the bottle). Again the result was the same, with one important difference. In the more advanced children the bottle elicited a clearly recognizable sucking movement, opening of the mouth, stretching of arms and legs toward the bottle, squirming and sometimes babbling. The smile, however, was notably absent in this series of reactions.

We consider the negative result achieved in this experiment fully as important as the previous positive ones, because it disposes of several extremely plausible hypotheses on the cause and the significance of the smiling response.

The first of these is that the smiling response is a conditioned reflex, established in response to the gratification of being satiated by food. Darwin (1872) and, after him, Freud (1905a) state that smiling appears for the first time in infants who, satiated, release the nipple. From our observations, smiling as facial movement appears independently of any peripheral stimulation. It does appear at a later stage in connection with the feeding situation; but whether as a result of feeding or of the other concomitant circumstances is a question which cannot be answered at the present stage of our knowledge. How are we to interpret, for instance, the behavior of an infant (Aurora), filmed during its nursing, who for several minutes nursed with complete absorption, then interrupted its nursing, smiled at its mother's face, started nursing again and repeated the behavior about a dozen times, relinquishing the nipple and taking it back in its mouth each time, making smiling a game between itself and the mother?

Gesell's formulation of the child connecting its mother with innumerable situations of expectancy appears to be more to the point. But in this statement the concept of the conditioned reflex is implicit. But, if response-smiling were a conditioned reflex, it would have to occur at least as impressively in response to the perception of the conditioner, food, as in response to the perception of the conditioned, the human face. Nothing of the kind occurs.

Translated into terms of Pavlov's dogs, it is as if the dogs who learned to salivate at the tone of the buzzer did not salivate when beholding the meat.

The other hypothesis we are now in a position to refute is the one which holds the smiling response to be the result of visceral excitation, the smile of another person being one of the adequate stimuli for such visceral manifestations (Murphy and Murphy, 1931). It is not evident from these authors' formulation whether by the visceral response they mean the response to food. If so, the hypothesis falls under the category discussed above. If, on the other hand, the authors mean by "visceral excitation" a syndrome of autonomous nervous system reaction plus glandular plus smooth muscle response, then we accept their hypothesis. In our opinion every emotional reaction of the living organism is concomitant with such visceral response, major or minor. In this respect the baby's smile is not different from that of the adult, and no precedence can be established at our stage of knowledge either for "visceral excitation" or emotional experience.

Since the mask experiment yielded positive results, it became apparent that another factor should be considered in its capacity to induce the smile: the similarity of the stimulus to a human being. Isolating this criterion presented something of a problem, however. As far as the mask experiment was concerned, the problem of size was the one factor which lent itself to modification. We, therefore, offered each of the children a small rubber doll (10 inches) or one of the current 12-inch dolls, porcelain-headed. Neither of these dolls elicited the children's smile. For the most part, they introduced the doll into their mouths up to the fifth month; after that, they played with it.

Another problem intruded itself at this point. The films taken of the mask and of the scarecrow experiments are extremely convincing. Indeed, the joy of the infants on beholding the nodding mask, which for the grown-up would be a repulsive object, is so impressive in the films that one might feel inclined to conclude that the children find the mask funny and that they laugh for this reason. This assumption is disproved by two observations: (1) The child becomes serious when the nodding head of the adult with the mask on it is turned into profile (continuing to nod all the while). A mask in profile is not less "funny" than a mask *en face*. (2) Knowing from the findings of this and other studies that at this age the child does not laugh at its toys and that, therefore, we could present a toylike object without risking spurious factors, we offered our subjects a hollow block ($3\frac{1}{2} \times 3$ inches), which had funny faces depicted on each of the four sides. None of the children laughed.

IV. Conclusions

We are now better prepared to answer some of the questions posited at the outset of our experiments.

1. It can be stated that the child at this age is incapable of understanding and still less of evaluating the *expression* of the human face.

2. It is not the *human* face—its human quality—which acts as a stimulus. The stimulus for the reaction is a configuration consisting of certain elements *within* the human face, combined with motion.

3. It was found that racial, cultural, and environmental factors have a negligible influence, if any, on the reaction.

4. The present set of observations do not shed any new light on the origin of the reaction. We will, therefore, abide by Gesell's formulation according to which expectancies of a highly varied nature are set up in the infant in connection with this stimulus.

5. The significance of the inception time of this reaction will also have to be explained in a tentative fashion. In a recently published article (Spitz, 1945a) I have presented the hypothesis that up to its third month the child's

perceptive system works along the lines of total perception, and that its perceptive organization follows the pattern of the autonomic nervous system's perception. In the course of its maturation and with the help of environmental stimulation, a progressively increasing number of elements are distinguished in the environmental perceptions. I have called this second mode of perception, which culminates in the adult's perceptive apparatus, the perception according to the diacritic system. The appearance of smiling in reaction to the human face and to the human only, is the first step in the development of diacritic perception. It is significant that this first step should be accomplished in response to social stimulation, in response to another person's face, and that it should be fraught with emotional significance. From our observations we can state that during the three to four months in which this reaction is present it changes imperceptibly in the direction of increased acuity of diacritic discrimination. Another way of expressing the significance of the smiling reaction is that its onset designates that level of the infant's development at which it becomes able to differentiate "I" from "You," the subject from the object, his own person from other persons (and incidentally from objects without emotional significance).

6. After the sixth month the smiling pattern as a response to anybody and everybody disappears. The significance of this extinction follows from what we have said. It is a further, and immensely significant, step in the differentiating diacritic discrimination. A similar view has been expressed by Murphy and Murphy (1931).[4] In our opinion, the disappearance of the indiscriminate smiling pattern marks the beginning of differentiation between "friend" and "stranger." With this step the reaction to the "human being in general" has progressed to a reaction to the emotionally welcomed individual.

7. Therefore, the smiling reaction is an indicator of the emotional maturation of the child during its first half year. It informs us that the child is not only achieving mastery of perceptive discrimination and neuromuscular coordination of its mimic musculature, but that it is also progressing toward a finer differentiation of emotional reaction. It has become capable of distinguishing, within the chaos of its reactions, *some* which produce something different in the way of experience than did either the unpleasure[5] reaction or the attitude of quiescence in the neonate. It has become capable of relating such expe-

---

[4] [The original text cited Murphy and Newcomb, probably in error. Ed.]

[5] We use the term "unpleasure" to describe the experience corresponding to the negative branch of the pleasure-pain principle. It seems to us that terms such as displeasure, pain, suffering, and discomfort which are currently used cover only narrow sectors of what is in reality one-half of all human experience. We, therefore, believe that a straightforward neologism like "unpleasure" stands a better chance of avoiding misinterpretation. This opinion is shared by Strachey (1943).

riences to external factors. These external factors are in some way connected with a human partner. The coloring of the child's reaction to them appears to be similar to what we call pleasure in the grown-up. We may, therefore, say that the child has acquired the capacity to distinguish and to experience positive emotions.

This disappearance of the indiscriminate smiling response after the sixth month is a sign of definite progress in environmental discrimination and it is also an indication of further emotional maturation.

8. This throws light upon the significance we can expect from deviant patterns in the smiling reaction. These deviant patterns will show a distortion of the average emotional maturation and will act as a signal of an emotional disturbance. It is in the light of this that in the ensuing section of this report we shall examine the deviations from the usual smiling pattern.

GENERAL CONCLUSIONS

We have demonstrated the phenomenological conditions of the smiling response of the baby. The rigidity of these conditions has misled one of the previous observers, Kaila, to postulate that the smiling response is a stimulus-response process to a stimulus of purely Gestalt character. In making this assumption, he has—as is the general tendency of formal Gestalt psychologists—neglected the fact that the phenomenon has a history. The significant point in our investigation is not the proof of the specificity of the stimulus and of its purely configurational character. The real significance is to be found in the deviations from the general pattern and is particularly well illustrated by deviation (in one case, that of Evamar), in which emotional disturbances of the child's mother result in a reversal of the reaction. It must not be assumed, of course, that every emotionally disturbed mother will induce the same kind of reaction-reversal in her child. Though the gamut of possible reactions in the course of the first year is very limited, still the infant has many other possible patterns for reacting to emotional traumata, such as eating difficulties; psychosomatic disturbances (in the nature of digestive troubles, skin diseases, etc.); developmental disturbances such as retardation or acceleration, as the case may be; tantrums; changes in the activity pattern; and so on.

We have also to explain why we call this phenomenon a "reversal" rather than a negative reaction. The smiling response of the baby is proof that it perceives and recognizes the stimulus offered to it. It recognizes the grown-up as an object which is somehow different from the other objects in its environment. A negative reaction takes place when it either does not perceive or when it does not react to the stimulus. When (as in the case of Evamar) the child begins to scream on perceiving the stimulus and permits itself to be reassured only on withdrawal of the stimulus, then it has both perceived and recognized the stimulus. We, therefore, cannot call the reaction a negative one. The stimulus still provokes an affect; it has merely changed from positive to negative. The screaming proves that the baby has distinguished the grown-up from inanimate objects of its environments just as reliably as if it had smiled. In other words, instead of pleasure, the stimulus evokes unpleasure. Therefore, we call this reaction "the reversed smiling response."

It was most impressive to observe that this reaction (in the case of Evamar) took place in response to the approach of any grown-up during the time the mother was emotionally unbalanced, that a brief psychotherapeutic intervention by the matron, relieving the mother from her emotional tension, resulted in a completely normal reaction within one week.

At this point the realization that the configuration stimulus fulfils only the role of a signal, the signal of an emotionally cathexed experience, becomes inescapable. That this experience is the signal of the approach of another human being and, therefore, belongs to the category of social experiences is not difficult to see.

The question now arises whether the concept "another human being" is an acquired one or whether it is preformed after the manner of an anlage. We have shown in our study that the infant manifests its recognition of "another human being" by smiling. When, therefore, we investigate what the concept "another human being" means to the infant, we will try to ascertain the function and origin of smiling. For this purpose we will have to divide the phenomenon of the infant's smile into two distinct categories. The first category is that of the motor pattern of the smile. The second category is that of the function to which the motor pattern of smiling is put in the service of semantic facial expression.

There can be no doubt but that the motor pattern of smiling is present, if not at birth, then at least as anlage which is manifested in the first days of life without any environmental stimulus for its provocation, as already mentioned.

The preformed motor pattern, however, is used by the child in a specific social situation beginning with the second month. At this point what was previously a motor pattern devoid of meaning takes on a new function. It is integrated on a higher level into a pattern syndrome embracing the motor pattern on one hand and a psychic pattern on the other. On this new level, a psychomotor level as it were, it becomes autonomous and independent from the previous motor pattern. On the psychomotor level the pattern syndrome invariably shows a vast preponderance of the psychic factor over the somatic factor.

On this basis we can say that the motor anlage of the smile after the second month is integrated into the nascent pattern of the child's emotional needs on the social level. In the course of this integration the purely motor pattern of the smile is endowed with the psychological meaning inherent in the child's emotional relations with its human partners. In view of this significance of the smiling pattern in interpersonal relations we feel justified in calling it a pattern used for semantic purposes, in short a semantic pattern.

A number of children, not large but still significant, do not smile at all in response to another human being's stimulation during the critical period of the third to sixth month.

This lack of response can be understood by a somewhat closer analysis of the concept "another human being" ("a partner"). As previously stressed, the early establishment of such a concept in the child's mind, the segregation of the human stimulus from the mass of environmental stimuli at an age when no other stimulus is so segregated, requires an explanation. In the nursery situation the stimulus "another human being" is provided exclusively by the mother or by the mother substitute; we will, for simplicity's sake, include also the latter when we use the term, "mother." This mother provides the child with all the pleasant stimulations and experiences without exception.

Of course, the relationship between mother and child does not start with pleasant stimulations. As mentioned previously, the neonate is incapable of perceiving pleasurable stimuli. The first stage of relations between mother and child is, therefore, the stage in which the mother provides relief from discomfort. This is of cardinal importance during the first weeks of life. Insensibly, the relief from discomfort merges with the experience that the mother's presence ensures security, freedom from suffering. From here, it is only one step to the stage at which the child perceives the pleasurable quality of some stimuli offered to it by its mother's presence. When this third stage has been reached, it becomes understandable that the reaction to the mother's presence will be the same as that which is produced from there on to all and every pleasurable stimulation in the course of life.

These three steps: relief from discomfort, assurance of security, and tendering of pleasurable stimulation are accomplished as a consequence, and with the help, of the mother's ministrations while nursing the baby, keeping it clean, washing it, diapering it, and fondling it. The situations in which the infant experiences the mother's proximity while looking at her face are literally numberless. The films we have made of nursing babies are very revealing in this respect. The nursing infant does not remove for an instant its eyes from the mother's face until it falls asleep at the breast, satiated.

This visual contact is however, only one sector of the total experience. There are the other senses also, of varying degrees of importance. We believe, for instance, that the sense of smell in the human infant has no deep significance—at least the experiments of Canestrini (1913), Hetzer and Ripin (1930), and Frankl and Rubinow (1934) make it appear so. What the situation is in respect to the sense of taste is as yet insufficiently explored. We feel that certain reactions of children in connection with weaning show that at the age of six months, at least, a very delicate discrimination in the field of taste may be present. The sense of hearing also plays an important role; according to other authors (Bühler; Hetzer; Gesell; Dearborn; Shinn, 1900; Jones, 1926; Brainerd, 1927; Tiedmann, 1927) acoustic stimulation is one of the earliest to provoke the baby's smile. Little or nothing has been done to investigate this area up to now.

SUMMARY

1. The infant experiences its relationship with its mother emotionally. The infant responds with a smile to this experience. From the third to the sixth month the signal of this experience is a configurational stimulus originating within the human face.

2. Disturbances in the emotional relations between mother and baby inhibit the development of the smiling response.

3. Normalcy of the smiling response becomes, therefore, one of the criteria of normalcy of the emotional relation of the infant with its mother.

4. The human being establishes its first social relations with its mother. This first relation is the basis of, and determines the pattern for all later social relations. The presence of the smiling response is a criterion of the normal inception of the infant's social relations. Therefore, it may be a prognostic indicator of the infant's later capacity for social contact and social relations.

Autoerotism Re-examined:
The Role of Early Sexual Behavior
Patterns in Personality Formation

GENITAL PLAY AND MOTHER-CHILD RELATIONS

In view of the evidence of the decisive role of mother-child relations in autoerotic activities, we compared three groups—the children in the penal nursery, those in the foundling home, and the children raised in their own families.[1] We used the mother-child relations as the independent variable, the children's autoerotic activities as the dependent variable.

We found that (1) where the relation between mother and child was optimal, development in the first year of life surpassed the average in all respects, and genital play was present in all cases. (2) In the case of the infants where the relation between mother and child was a *problematic* one, genital play was much rarer and other autoerotic activities tended to replace it, while development, satisfactory on the average, was rather erratic. (3) Where the relation between mother and child was absent, general development dropped below the average, and genital play was completely missing.

These data confirm that during the first year of life autoerotic activities vary as a function of the prevailing object relations. This was indeed an unexpected finding. It has been somewhat surprising to me that it was not challenged in the course of the 12 or so intervening years. The single statement

---

Reprinted in slightly abridged form from *The Psychoanalytic Study of the Child,* Vol. 17. New York: International Universities Press, 1962, pp. 283–315.

[1] In a paper written some fifteen years ago, the late Ernst Simmel (1948) adumbrated some of the ideas which I am developing in the present paper. He wrote:

> In the stage of developing its object relationships, masturbation may be regarded as the infant's first social activity. For through this activity the child withdraws from the disappointing object which rejects its love and stimulates aggressive destructive reactions. In its own body, the child finds a substitutive gratification for the narcissistic trauma, replacing the object by its own genital as an object, and finding in itself a way of discharging object-directed erotic and aggressive tendencies. It has thus renounced direct instinctual gratifications from the real objects, but keeps an ideational relationship with them in masturbatory fantasies. Through masturbating the child begins to resolve its instinctual conflicts within itself without, I might say, bothering the objects; but it is forced again secondarily into conflict with them if the parents interfere with this masturbation which is the child's struggle for a pleasurable release of instinctual tension.

on the subject which came to my attention was that of Jeanne Lampl-de Groot (1950) who in a critique stated that this was not the whole story. I agree; indeed, in the introductory remarks we stated that our study was more in the nature of a description than that of classification; that it was an attempt at illustration; that our interpretations were tentative, and that the regularities found by us were to be considered in the nature of approximations; an orientation, as it were, within the map of the ontogenesis of sexuality and of its phenomenology.

That is my opinion to this day. I believe that longitudinal studies should enable future observers to connect the form which infantile autoerotism takes from its beginning, not only with the relationship between mother and child, but also with the behavioral patterns which will develop later; and in particular, with the patterns of defenses developed subsequently by the individual child.

Indications on this subsequent development are contained in observations made by me during the follow-up of the 61 infants housed in a foundling home. These children were studied intensively for four to six hours per day up to the end of their second year (Spitz, 1945b). In the following two years we visited them at half-yearly intervals in order to record their further development, on which I shall report further on. As usual in longitudinal studies, the follow-up years brought a drastic reduction of this population. But 21 subjects, one third of the original population, could be followed for somewhat more than two additional years, bringing the older of these children into their fourth year. Regrettably enough, we were unable to follow our subjects further, so that we lack information on their development in latency and puberty.

Still, our follow-up visits yielded some data on the development of these children's autoerotic activities in the first four years of life. For reasons to be discussed later, I have not published these in my original report (Spitz, 1946b). Recent experimentation on infant monkeys has yielded results which are strikingly parallel to these unpublished findings.

However, the direct application of conclusions drawn from animal experimentation to human psychology is not permissible. Caution must be exercised to avoid explaining the psychological processes of one species (e.g., man) with the help of insights achieved from experimentation with another species, particularly when the latter is on a level of minor complexity of organization. Therefore, when in what follows some animal experimentation is reported, it will not be for the sake of *explaining* conclusions I have drawn from my own findings in man. It will rather be as an illustration of a principle which I have always maintained, namely, that the convergence of findings in two or more different lines of research reinforces and validates conclusions reached independently in each of them.

In the present study I will avail myself of experiments performed by Harry

Harlow (1959, 1960a, b, c, d, e) on rhesus monkeys and of the striking parallels between his findings and those which I have published on infants deprived of emotional supplies.

Here the convergence of the findings sheds additional light on the problems surrounding masturbation and on its role in the development of man. This convergence of the findings in two independent lines of research permits us to draw further conclusions from them. These conclusions may throw additional light on the problems surrounding masturbation and its role in the development of man.

The fact that Harlow does not speak of masturbation in the surrogate-raised rhesus monkeys permits us to assume that it cannot be very conspicuous. We may then ask ourselves what the nature of the disturbance of these animals could be. Actually, their behavior is reminiscent of psychiatric disorders in man: incapacity of contact, of expressing appropriate emotion; anxiety when confronted with specific emotion (sexual); heterotope[2] sexual attempts; and anxiety, hostile aggression, and destruction in response to sexual advances.

This, however, is not the problem which Harlow is investigating. The question he sought to answer was: what has the mother to offer the infant besides food and physical comfort; and what, if anything, is missing in the surrogate mother?

The best answer I can give to this question (and Harlow may not agree with me) is that food and comfort are needs which *must* be gratified. However, they provide only the immediate elements for barest survival. But if survival is understood beyond the immediate, beyond even the life of the individual and includes the survival of the species, then the indispensable element which is so paramount in the real mother and is missing in the surrogate is *reciprocity:* the circular exchange of affectively charged actions between mother and child.[3]

Any observation of the interaction between a mother and her baby makes this self-evident. Take a film I have of a mother putting the nipple of the milk bottle into the mouth of her seven-month-old. He reciprocates by putting his fingers into her mouth; she answers by moving her lips on his fingers, whereupon he twiddles his fingers, and she responds with a smile; all the while he stares at her face with rapt attention. Such little scenes can be observed in endless variations in any mother-child couple. They are the paradigm of what is missing in the surrogate mother.

---

[2] *Heterotope* and *orthotope* are terms introduced by Sandor Rado in a paper given before the Berlin Psychoanalytic Society in 1930. Rado designated "orthotope" sexual activity which takes place between male and female sexual organs in a manner suitable to lead to impregnation. He called "heterotope" sexual activity in which organs other than the genital of one or both of the partners were involved.

[3] Reciprocity is a major sector of object relations. Some of its aspects will be discussed in several of my forthcoming papers.

Harlow in effect introduced the factor of reciprocity in an experiment in which two baby monkeys of the same age were raised together in a cage on a cloth mother. As a result, these monkeys closely clutched each other all the time and were unable to form any other relations, to engage in any play, sexual or otherwise, with monkeys on their age level or older. Harlow calls them the "together-together" monkeys. What is missing here? Surely not reciprocity—if anything, there is too much of it.

Aspects of Anaclitic and Diatrophic Relations

It is this "too much" which offers the key to our problem. The difference between the same-age monkey and the mother is that two same-age monkeys have identical needs and reciprocally fulfill these completely. Thus they form a closed system, an isomorphic equation in which one side completely offsets the other. The result is stasis, complete paralysis.

The relation between child and mother is not like this at all. The two sides of the equation—the needs of the child versus the needs of the mother—are completely dissimilar, though in certain respects complementary. To express it in my own conceptual framework, that is in terms of object relations: from the dynamic point of view the baby's attitude and behavior are anaclitic. The mother's complementary response is what I called the diatrophic[4] attitude (Spitz, 1956a). Due to the infant's helplessness, the anaclitic relationship encompasses the totality of the infant's commerce with the surround. Initially the anaclitic relation is an offshoot toward the periphery of the infant's primary narcissistic cathexis of his own person. Quanta of primary narcissistic cathexis attached to the gratification of the infant's needs are centered through the mediation of the oral zone on the mother to the exclusion of all the rest. This is a restatement, using different terms, of the proposition that in the first months of life the infant experiences the mother, and in particular her breast, as part of himself.

Not so the diatrophic attitude and relation. The mother's relation to her baby, while paramount, is only *primus inter pares*. In the nature of things the mother's relations to her husband, to her other children, her duties and responsibilities claim their share. Her relation to her baby comes first, of course, but share it must. And the mother, being a responsible adult, will also have to devote thought, attention, and time to a multitude of other activities.

Actually this does not work to the detriment of the infant, for the diatrophic attitude is a need-gratifying one and, though ever-present, it is *implemented*

---

[4] Diatrophic—to maintain, to support.

only in response to the infant's anaclitic needs. In the first weeks of life these arise intermittently in a circadian rhythm,[5] and mesh with the widely spaced, relatively short waking periods. Indeed, one might think of the first weeks of life as an alternation of modes of being in the circadian rhythm—relatively more narcissistic periods of sleep alternating with relatively clear-cut anaclitic waking periods. In the human mother the implementation of the diatrophic attitude can therefore be discontinuous and can be compared to the operation of a circular feedback process.

In the rhesus baby the picture is quite different. While the human neonate expresses anaclitic *demands* during very few hours of the day only, we find Harlow's surrogate-raised rhesus babies (as a consequence of their incomparably longer wakefulness periods) clinging anaclitically to the surrogate mother 17 to 19 hours daily. They interrupt their clinging only for 1 or 2 hours to suckle at the feeding place—there remain few hours of the day when they are not behaving anaclitically.

Accordingly, two rhesus babies of equal age and raised together will have identical needs, namely, to cling to a warm, furry, living being. Therefore, they will cling to each other day and night, the anaclitic need of the one satisfying the anaclitic demand of the other and vice versa.

In contrast to the surrogate mother, a living rhesus mother has many other needs besides the implementation of the diatrophic attitude. These range from food-seeking to playing, from grooming her baby to grooming other monkeys; and all the other business, social calls, and whatever else occupies a grown rhesus monkey. Therefore she offers her baby, besides food and the opportunity to cling, a wealth of action, shifting over a wide scale from approach to retreat, from embracing to rejecting, from gratification to frustration. The rhesus baby partner does nothing of the kind, for he has exactly the same needs as his age-equal counterpart. In the overwhelming majority these consist in clinging. In contrast, the rhesus mother incessantly provokes through her activities and initiatives adaptive responses to constantly varying situations from her infant.

Moreover, she is also constantly responding to the baby's initiatives with a whole gamut of different actions, which in their turn require a variety of appropriate responses. Partly through other-directed activities, and partly through activities aimed at her baby, the rhesus mother frustrates and often disciplines her baby, cuffing, scratching, and even biting him.

The circular social interactions which develop in the normal course of these mother-child relations are numberless and infinitely varied. Each requires a

---

[5] Circadian is derived from *circa diem,* and could perhaps best be translated as "around the clock," to be distinguished from *diurnal,* meaning occurring each day in the daytime, not at night.

different adaptive response from the baby. To these responses the rhesus mother in turn will respond in a novel and, for the baby, unpredictable manner. Each of her responses represents a push in the direction of the developmental unfolding of the infant's personality—each of them bringing him nearer to autonomy from the mother and to seeking contact not only with the "other" but also with the "generalized other."

Where in this picture the implementation of the sexual drive starts, is something which we can only guess; a great deal of further observation and experimentation will be needed to provide specific data. But we can guess that licking in the vertebrate, grooming in the monkey, fondling, cuddling, handling, primping, fussing, bathing, and washing in the human child may well have *something* to do with it.

However, I am *not* ready to believe that bathing or washing, for example, becomes effective for the human child as an isolated action-interaction sequence. It becomes effective only as an action sequence imbedded in the whole variegated pattern of the individual mother-child relations. A good example for the wide-ranging interconnections of such an action sequence is to be found in nonprimate mammals. Rat babies will die if the mother does not lick their genitals for a number of days after birth; otherwise they are unable to urinate. How little we still know of the interdependence of the various systems, somatic and otherwise!

Coming back to Harlow's monkeys, I submit that the surrogate-raised rhesus babies are arrested on what in man we would call the primary narcissistic level; they clasp their own bodies; they clasp their mother. When older, they carry the cloth mother with them in all activities, and she becomes an obstacle to initiating social activities with other monkeys.

If it is permissible to reverse Mahler's (1952) felicitous concept of the symbiotic-parasitic relationship, we might say that these rhesus babies have transformed the cloth mother into a symbiotic host. This relation is strongly reminiscent of Winnicott's (1953) transitional object relation; but in effect it falls far short of it. For the transitional object really serves as a mediator, as a bridge leading to object relationship. The reason for this is that the transitional object is used only as a temporary substitute when the real object is unavailable. Not so the cloth mother symbiote; she has become exclusive, she really *dis*places and *re*places the libidinal object—and this bars the road to all other relations.

The same applies to the "together-together" monkeys, where each partner becomes an obstacle to the true object relations of the other, as a result of the anaclitic gratification offered in the together-together relationship. If object relations proper are to become effective, anaclitic gratifications of a narcissistic nature must be abandoned. This is the kind of narcissistic relation which monkeys raised on the same surrogate mother with an age-equal partner establish and maintain; there is no frustration and therefore neither incentive nor push to form different relations.

The surrogate-raised monkeys who, when grown, carry the cloth mother around, obviously must provoke in us some speculation about the role of the transitional object, the well-known "protective" animals, blankets, pillows, of human children, exemplified in the popular comic strip called "Peanuts." This features Linus, a little boy, dragging his blanket with him in every activity, mouthing it. One wonders whether children reared in less sophisticated cultures than ours do this also. Little Linus, presumed to be funny, is in effect an indictment of our child-rearing practices. For our children the wire mother in the form of a bottle-propper has practically become the rule. Through the centuries, we have progressively inhibited all body contact between child and mother, through clothing, through the crib, through the campaign against breast-feeding. Our most recent achievement in the endeavor to deny any relation, physical or casual, between mother and child is to deposit newborns in hospital checkrooms, instead of keeping them next to the mother's bed or, perish forbid, in mother's bed itself. This seems to me a signal victory on the road to abolishing the link between sex and survival, a major step toward Aldous Huxley's *Brave New World*.

Harlow's findings prove experimentally what I have stressed for a quarter of a century: the importance of breast feeding in establishing object relations does not lie in the fact that it assuages hunger and thirst. That it stimulates the primal cavity, the oral region, is also only part of its significance. As I see it, the major role of breast-feeding in the establishment of object relations lies in the fact that it enforces the most consistent, the most multiform contact with the mother's body. It takes all the perverse imagination of the human animal to circumvent this necessity, as in the Balinese (Mead and Macgregor, 1951) who nurse their babies holding them in a riding position on their forearm; or in the case of the Albanians, who nurse the baby tied to a cradleboard by bending over him and hanging the nipple into his mouth (Danziger and Frankl, 1934). This is not to say that the manifold stimuli provided by the breast-feeding situation are experienced as isolated from one another. I consider the widely different, but simultaneous sensory percepts during breast-feeding part of a total experience (Spitz, 1955c), from which single sectors may or may not be segregated in the course of development.

Breast feeding thus reestablishes for a while the union with the mother, which was lost through the precipitous process of birth, and through the sudden cutting of the umbilical cord. It makes possible the phylogenetically acquired slow and progressive achievement of autonomy from the mother by imposing and facilitating massive interchanges between the actions and sensations of the baby's body and those of the mother's body.

I have pointed out earlier that at the adult level the picture presented by Harlow's surrogate-raised monkeys is one of severe disturbance, both in the social and in the sexual sector. Any attempt to assess these disturbances in monkeys is strictly limited to the observation of the animals' manifest behavior. That is a rather crude indicator of deviations from the norm. The information afforded us by this indicator therefore can only point up the more spectacular disturbances. In man, verbal behavior and introspection provide us with far more detailed, more numerous, and more sensitive instruments of investigation.

Moreover, we have nowhere as complete an inventory of the average behavioral development of the monkey baby as that available to us for the human infant. Furthermore, because of his lower evolutionary level, a number of highly complex, specifically human achievements are missing from the monkey's behavioral inventory. These particular achievements not only are of great diagnostic reliability, but represent also highly sensitive indicators of development and psychic process.

A human child who, e.g., in the second or third year of life has not yet acquired speech evokes our concern. He will be considered seriously disturbed if, in the absence of an organic defect, he does not acquire speech in the subsequent years. Thus the acquisition, the level, the proficiency, the form, and the content of the child's verbal communication are all obvious, exceedingly sensitive and informative indicators of the child's normal psychological development and of any deviation therefrom. Nothing comparable is available in the monkey.

Conversely, normal behavior patterns which the human child abandons at a certain developmental stage must remain part and parcel of the monkey's normal adult behavior. We would be gravely concerned if a human child continued his biting behavior, which is normal below the level of 12 months, into his fourth and fifth year. And we would be equally concerned if he were to continue at that age to revert consistently to locomotion on all fours. We would justifiably consider the survival of such archaic behavior an indicator (or a symptom) of serious underlying psychiatric disturbance—and it is irrelevant here to distinguish between its being endogenous or not. In the adult monkey, however, both behavior patterns belong in the animal's normal behavioral inventory.

Thus in evaluating the monkey's level of development, social and otherwise, we are limited to a few gross behavior patterns, manifest sexual behavior being among them.

The fact that sexual development is only a crude indicator does not detract, however, from its value for our orientation. In the human we usually can detect disturbances of object relations and of development long before sexual activity becomes disturbed. When it does become disturbed, it indicates spectacularly that other sectors are also damaged. In my own infant observations I have noted that deviant sexual patterns were highly correlated with severely disturbed or completely absent object relations.

Indeed, it is my contention that in the first 18 months of life, autoerotic activity (in the form of genital play or its absence) is a reliable indicator of the adequacy or inadequacy of object relations, just as age-adequate sexual activity (or its absence) would be in the adult.

Obviously, sexual activities will be different on these different levels. We do not yet possess sufficient objective data to be able to make systematic statements on the subject, *pace* Kinsey. However, in this behavioral sector of the personality we can discern something in the nature of the developmental lines of which Anna Freud speaks; we can trace a line of the unfolding genital behavior patterns. This line should not be confused with the successive stages of libido. The libidinal stages and the manner in which they are reached and mastered exert a decisive influence on the form which genital behavior takes at any given age. The following remarks, therefore, refer simply to the normally expectable genital behavior from birth to maturity.

INFANTILE GENITAL PLAY AND DEVELOPMENT

In a general way, one might say that some genital play should be expected in the infant by the end of the first year of life. In the toddler or the preschool child, a transition from genital play to masturbation is to be expected, the details of which have not yet been investigated either quantitatively or qualitatively.

I do not know enough about the latency child to pronounce myself on what to expect there; I believe that the forms and behavioral patterns of genital activities during this age period will vary considerably, for they are even more highly culturally determined than during the preceding stages. In puberty, masturbation should be considered a normal sexual activity, while in late adolescence the transition to intercourse will be considered as such.

Actually, as psychoanalysts, we have, I believe, become aware that a special pathology is present in those of our patients who assure us that they discovered masturbation only in their twenties. I have had occasion to study several cases of this kind; they were, on the whole, rather severely disturbed. As yet I am not prepared to say what particular form of pathology, or rather, what structure of the defenses, is responsible for this developmental retardation. I need hardly say that I am not speaking of those cases in which amnesia has obliterated the memory of masturbation.

I am aware that I will provoke many objections when I state that reasonably

satisfactory object relations are among the conditions which make masturbation possible. It should be remembered that normal object relations do not
create the drive. They channel it into its behavioral implementation, beginning
with the means available on the own body and continuing on the "other's"
body. Here again cultural influences play a major role in determining the
measure in which the sexual drive is permitted satisfaction on the own body
or on the "other's" body.

It should be added that when object relations do not channel the drive into
its developmentally natural implementation, or when this implementation is
inhibited, a variety of other solutions becomes necessary. The most elementary, the most undesirable solution is regression to archaic behavior patterns
on the anal, oral, or even on the primary narcissistic level. We are all familiar
with these regressions in neurotics, and particularly in psychotics, where in
the more extreme cases infantile rocking and thumb sucking may be in evidence.

More desirable solutions compatible with genital play and subsequent masturbation are available. They may consist in the elaboration of specific defenses, such as reaction formation, sublimation, etc. In this process cultural
forces become effective and significant.

It seems that so far there has been no systematic attempt to investigate the
relationship between the age-adequate form of genital activity and the successive stages of development. It is true that this question has been approached
by psychoanalysts at one time or another in a somewhat random fashion.
Little has been published also about the influence of premature sexual gratification on the level of sublimation and of cultural achievement. Some of
us do have the impression that in cultures which permit the unrestricted
gratification of the sexual urge already in latency or prepuberty, the level of
personality development is generally lowered and the activation of higher
intellectual functions impaired.

This would not be surprising; I have always maintained, and Harlow appears
to have demonstrated this, that the frustration of the drives is an indispensable
prerequisite for developmental progress. By that I do not mean absolute
frustration, but an optimal level of frustration, a middle road, as it were.
"Optimal" applies to the age level at which frustration is imposed, to the
duration of the frustration, and to the forms which it takes.

The problem of the frustration of the drive brings us back to the decisively
important role of the sexual drive in the formation of social relations.

In Harlow's monkeys we have seen that the nature of object relations
determines subsequent social relations. Normal mother-child relations will
permit the monkey baby to develop normal relations with other monkeys of
its kind—that means to acquire the capacity and the desire to deal with a

whole spectrum of social relations with shifting and ever-changing roles. Being raised on a surrogate mother deprives the rhesus baby of those exchanges which make it possible to acquire this capacity. Being raised together with another monkey baby of equal age on a surrogate mother leads to mutual clinging of the two babies. An indissoluble closed system is formed which excludes all relations with others of one's kind.

Harlow's experiments show that a cloth surrogate is not enough. If the rhesus baby is to achieve normal rhesus maturity, a living individual, a real rhesus mother, is needed. Her interaction with her baby opens the road to individuation, to social relations, and to sexual relations.

The findings made on monkeys are very similar to the findings made on infants totally deprived of object relations. Therefore we are justified in assuming that the presence or absence of age-adequate genital behavior patterns, and masturbation among these, are indicators of the nature of the object relations which preceded them. But their role is not limited to that of an indicator of what went before. Even more importantly, genital behavior and masturbation will influence the future personality. For their presence will interact with other developmental influences and have a significant role for the individual's relations to others.

Therefore, we have to investigate the possibility that in the human the defense mechanisms may undergo significant modifications when the sexual drive is not implemented in infancy, at the toddler age, or later.

Psychoanalytic theory rests on Freud's concepts of conflict and defense. The conflict arises between the demands of the instinctual drives and the obstacles to their gratification imposed by the environment in the form of external restrictions or internalized controls. The defenses are elaborated by the ego in the course of the process of domesticating the instinctual drives. In schematic terms: the domestication has to reconcile the demands of the drives with two factors, an outer one and an inner one. The outer one is reality, including environmental restrictions. The inner one is represented by the demands of the superego (that is, internalized reality). In both cases the outcome may be a compromise formation of one kind or another; in extreme cases, when there is no other way of simultaneously satisfying the drive, the environment, and the superego, the conflict may enforce the suppression of the demands of the drive.

Sublimation is a good example of compromise, hysterical anesthesia an example of suppression. Between the two, compromise and paralysis, there exists a whole gamut of solutions, the majority of them highly constructive. These solutions are attempts at adaptation and include the defense mechanisms of the ego.

Defense mechanisms are psychological devices for dealing with specific conflicts. They arise therefore in the wake of conflicts, and we may ask ourselves what will happen when one of the major reasons for conflict, namely, autoerotic behavior, is absent from the child's behavioral repertoire. What will happen if the main developmental line, which normally should proceed through the successive stages of libido development, is eliminated?

In our Western Protestant culture, this developmental line is the central axis of conflict and repression; it is the motor of the Oedipus complex and of the formation of the superego. It is, I believe, worthwhile to speculate how different the structure of the system of defenses, of object relations, of oedipal development, and superego formation would be if sex activity in the toddler presented no educational problem because it was absent. Obviously this is a question which should be approached observationally, for instance, through the longitudinal study of orphanage-raised children. It should be checked whether such children achieve masturbation and when they achieve it, what its phenomenology is, its frequency, etc. At the present stage of our knowledge, we can offer only hunches in regard to the possible deviations to be expected when masturbation is absent or the tendencies to masturbate are missing in the toddler.

The "Good, Quiet Boy" Murderer

I wonder, for instance, about the overly docile, overobedient, the quiet, angelic, "no-trouble-ever" child. Even during the most turbulent years of latency and puberty, he never presents educational problems to parents or teachers, except for his distressingly inadequate learning performance. Could this be a concomitant of a history of absence of infantile sexuality? Everybody, the teachers, the school, the parents, the neighbors, consider such a child as particularly good, obedient, and problemless. He tries so hard in school, but does not seem to get anywhere. He does not have many friends either, and may be taken advantage of by the more domineering of his age mates, by those who relish an adoring, devoted slave. And then, one day, we read of the sudden, incomprehensible, murderous outbreak of an adolescent who had been this "good" boy.

In school he sat through classes meekly, friendless, without participating in group activities, unless so directed, and without appearing to absorb anything of the scholastic material. He was promoted, because he "tried so hard" (and because our school system considers it undemocratic that any child, however inadequate, should not be promoted like all the others). He ended up with a low I.Q., as a "dull normal," suitable for a trade or for menial occupation. Frequently he was rejected by the draft board.

It is quite probable that the I.Q. potential of such children is not as dim as routine testing results and school reports seem to indicate. But our ordinary educational methods are not equipped to deal with this kind of deficit, where deviation sets in too early to permit the school to reclaim such contactless children for society. Moreover, at the elementary school level, these children do not attract the attention of their educators. For they are colorless, inconspicuous, and do not even come into conflict with society, i.e., with their classmates. Conflicts arise from relatedness, not from lack of relation.

The "Good Little" Prostitute

At first glance, it appears that the "good boy" murderer has no real counterpart in the female adolescent. I believe that he has, in the form of the "good little" prostitute, the classical female delinquent, who often tests as dull normal or below, and who is such a favorite heroine of our avant-garde, angry, Beatnik poets.

I have had the opportunity to study a large population of such female delinquents in the course of a five-year research in the nursery of a penal institution housing delinquent minors and their illegitimate infants. The former clergyman of this institution had reviewed the records of the 200 delinquent girls committed there in the course of a three-year period. He found that over 90 percent of them came from broken homes. We may infer that the overwhelming majority of the delinquents housed in this institution had been deprived in one way or another of the opportunity to form normal object relations during infancy.

My own findings on these delinquent girls also support my proposition that normal object relations in infancy and childhood are of decisive significance for the development of the personality. By and large, these were harmless, not very bright girls, convicted under the Wayward Minors Act.

According to the proposition I voiced above, in their case, sexuality should have been conspicuous by its absence. Were these not individuals who had been deprived of object relations during infancy? Yet here we have girls who not only had achieved sexual activity, but whose downfall was caused by this very activity! The contradiction is only apparent. In Harlow's monkeys also it is females who ultimately are brought to sexual activity, even though, to quote him, "without enthusiasm or cooperation." One or two of them finally submitted relatively passively to active normal males.

It seems to me that in our delinquent subjects, the picture is that of the slightly stupid puberty girl, who does not know "what it's all about," but obediently does what she is told to do.

Any institution for delinquent girls houses a large number of such mentally and emotionally underprivileged; their absolute unselectivity and promiscuity in regard to their sexual partners are matters of common knowledge.[6]

ABSENCE OF INFANTILE GENITAL PLAY AND PERSONALITY FORMATION

Accordingly, I have postulated that a specific socially deviant behavior, in both boys and girls, is associated with early lack in object relations. This deviant behavior becomes conspicuous in a manner disturbing to the community only when the subject reaches puberty. At that age level an increased autonomy is expected from the individual; he is expected to give up his need for anaclitic support. At the same time, in exercising this autonomy, he is expected to show a modicum of conformity with social usage. In the case of the deviant boys, this leads to conflict with the need-gratifying objects; in the case of the girls, to an infringement of social mores through lack of object constancy and through the attempt to cling to ever new need-gratifying objects.

How are we to understand the psychic structure of such beings and the dynamics which lead to it? I have indicated earlier that with the absence of masturbatory practices a major source of conflict between parent and child has been removed. The sexual drive implements many of the child's activities, both manifestly sexual and nonmanifestly sexual, such as play, games with his age mates, etc. With the disappearance of sexual activity from manifest behavior, the child is not "bad" any more; not bad in "playing with himself," nor bad in playing with other children, for he does not even get that far. He does not form attachments or friendships. He may be a bit dull; but for the elementary rewards of food, warmth, closeness, he will do what the parents want him to do, and he will cling and be described as a "loving child." He is good in the sense of "Be good, sweet maid, and let who can be clever." But of such is not the Kingdom of Heaven.

When conflict is removed, so is frustration; with that, the incentive is absent for the adaptive development of the prismatic variety of sectors in the child's psychic apparatus. There are no problems to be solved, there are no obstacles to be overcome; there is just the road of least resistance, and the least resistance is to be a "good" child.

---

[6] I am not implying that every promiscuous girl, every prostitute, has subnormal mental equipment—even history would prove me wrong. But the personality of the intelligent prostitute, of the promiscuous intellectual, is a neurotic one, and has its origin in neurotic conflict. That is situated at a more advanced developmental level, at a later age, than that at which the "good little" prostitute was damaged. Neurotic conflict hardly arises in the absence of autoerotic activity. In this respect, the population of the penal nursery was moderately skewed, thus giving me the opportunity to observe a relatively large number of mentally somewhat underprivileged delinquents. Our laws and social institutions favor the commitment of the unintelligent. The intelligent prostitute will elude the police more easily; and it is not the bright girls, but the "dull normals" and the somewhat feeble-minded who get trapped by pregnancy.

A major problem of these children is that the question of the defenses hardly arises. For the defenses are a powerful tool, perhaps the most powerful of all, in the instrumentarium of human adaptation, development, and progress. In these "good" children without sex activity, there is little to defend against, and at the oedipal stage no Oedipus conflict is provoked.

For these "good" children the defense mechanism of choice is that of identification; it would probably be more correct to speak of introjective and projective mechanisms in the sense of "magic participation" as discussed by Edith Jacobson (1954). Her lucid analysis of the dynamics of becoming part of the omnipotent object covers many aspects of what I am describing. Perhaps Sperling's (1944) concept of "appersonation" should also be considered in this context.

Similarly, what the Kleinian School calls "projective identification"—the object exists simultaneously externally and internally (Klein, 1948) and the ego may become completely submerged at times—is also relevant to our topic. Here, however, Edith Jacobson clearly demonstrated that these Kleinian concepts refer only to prototypes which operate in earliest infancy. The mechanisms to be developed from them appear later; while processes analogous to the prototypes themselves can be observed only in psychotics and borderline patients. This is in good agreement with my own ideas. Though the later development of the subjects I have been discussing rarely falls into any of the conventional categories of psychosis, one surely would consider them borderline.

Of the other defenses, the mechanism of regression is obviously available from the beginning, as it is so close to the physiological prototype. How far introjection and projection operate, and whether repression is available, will have to form the subject of a special study.

It should be clearly understood that I am discussing only the extreme cases of mother deprivation in man, those which are comparable to Harlow's surrogate-raised monkeys. Bowlby (1960) recently alleged that such cases are no longer seen—an optimism which I cannot share. Man's inhumanity to man has not decreased that much. After all, the term which German ethologists are using for their "stimulus-deprived" animals is derived from human experience. They call them "Caspar Hauser animals"—a doubtful compliment to humanity.

Obviously the overwhelming majority of the cases which come to the psychiatrist's attention are less extreme. According to the amount of deprivation, its duration, and the age level at which the deprivation began, such cases present a wide spectrum of deficit ranging from the extremes of hospitalism to relatively inconspicuous defects.

I am, of course, not speaking of those cases in which the surround suppresses or restricts genital play and masturbatory activity. I am speaking of the *nonachievement* of genital play and masturbatory activity at the age-adequate level, as a consequence and an indicator of a significant deficit in mother-child relations. It is a symptom—and not the only one—of the deficit. The nonachievement of genital play and masturbatory activity is a developmental disturbance which damages, or does not permit, the emergence of one specific sector of the personality. This is a sector acquired through development (in the sense of Hartmann, Kris, and Loewenstein, 1946). The picture of this deficit has often been described quite unspecifically as developmental arrest; I am trying to be more specific. That is why I have at this point taken up the question of the defenses, which I consider as adaptive structures of the most far-reaching importance in the development of the ego.

From this point of view we have to ask ourselves what defensive mechanisms (beside the more primitive ones of regression, introjection, projection, repression, and denial) become available to the children who do not achieve manifest sexual behavior. This obviously depends on the severity of the case, and more precisely on the etiological factors already mentioned: on the degree and duration of the deprivation and on the age level at which it took place.

However, the degree of this impairment does not concern us here. Our problem is whether defense mechanisms will be produced in the absence of conflict. I believe that in these cases of impairment, defense mechanisms which ordinarily develop *after* the first year of life (reaction formation, isolation, undoing, even identification with the aggressor, etc.) will not be achieved.[7]

---

[7] My distinction between primitive defenses and those developed later is based on a division of the concept of defenses into: (1) prototypes of defenses, (2) precursors of defenses, and (3) genuine defense mechanisms. (1) Prototypes of defenses I consider to be physiological behavior patterns and functions which serve, so to say, as models of later psychological processes. (2) Precursors of defenses are psychologically regulated behavior patterns. Unlike the prototypes, they involve psychological conflict either between the drives themselves or between the drives and reality. However, they do not yet involve structural conflict. (3) Defense mechanisms proper involve structural conflict. This structural conflict does not necessarily require the presence of a superego or even that of a forerunner of a superego. In its most archaic form the conflict may take place between ego and id.

In my opinion, defense mechanisms originate as adaptive devices. However, the adaptive function is not a useful criterion to distinguish defense mechanisms from their precursors or their prototypes. Both precursors and prototypes perform their adaptive function already in the first year of life, and often long before the psychological development of some of the true defenses.

I find unconscious processes the most useful criterion for establishing whether a given phenomenon involves defense mechanisms proper or only one of their forerunners. If what we observe is the outcome of an unconscious process; if it represents an attempt at psychological resolution of a psychological conflict, that is to say, a conflict between the drives, or of a conflict between drive and reality (for instance, a conflict with the love object) and the outcome of this attempt is a device which from then on will serve as a model for dealing with comparable psychological conflicts—then we are dealing with a defense mechanism.

These are genuine ego defenses and contribute permanently to the structure of the ego and to personality formation. But the adaptive devices we can observe in these impaired children are not genuine, permanent ego defenses. They are impermanent identificatory maneuvers, pseudo defenses, transitory attempts at dealing with immediate situations. Accordingly, they are as easily abandoned as acquired and do not exert a lasting influence on psychic structure and character.

Therefore the problem I am discussing is the role of genital play and masturbation in ego formation on the one hand; the arrest of ego development, as manifested by a deficit in the implementation of the sexual drive and in the formation of the defenses on the other. One may well ask how the individual survives such deficits when they become massive.

In the animal world, at the level of the primates, the individual obviously will not survive, unless it be through fortuitous circumstances, such as being raised in a laboratory. In man, Western culture ensures such survival up to the point where the individual can become self-supporting. In the extreme case, we have then the picture of the individual to whom the autonomous functions of the ego are available, but in whom some of the functions on the level of secondary autonomy may be absent and in whom the higher, psychological functions involving control (defenses, Oedipus complex, superego) are lacking.

In these individuals, ego identity may be achieved, but only to a certain extent. It is questionable if identity of the self can be reached—again, it should be remembered that this applies only to extreme cases. In such cases, but also in many of the milder ones, the boundaries of the personality remain fluid and shadowy. In my opinion, the identity of the self is worked out through a delimitation of the self from the nonself. That segregation is achieved through cathectic displacements and investments within the systems of the ego. The memory systems and the thought processes are particularly important in this respect. The absence of firm boundaries between self and

---

However, the various defense mechanisms do not develop at the same age level. When I speak of the primitive defenses, I am referring to those which in their whole structure are closer to prototypes and precursors than the later and more sophisticated defenses. From this point of view, regression unquestionably belongs among the primitive defenses, for not only is it present already in the first year of life, but it is also the most readily available device for dealing with archaic ego-id conflicts. Both incorporation and what I would call "ex-corporation" certainly are adaptive processes. But whether introjection is already operating at the early stages of ego development, toward the end of the first year of life is as difficult to decide as the question of whether projection is in evidence at the same age level. But denial most probably is available at this early level; and it will be a question of personal opinion whether one wishes to posit the presence of repression at this early developmental level, or whether one should not rather situate it somewhere in the second year of life, as seems more probable.

[See more extensive discussion in "Early Prototypes of Ego Defense," this volume.]

nonself, between ego and id, and the inability to achieve object constancy explain the compliance, the "goodness" of many such individuals. Without having achieved a self, they, pliantly and complyingly, become an extension, as it were, of the need gratifier.

But it should always be remembered that these individuals, who become an extension of the need gratifier, do not have true object relations with him. True object relations are the outcome of a prolonged developmental process. The vicissitudes of the drives, the stages of libido, the crucial points of development, such as the Oedipus complex and its dissolution, latency and puberty—each of these contributes in its own way to the capacity to form object relations and to the durability of the relations thus formed.

The lack of sexual striving proper, the lack of masturbation, or the lack of fantasies connected with it, already preclude the oedipal conflict and modify the later vicissitudes of the drives. The clinging attitude of such children to the individuals of both sexes surrounding them should not be misinterpreted as object ties. It often becomes cloying, and it is precisely this cloying-clinging which precludes the Oedipus relation. The need gratifier can be anyone—father, mother, aunt, uncle, brother, sister. The relation can shift from the one to the other; there is no competitor to take the object away, for our subjects have the capacity to become a part, an extension, of any individual toward whom drives or needs are directed, as long as the individual permits it.

Of course, it is rare to observe this picture fully. There are many variations and modifications; these result from the individual history of the child. The essence is that the sexual drive is either not implemented in terms of the genital organ, or, when it is, it is a secondary implementation in the nature of a drive discharge without concomitant psychological content, as would be infantile incontinence or a sneeze. Without such psychological content the Oedipus situation does not arise.

In the absence of the Oedipus complex, the formation of the superego cannot be expected. There are no imagos to be lost, and therefore none to be introjected. Indeed, the introjects are already there, primitive ones, and therefore not firmly anchored. They remain on the level of need fulfillment and are relinquished when they become frustrating. This explains the extraordinary ease with which such children accept new situations; it explains the shallowness of their attachment and, of course, the ineffectiveness of transference (Bender, in a discussion, remarked on what she calls the schizophrenic child's ready, anxietyless acceptance of a new environment). I have described one such individual in another context in "The Case of Felicia" (Spitz, 1955a). Evelyn, Felicia's mother, shifted without an instant's hesitation to that person who at the given moment offered her greater gratification.

That also explains the "good" little prostitute—without hesitation she shifts to the person who will offer her gratification, be that in the form of a drink, money, fondling, command, or a cup of coffee.

So much for the "good" little girl who becomes a "good" little prostitute. But what of the boy murderer? That does not seem a difficult question to answer. In most such cases, as reported in the papers, we find that a gratification, often trivial, had been denied. The boy was not permitted out of his room; he was denied the use of the car; he was scolded—time and again one is puzzled and bewildered by the incongruity between the frustration and the murderous response.

The answer, as I see it, is that the level of object constancy achieved by these individuals is and remains inadequate, and that their superego development is only rudimentary or nonexistent. The inadequacy of their object constancy becomes manifest in their readiness to change their ego ideal. Their rudimentary superego is a poor guide in making choices. As a result, they are unable to establish a hierarchy in their goals and to relate their actions to the decalogue of the surround.

The mode of their drive gratification fails to advance much beyond the level of the pleasure-unpleasure principle, and frustration tolerance remains low. When a prohibition is imposed, the resulting frustration is experienced as a total one. As soon as the need gratifier frustrates them, he loses his object attributes, such as they are. From a need-gratifying object he turns into a need-denying frustrator, an aggressor, and as such he becomes the victim of the delinquent boy's aggressive, destructive drive.

Conversely, in the girl, the moment the partner offers a gratification, he is accorded access to what he desires, though he does not become a true libidinal object on the genital level, but only a need-gratifying object. And the need to gratifies is not the sexual need, for the "good" little prostitute is frigid.

These considerations have carried us away from our original topic, the question of masturbation. If my speculations can be validated, some revision of our views on masturbation is in order. We will have to accept genital play in infancy as an indicator of satisfactory object relations. This implies also that masturbation during the preschool age, during latency and adolescence, is to be regarded as a necessary and logical developmental elaboration of this beginning. But, as we know from Freud (1905b), the role and significance of infantile sexuality is vastly greater than that of being a mere indicator.

This becomes immediately clear when we remember that the child's urge to implement his sexual drive in the form of genital play provokes opposition from the surround and brings him into early conflict with socially accepted repression of sexuality. This opposition ranges from mild, loving "under-standing" to harsh and sadistic measures (Spitz, 1952), with the avowed aim of eliminating the child's sexual activity. The child responds to this pressure with a variety of adaptive measures, ranging from superficial compliance to open rebellion, from latent pathology to severe personality disturbances. We are all familiar with the manifest behavioral changes so frequent at this age level. Occurring, as they do, in the period of anal stubbornness, they are bound to be fairly conspicuous; they may be, and they mostly are, manifested in sectors other than the overtly sexual one.

At the same developmental level, at the transition from the oral to the anal stage, a major dynamic shift takes place in the psychic economy. This is initiated by a maturational surge which increases powerfully the quantities of drive energy requiring discharge. The developmentally elaborated drive controls are still inadequate to cope with the increased drive pressure which arises from the newly invested anal zone and also from the harbingers of the incipient genital phase. The drive pressure is reinforced through the resistance offered by the environment's countermeasures to its manifestations.

One of the consequences of the conflict between drive pressure and environmental resistance is that it provokes a variety of fantasies, in which libidinal and anal-sadistic elements participate, the anal-sadistic ones predominating. The conflict between aggressive and libidinal fantasies provokes guilt feelings and concomitant anxiety. Attempts to deal with the latter lead to the elaboration of defense mechanisms, such as identification with the aggressor, reaction formation, denial, etc. On the pathological side, these conflicts are liable to lead to eating disturbances, infantile insomnia, and nightmares; pavor nocturnus belongs among these disturbances: it is my opinion that there are several developmental levels at which pavor nocturnus is common. Of these, the level of the second year of life appears to be the earliest.

These stormy intrapsychic processes contribute importantly to the shaping of the elements which enter into the still rudimentary organization of the ego. They mark the transition from the achievement of secondary autonomy in the ego to the stage in which defense mechanisms are elaborated; and through them, the character and personality of the individual are determined. At this stage one can observe identifications which represent the earliest outlines of the ego ideal, and when probably even some dim rudiments of the superego come into being. It is the stage at which the earliest archaic images are conceived, the imagos destined to become the content of the ego ideal on the one hand, and later to be introjected as the formative elements of the superego.

These all too schematic comments on the vicissitudes provoked in the psychic economy by the child's implementation of his sexual drive indicate what a powerful force the child's early sexual activity represents in the advancement of his development. This is a force which transcends the individual's personal development, for it also exerts an influence of the first magnitude on the individual's emerging social relations and on his adaptation to society.

Lest these comments be misinterpreted, I am not in any way suggesting that masturbation should be encouraged. It must have become clear that masturbation *as such* is not the prime force in question. Far from it; I am stressing the role of masturbation in eliciting the fantasies connected with it, the conflicts which it inevitably provokes, and the defense mechanisms which result from these conflicts. I consider this process to be among the most potent in making man into a social animal. With the help of the oedipal conflict and its outcome, the superego, he is enabled to form social relations and to integrate himself into the social order.

Looking back at my argument, I find that it has led me onto the horns of a dilemma. On the one hand, I found that genital play in infancy (or its absence) is an indicator of the nature of the child's object relations. Genital play will lead to infantile masturbation and to the fantasies connected with it. These fantasies contribute powerfully to the process of personality formation and to the elaboration of social relations. Both my own observations and animal experiments showed the undesirable consequences of the absence of sexual behavior in infancy and early childhood.

On the other hand, I am well aware that unrestricted permissiveness in regard to masturbation and sexual manifestations in childhood does not contribute to developmental progress. On the contrary, our psychoanalytic experience and knowledge indicates that it is the restriction of sexuality, and in particular of masturbation, which leads to such social and civilizatory human achievements as the superego.

Obviously, as always in evolution, a compromise must be found. From the viewpoint of our civilization, the consequences of masturbation without restriction are probably as undesirable as those of restriction without masturbation. Both lead to sterility, be it mental or reproductive.

We have no easy formula for the amount of frustration which should be applied in child-rearing, beyond the basic principle *"est modus in rebus."*

Man is a unit born of compromise. But this unit cannot be divided from the larger totality, from society, from culture—which in their turn depend on man's individual development. In essence, man and his future, his survival as an individual, as well as mankind's survival as society and civilization are as dependent on the child's relation to his mother as they are dependent on the way in which the individual deals with his drives. Ultimately, mankind and its works depend on how man deals with his offspring, with his children.

Paraphrasing the words of the poet: Man, "a stranger and afraid in a world he never made," can survive and achieve his destiny only if he is led by the hand into society by the twin gods of Eros and Aggression.

Life and the Dialogue

Those among you who are old enough to have lived part of their conscious life before the advent of motion pictures, and perhaps even before the flickers in the penny arcades, may remember visiting a then popular entertainment, the waxworks. It is a long time since I have seen waxworks announced anywhere; the last one was that repository of Victorian tradition, Madame Tussaud's in London. I do not know whether any of these spooky, slightly sinister, and somewhat monstrous museums still exist. If so, it might repay the student of the human mind to visit them and to make a few observations.

For these waxworks were not, as one might assume, just galleries of the portraits of celebrities and oddities. They did not consist only of wax portraits of public figures in their official roles or in the midst of their family, and, conversely, of the gory waxen puppets scattered on the re-enacted scene of a sensational murder. They also exhibited wax figures which, with the help of a mechanical device, moved and tried to create something approaching a lifelike illusion. And, most intriguing, here and there a wax figure was smuggled into the path of the gaping yokel, who mistook the puppet for one of the spectators, until he knocked against it. Inevitably, it came about that one or the other among the spectators, usually an unmarried gentleman between 20 and 40, had a flash of inspiration and would freeze in a rigid posture, pretending to be a wax figure; and when the kids touched him, he would "come to life" and scare them out of a week's growth.

There is a strange fascination about the idea of the inanimate creating the illusion of life; and also about the living posing as inanimate. This fascination permeates a great deal more of our thinking than we are usually aware. Were a waxworks available, I would have photographed it, to show you a really good illustration of the subject which will occupy us today. For I will discuss how we come to distinguish the animate from the inanimate, how we discriminate between the living and the things.

Recently, in a magazine illustration, a little girl was shown kissing a very lifelike doll nearly her own size—with the caption "Which one is the toy dolly?" The caption obviously is intended to be "cute." But the photograph

Reprinted from *Counterpoint: Libidinal Object and Subject,* ed., Herbert S. Gaskill. New York: International Universities Press, 1963.

147

fools nobody: even though absence of color, lack of motion, and two-dimensionality, handicap photography in conveying meaning, we "know" the child from the doll immediately.

It seems licit to ask, and it is a valid psychological problem to investigate, how we manage to distinguish the living from the inanimate. How this takes place in the adult is something which I must leave to the study of others. Today I will only discuss how this distinction is made by the infant, and more specifically: when does it begin?

For begin it must. I think we may safely assume that a visual distinction between living and inanimate is not present at birth. If this is correct, then we have the further obligation to investigate the process and the steps through which the human infant acquires this highly specialized variety of discrimination. And why, from an early age, the child prefers the living to the inanimate.

Why is it that, beginning with a certain age, every child will without hesitation be more interested in a live puppy than in the most clever mechanical one, or (if we but permit it) in a live baby more than in the most elaborate doll, whether that doll be able to cry and talk or not, whether it goes to sleep or not, whether it wets its diapers—as present-day dolls are able to do.

In psychoanalytic literature, Winnicott (1953) in his important paper "Transitional Objects and Transitional Object Phenomena" comes closest to the problem of differentiation between the animate and the inanimate. I believe I interpret him correctly in stating that he considers the child's continued relationship to an inanimate "thing," cuddly toy or otherwise, as a device used by the child to make possible among other achievements that of autonomy from the libidinal object on the one hand; on the other, to enable the child to master conflicts and problems in his relations with the libidinal object with the help of fantasies enacted on a transitional, an inanimate object.

Mahler (1960) approaches the problem from the opposite direction. She introduces the concept of *dedifferentiation* and describes how ego regression in the schizophrenic child goes to a level of *perceptual* dedifferentiation at which primal discrimination between living and inanimate is lost. This means that Mahler posits that at a given point in infantile development such a discrimination is acquired; she ascribes the first mention of this process to Monakow—wrongly, I believe, because what Monakow described occurs long after infancy and has little relation to our present-day concepts of the inception of perceptual discrimination. It is Mahler's and not Monakow's merit to have called attention to the fact that differentiation between the living and the inanimate is not present from birth but undergoes a process of evolution. It will be our task to attempt to describe some early stages of this process in regard to the special sector of discrimination between living and inanimate.

I will begin with a brief review of our knowledge regarding the preliminary stages of visual differentiation between animate and inanimate during the first year of life.

Already a few weeks after birth we can isolate two visual stimuli which reliably provoke the infant's attention and his response to the living. First, the percept of the human face and eyes, to which the infant reacts already at four to six weeks of age by following them with his eyes. The other such stimulus is the perception of movement of any kind. I have stated elsewhere (Spitz, 1959) that in my opinion, both these responses are probably inborn; to be exact, inherited. They appear to be in the nature of an IRM,[1] though at this stage of our knowledge no proof for this can be presented.

In the course of development, these stimuli combine with others, acquire cohesion, and become part of a Gestalt which, at the age of two to three months, elicits the infant's first social response and initiates his perception of the difference between I and non-I.

At this stage, as shown elsewhere in a series of experiments (Spitz, 1946d), there is no difference between the child's reaction to the living human's face and that to an inanimate artifact, as long as they both fulfill the conditions of the privileged Gestalt plus movement. This state of affairs continues up to the sixth month—with the usual age variations observable in individual children.

However, at the next stage, beginning around the sixth month of life, the child will no longer accept the inanimate object in place of the living partner, however briefly. Endowing the inanimate with the privileged Gestalt and with movement is of no avail. Indeed, it would seem that, the more the inanimate artifact approaches the living prototype, the more anxiety-provoking it becomes.

I have advanced the proposition that, at this age level, a transitional period is situated in which an adaptation to the inanimate on the one hand, to the living on the other, takes place. This adaptation involves discriminatory processes with survival significance. I arrived at this assumption because I observed in the human infant at this age a variety of unexpected and unpredictable responses to the living as well as to the inanimate. Furthermore, similar observations were reported by ethologists about the young of a number of animal species at a comparable developmental level.

---

[1] [Innate releasing mechanism. A brief discussion of this concept is given by Spitz in "The Primal Cavity" (fn. 1), this volume. Ed.]

I presented my findings on the infant's responses to the living, familiar or unfamiliar, in a number of publications (Spitz, 1950a); I have called this response the *eight-months anxiety,* for this is a response of anxiety which the child manifests in the second half of the first year when confronted with a stranger. I postulated (Spitz, 1959) that this response to the living, specifically the differentiation between the libidinal object and the stranger, represents an indicator of the appearance of the second organizer in the infantile psyche.

I have only hinted in my publications at similar reactions to the *inanimate* on the part of the infant (Spitz, 1950a), because my observations of such reactions were rather scattered at first. For a long time I was not able to find an explanation for them. But in the course of my work it became evident that, around the time at which the eight-months anxiety appears, a number of infants show anxiety reactions in response to toys and other inanimate objects. These reactions do not appear with the same regularity as the eight-months anxiety—they are more erratic, less reliable. But once our attention has been drawn to them, we may perhaps find laws governing this response also.

My attention was drawn to this phenomenon for the first time when I offered a 12-inch doll to infants who had never before seen one and they reacted to it with anxiety. This reaction varies of course from child to child, just like the eight-months anxiety. It ranges from mild unwillingness to touch the doll to screaming panic.

I was not very successful in correlating the presence of doll anxiety with the history of the individual child or with the presence or absence of eight months anxiety. However, the phenomenon appeared to be reinforced in children who had undergone separation, though this is only an impression and will have to be tested with much greater exactitude.

In the further course of my experiments, I discovered that, though the doll provokes the most spectacular negative responses, such responses can also be elicited by other inanimate objects at the same period, though not necessarily in the same children.

These observations led me to the conclusion that the second organizer of the psyche marks the period at which the infant goes through a development as the result of which, among other achievements, he becomes capable of distinguishing not only the love object from the stranger, but also the living from the inanimate. You notice that I am hinting here at a momentous development in the infant's thinking processes. I believe that this is the *precursor* of the inception of the concept of "alive," of life.

Like the capacity to distinguish the libidinal object from everybody else in the world, distinguishing animate from inanimate is an achievement of major importance and as such fraught with conflict, sometimes manifested by anxiety. I suspect that in this conflict the aggressive drive plays a significant role. But of this later.

Anxiety reactions of infants before this or that inanimate object have hardly provoked the attention of child psychologists, though in the last decade psychoanalysts have become aware of them in clinical cases. Ethologists have become alerted to these reactions to the inanimate, which appear to be rather spectacular in primates, but have been also observed in various other animal species. I had the opportunity to discuss this problem with Konrad Lorenz, with Eibl, and with their associates, as well as with Donald Hebb and his staff. They all consider the phenomenon to be a reaction to strangeness, but to strangeness of some particular kind.

Already Yerkes observed that, when the personnel of the laboratory happened to carry a dead monkey past the cage of the other monkeys, these were apt to panic or to get furious, or both, and might attack the personnel. Hebb discovered, furthermore, that the plaster model of a monkey's head produces similar reactions. They called this phenomenon "ghost reaction."

Lorenz observed that rooks, and also other birds, will attack a person carrying a dead bird of their own kind. And in one of his characteristically impressive observations, Lorenz relates that returning from his swim, his black swimming trunks dangling from his hand, he was "dive-bombed" by a flock of rooks which had perceived the dangling black trunks as a dead rook. (The seemingly unmotivated attacks on unsuspecting persons by birds, reported from time to time, may well have a similar explanation.)

Experiments made by Hebb (Hebb and Riesen, 1943) also appear to be related to our problem; he offered monkeys a number of artifacts, among which the most anxiety-provoking were those which represented the head of an animal of the same species. Hebb remarks that some strange variation of something familiar, a familiar object in a new context is particularly potent.

(Obviously, this is a phenomenon with more than one facet. Most of the animal observations appear to involve IRMs which are somehow linked to survival. They are the defensive measures against the common enemy and, in connection with this, the intraspecies protective measures. There is that most surprising phenomenon, the anxiety in front of a deviant stranger of the same species; and finally, there is the response to the mutilated or dead of the same species.[2])

---

[2] It is characteristic that strangers of another species do not produce the same kind of fear. Fighting in animals also (outside of fighting for food) is always an intraspecies behavior and not an interspecies one.

The intraspecies protective measures manifested in the "dive-bombing" attacks of birds are of the same nature as the ganging up of small birds against a larger common enemy, like the owl. In the Middle Ages, and until quite recently this trait of small birds was used for hunting. A live owl, and sometimes a stuffed one, would be placed during the daytime in the open, while the hunter remained hidden, throwing a net over the small birds which attacked this decoy in swarms.

What has all this to do with our specific problem, namely: how the child learns to distinguish the animate from the inanimate? Obviously, this distinction plays a major role also in the behavior patterns of animals just discussed. Animals are probably endowed with those behavior patterns through phylogenesis.

But Man?

When I arrived at this point in my thoughts, another experiment with the inanimate suddenly came to mind. This was Harlow's large-scale investigation on what he called "The Nature of Love." In discussing his findings (Spitz, 1962), I had also unwittingly dealt with some of the major aspects of today's problem. In that paper I discussed extensively Harlow's experiment of raising rhesus monkeys on surrogate mothers made of wire and terry cloth—of course, inanimate; and more specifically I discussed the consequences of this procedure. In a nutshell, these consequences are that the surrogate-raised monkeys cannot develop play or social relations. They are subject to uncontrollable anxiety and to outbreaks of violent agitation, hostility, and destructiveness. When grown up, they have no sexual relations and show no sexual behavior of any kind.

Certain conclusions which I had drawn from these findings and from my own observations provide also an answer to our present problem.

Let me repeat the proposition I advanced at that time: I asked: what factor, present or absent, in the inanimate terry-cloth surrogate mother exerts such a destructive influence on the baby monkey's development? I came to the conclusion that this factor is the lack of *reciprocity* between the surrogate mother and the rhesus baby.

Today I feel inclined to be more specific and to say that the missing factor in the inanimate surrogate mothers is the capacity to conduct a dialogue with the baby. This dialogue is, of course, not a verbal dialogue. It is a dialogue of action and response which goes on in the form of a circular process within the dyad, as a continuous mutually stimulating feedback circuit. I am willing to make a concession to the purists among you and to call it a *precursor* of the dialogue—a discussion—an archaic form of conversation.

For I realize that in speaking of "action and response" I am guilty of an almost impermissible oversimplification. Emotion enters the picture. The action can be and mostly will be invested with emotion, but the same applies, of course, to the response. The action may involve a minimum of emotion; the response may be emotion alone, as easily as emotion-charged action. The action may be directed or nondirected, and so may the response. That will make the difference between its being an expression of an internal state or an appeal to the partner of the dyad—and so forth *ad infinitum*.

Of course, this is not a repetitive process. On the contrary, the reverberations provoked in the mother by the child's initiative and those in the child by the mother's resulting behavior (and vice versa) produce ever new constellations of increasing complexity. It should be added that these are constellations and structures resulting from energy displacement. Each of these circular processes will achieve some sort of gratification, or frustration, and then subside. Traces will be left in their wake in the psyche and in the memory systems of each of the two partners. These traces will modify the next circular process in its inception, or in the form it takes, or in its unrolling, or in the way it achieves its goal; thus adding to the increasing complexity of the dialogue.

It is evident that only between two living partners can such processes take place. Therefore, they are suitable to serve to distinguish the living from the inanimate.

Obviously, the inanimate cannot engage in a *dialogue* with the child. Even when provided with highly sophisticated mechanical devices, it cannot engage in circular action-reaction response exchanges. For the inanimate, although it may occasionally lend itself to the child's needs, e.g., provide food, warmth, or serve as a target for the discharge of aggression, will present an unresponsive "outside." It will leave the child to deal, unaided, with his drives and with his needs; and that at a developmental level at which he does not yet have the means or the devices for doing so.

The relation to the inanimate must of necessity remain unilateral—the child acts, but the inanimate does not react.

I consider it highly probable that this lack of feedback is the main criterion through which the child learns to distinguish the animate from the inanimate. It follows from the fact that the child prefers the living to the inanimate that the feedback must represent a gratifying experience.

It is licit to speculate whether this gratifying quality is derived from the memory of gratification experienced from the mother in a variety of situations. I for one am not inclined to believe this. I think that the gratification obtained from the dialogue with the living has not only one single, simple origin, but that it is the result of multiform processes. I believe that gratification *and* frustration, libido *and* aggression are involved in making the living so much more appealing than the inanimate. As you may remember, Harlow tried to add a number of devices to his surrogate mothers to render them more attractive to the rhesus babies—warmth, movement, food—all to no avail. The inanimate surrogates could not compete with living rhesus mothers.

The one function to which inanimate objects appear to lend themselves well is the discharge of the aggressive drive. Since the inanimate does not respond or retaliate, it becomes suitable for hitting, chewing, breaking, smashing, throwing without limitation of the number of times and the extent to which the baby carries these activities.

Conversely, the live partner is more suitable for the discharge of the libidinal drive. For he provides the inexhaustible resources of the dialogue and, at the same time, offers to the child not only a manageable discharge of libidinal—*and* aggressive!—energy, but through the very nature of the dialogue opens up new and tempting avenues for expanding these discharges and at the same time reaping from them the rewards of affective gratification.

Furthermore, the unrestricted discharge of the aggressive drive does not lead anywhere—the repetitive destruction of the inanimate remains always the same—it is, literally, a dead-end street. With a living partner on the other hand the feedback is bilateral, and different in each of the partners. It takes place in a progressing continuum; ever-new, ever-changing answers arise within the dialogue, on progressively higher levels, offering ever more sophisticated gratifications.

Rigid unresponsiveness then will become one of the important criteria each child uses to recognize inanimateness. Once the child becomes able to apply this criterion, anxiety reactions to this or that inanimate object may appear in some children. Our observations show that a history of handling inanimate things on the one hand, of object relations with the mother on the other, precedes the stage at which the living is differentiated from the inanimate.

However, this does not explain why some children—and by no means all!—make a seemingly arbitrarily selected inanimate thing into an object of fear. I have already mentioned that I was unable to discover in the history of these children a satisfactory explanation either for the choice or the anxiety.

It is here that the animal psychologists' explanation of the anxiety-provoking effects of the familiar in an unfamiliar setting throws some light on our problem. If we look at the infant's anxiety response to the inanimate, we find that the common denominator in all of them *is* an element of strangeness, of unfamiliarity in the inanimate itself or in the setting in which it appears. Accordingly, a doll which *does* possess a human face, that most important distinguishing attribute of the love object, *but* which is quite small and inanimate, may become the most threatening anxiety provoker for the eight-month-old. And the ball which rolls—it shouldn't move!—and the drum which gives tongue, the spinning top which hums—they are all strange, uncanny, potentially dangerous.

The really threatening things are those which resemble the familiar animate most closely. That is also what Hebb found. And he further remarks that, in his opinion, "many fears depend on some degree of intellectual development . . . and that the range of such fears is characteristic of 'higher' animals, like man and chimpanzee'' (McBride and Hebb, 1948).

The child begins to distinguish the animate from the inanimate toward the end of the first year of life; this is in good agreement with Hebb's postulate that these fears depend on some degree of intellectual development. For this is the developmental level of the second organizer of the psyche, at which so many other signs of spectacular psychological progress become visible. Furthermore, this is also the age at which erect locomotion begins and therefore the one at which the ability to distinguish between animate and inanimate gains in importance from the viewpoint of survival.

Both stranger anxiety and the anxiety in some children before one or the other inanimate object appear mostly around the same age. However, I was not able to demonstrate a relation between the two. Elsewhere (Spitz, 1950a) I have advanced the proposition that stranger anxiety is the counterpart of the child's close relation to his mother. Such an explanation, however, does not appear to be applicable to anxiety before the inanimate. Could it be that anxiety before the inanimate is related to the child's unrestricted discharge of raw aggression on inanimate objects?

I have observed that this anxiety occurs primarily under the following conditions: (1) when the inanimate looks like a human being, but is different in size; (2) when the inanimate is in motion; (3) when the inanimate produces sounds.

The last two conditions suggest that the inanimate has the obligation to *remain* inanimate and not to move, and not to produce sounds; because if it does, what is it? May one perform aggressions on it? Will it not retaliate? Has it a volition of its own? Will it take the initiative? This animistic kind of thinking is particularly evident in some of my films on doll anxiety. In one of them the child, 11 months and 26 days old, looks searchingly at a baby-sized doll, cocks her head as if to look at it from a different angle, then looks at the doll straight on and considers it. She is unable to come to a decision. After a few seconds she approaches the doll, pokes her head at it, touches it with her face and then retreats, watching the motionless doll all the time. After a few moments of contemplation the child begins to show unpleasure, becomes restless and cries. (Film WF No. 207).[3]

This behavior looks as if the child were testing some quality in the doll and finding it lacking: the doll does not behave as the child seems to expect. The child concludes that it does not like the doll, does not want to have anything to do with it and is afraid of it.

---

[3] [These films are available for viewing in the René Spitz Film Archives. See Part 7. Ed.]

In another film the experiment is continued with a small (12-inch) doll placed in the child's lap. The child acts terrified, goes into a screaming panic, tries to retreat and at the same time to kick away the small doll, as if it were a loathsome something about to crawl onto her (Film WF No. 202). One is reminded of Yerkes' and Hebb's monkeys which would panic and then go over to attack. We may speculate whether our subject's kicking is the hostile outcome of her panic.

How does the discharge of aggression on the inanimate differ from its discharge with a living partner? After all, it is not as if *no* aggression were being discharged in the child's relations with his mother, with the libidinal object. But in these relations the mother does not permit the unrestricted discharge of aggression; she insists on keeping it within acceptable bounds. Why then does the child prefer the restrictive animate mother to the unrestrictive inanimate thing?

It seems to me that the mother compensates the child for her restrictions in two distinct ways: first, and most obviously, through her gratification of his libidinal drive, in immediate temporal proximity to her restrictive action. Second, the restriction itself permits the child to elaborate a variety of devices which enable him to lower the level of his aggression. Unmanageable quantities of raw aggression provoke anxiety because they threaten to disrupt the integrity of the child's ego. Therefore, reducing the level of aggression potential, domesticating it by channelizing parts of it into ego-syntonic performance, lowers at the same time the threat of anxiety.

In terms of the pleasure-unpleasure principle, achieving the *aim* of the raw drive should represent complete gratification. This is a purely theoretical postulate. In the months following birth, the dictate of the pleasure-unpleasure principle is increasingly restricted through the operation of the reality principle and through the emergence of the ego. After all, a number of drive gratifications are in themselves neither reality adapted nor ego syntonic. Moreover, as long as the ego is not firmly established, it is exceedingly vulnerable to influences which could lead to the breakthrough of the stimulus barrier and to the disruption of the ego's still weak cohesion. This weakness of the ego exposes the child to unmanageable anxiety. Such is the case in the first year of life and for a long time afterwards.

This may be the reason why at the end of the first year of life the child prefers the restrictive animate which helps him to maintain the integrity of his ego, of his autonomy, of his mastery over the drives. On the other hand, we may well imagine that at a certain point of development, at a certain specific age level, the inanimate, fraught with memories of destructive and ultimately frustrating drive discharge, may create anxiety, particularly if it is unfamiliar and therefore represents unexplored perils.

But the inanimate may provoke anxiety even more when it has the attributes of the living—physical resemblance, movement, sound—when, in other words, unrestricted hostility is provoked by the inanimate, but the resemblance to the animate reminds the child that this discharge is prohibited.

These are speculations; they cannot be validated. Yet, how should we interpret our film No. 206, in which a large baby-size doll is offered to one of a pair of identical twins, nearly twelve months $(0;11+26)$ old. The child goes through an extensive pantomime, apparently comparing the doll with her twin. She looks searchingly at the doll, makes a movement toward it and when the doll does not respond, her glance shifts back and forth between doll and sister. She ends up by first touching the doll, then her twin's shoulder with her lips, then the doll's face in a kissing motion; at this point, she turns away and makes a few tentative *biting* movements on the railing of her bed. I leave you to draw your own conclusions.

What are the consequences when the capacity to discriminate between animate and inanimate is not achieved? Or when this capacity is achieved inadequately and the boundaries between the living and the inanimate remain uncertain, unreliable, and shifting? You are all aware that this uncertainty of boundaries provides the devices used in ghost and horror stories, in myth and legend, since time immemorial, including the myth of Oedipus. It cannot be accidental that we have gone to such length to prove in our so-called "age of reason" that the supernatural, that the ghost stories, are untrue, a pack of lies, that they cannot and must not be. Are we by any chance whistling in the dark?

In the adult we are quite familiar with conditions in which the boundaries between animate and inanimate become uncertain. Then these boundaries become subject to the whims and the momentary shifts of the individual's emotional economy; then major psychiatric disturbances are bound to result.

In the child the failure to achieve the discrimination between animate and inanimate is one of the factors which perforce leads to the misinterpretation of reality, with resulting developmental maladaptation. Adaptive measures are taken by the child against nonexistent perils. The usual defenses of the ego, which are normally established in response to an expectable environment, are either not developed at all or aimed at the wrong targets, be these outside or inside. Extravagant demands for protection against imaginary adversaries and perils (in reality these represent the demands made by the drives on the child's ego), are made on the surround. The normally available supplies of constructive energy, both libidinal and aggressive, are drained by the misdirection of defensive measures. The growing child is left impoverished of emotion and incapable of dealing with the requirements of normal life and social relations. An outstanding example of such a process is the obsessive-compulsive's affective impoverishment.

It is not necessary to enumerate here the consequences of such processes, the anxiety readiness, the insomnia, the night terrors, the dereistic thinking, the magical ritual, denial, withdrawal. When these emergency measures fail the child, he will regress to the irrational, aggressive, destructive violence of early infancy.

From these consequences of the failure to acquire the capacity to discriminate between animate and inanimate, we may conclude that this discriminative capacity is one among the more important ego functions and has a major adaptive role.

These considerations have led us beyond the immediate framework of today's communication. We had asked ourselves by what means the capacity to distinguish animate from inanimate is acquired in infancy.

Not through anxiety. I hope I have made it clear that anxiety before the inanimate is not our essential problem; it is but the indicator of the miscarriage of a normal developmental process and therefore possibly the exception rather than the rule. Our essential problem is the developmental process through which the understanding of the difference between animate and inanimate is achieved and the method by which this is achieved. This developmental process is only a special instance of gradually progressing reality testing, applied to a particular aspect of reality, namely, to the animate and the inanimate.

The means by which this understanding comes about are contained in the dialogue. But that, of course, is not the only function of the dialogue. Ultimately, as I have indicated to you in the course of my presentation, my use of the concept of dialogue is an attempt at a more sophisticated approach to our usual concept of object relations. Terms like *object relations* tend to lose their impact with time. They have to be spelled out and illuminated from different angles, to make them come alive. What I have presented to you today is one such attempt.

For when you speak of "object relations" you are moving in the shadowy realm of abstract terminology. To visualize what one means by such abstract terms, one has to remember definitions. And visualizing them one realizes that the term *object relations* covers more ground than we are conveniently able to encompass at any one time in our imagination. It has to be broken up into smaller sectors with which we may be able to deal more easily. That is what a distinguished colleague meant when she remarked in a discussion some 30 years ago that much of our job consists in filling in the spaces between the lines Freud wrote.

In dealing with these smaller sectors I would like to try to use terms which require no definition, because they belong to our everyday speech. *Dialogue* is such a term. When we say "object relations" nothing compels us to visualize a process going on between a child and a live partner. But when I say "dialogue," then you will inevitably think of some meaningful conversation between two real persons, in which you have participated or to which you have listened. In other words, you think of something with which you are familiar from your everyday life.

Conversations with the inanimate do not belong in the realm of reality, for the partner in them is imaginary. And furthermore, a conversation with a living partner, a dialogue or, to be exact, the precursors of the dialogue with a living partner must of necessity precede any conversation with an imaginary partner: *nihil est in intellectu quod non prius fuit in sensibus*. The dialogue between the child and a living partner has to precede not only all meaningful relations with the animate, but also all imaginary exchanges with the inanimate.

That part of early object relations which I have spoken of as dialogue and which could be thought of as precursors of conversation already contains elements of all later dialogues: statement and counterstatement, discussion, argument, agreement, synthesis. The synthesis, the compromises reached in the course of the precursors of the dialogue are of major significance for ego formation; they represent splitting of the drives into manageable fractions, leading among others to neutralization. Therefore, the dialogue constitutes the contribution of the surround to the inception, the development, and the subsequent establishment of ego, self, character, and personality. Can one claim more?

With this I am placing myself on record that I consider the dialogue the source and origin of species-specific adaptation.

In man that includes the domestication of the drives and the development of the defenses of the ego. Without dialogue—and it is the dialogue through which the animate is distinguished from the inanimate—maturation may proceed, but development will be arrested.

In the monkey this leads, as Harlow has shown, to an impoverishment of the individual's personality and ultimately, through the deterioration of sexual activity, to the extinction of the species.

Man, when he is deprived of the dialogue from infancy, turns into an empty asocial husk, spiritually dead, a candidate for custodial care. But life in the human sense cannot be asocial—it has to be social. Life, as we conceive of it, is achieved through the dialogue.

Permit me to conclude with a few personal words. When, a year ago, I learned that you were preparing this celebration for me, I had thought of giving a very different paper. I wanted to tell you of my beginnings in psychoanalysis and how my psychoanalytic work developed in the intervening

53 years. But that would not have been a story of myself only. Interwoven and ever present in these years is the one whose loss makes me unable to tell you my story. Therefore I chose a new, an unrelated, a scientific topic.[4]

But toward the end of my talk, I gradually became aware that it was not by accident that I had chosen my new subject. In these last minutes I began to realize that this choice was meaningful. As a psychoanalyst I can well understand the decision my unconscious made. It is not surprising to discover that the topic which replaced the story of our life should be the difference between the animate and the inanimate.

Thank you.

[4] [Spitz is referring to the loss of his wife Ella, who died in June 1961. Ed.]

The Derailment of Dialogue: Stimulus Overload, Action Cycles, and the Completion Gradient

Since I first published the papers "Hospitalism" and "Anaclitic Depression" (Spitz, 1945b, 1946a), a great deal of experimental work has been done on affect deprivation in infancy both in animal and in man. It became possible then to divide the syndrome of affect deprivation into total and partial deprivation and to study the consequences of each (Spitz, 1951b).

This work has led not only to the better understanding of the consequences of affect deprivation but also to measures which have decisively reduced the frequency with which it occurred in the past and the severity of its consequences. Now that the more spectacular forms of maternal deprivation have lost their urgency, other problems, more obscure, more difficult to investigate and also to deal with, and perhaps even more urgent for humanity in general, claim our attention. One of these, for example, is damage suffered by infants who, while remaining under the uninterrupted care of their mothers, receive what appears to be the "wrong" kind of mothering. Such treatment leads to what I have called "psychotoxic diseases" (Spitz, 1951b).

Recently I was struck by the obvious: in the etiology of all psychotoxic disturbances the *wrong* kind of emotional supplies is conspicuous. Some of the psychotoxic disturbances (three months colic, infantile rocking, etc.) show in addition a specific etiological factor, in essence the diametrical opposite of emotional deprivation, namely, a surfeit, an overdose of affective stimulation.

After years of trying to formulate this problem of "too much," I now suggest to call this factor *emotional overload*. An example of this, for instance, is encountered in undisciplined parental behavior, one that is unlike genuine object relations, because it is the outcome of the parent's own unresolved emotional problems, such as repressed hostility, guilt feelings, narcissistic needs, etc.

Some aspects of the problem of "too much" in providing the infant with emotional supplies underlie the literature on what is known as "maternal

Reprinted from *Journal of the American Psychoanalytic Association*, 12:752–775, 1964.

overprotection.'' However, over the years that concept has taken on the character of an ''omnibus'' term, so that it now refers to a wide variety of mother-child relations. Today I am concerned specifically with the overloading of the infant's still inadequate perceptive system with stimuli, and of the infantile psychic system, such as it is, with quantities and qualities of emotion with which it cannot deal, for as yet he has no way to process them.

The findings on emotional deprivation in man have inspired a large number of experimental studies on animals. By contrast, the consequences of stimulus overload have been studied only in animals with the help of experiments. For obvious reasons it is not possible to duplicate such studies in man. Furthermore, as pointed out in a previous publication (Spitz, 1955b), phenomena observed in animals are not applicable to man without qualification. Of this also later.

Stimulus overload plays a conspicuous role in an extensive experimental study recently reported by John Calhoun (1962) in which the consequences of greatly increased population density among rats were explored. He raised from weaning six populations of 32 to 56 rats, evenly divided between males and females, with an abundance of food and drink, with predation and disease eliminated, in adequate living quarters. They were then permitted to multiply to approximately twice the number which would occupy the same space under natural circumstances in the wild.

This overpopulation generated social stress. A further biasing factor was introduced by the topological design of the living quarters, in that the four intercommunicating pens housing the population of the rats were provided with access paths so arranged that traffic was concentrated in some passages and diverted from others.

Topologically the pens were arranged in a row of four, the two central pens having access from both sides; the pens at the end of the row, access from one side only. The setup mildly discouraged the use of the pens 1 and 4, encouraging the use of 2 and 3, thus further increasing social stress. As a result of this arrangement the rats in pens 2 and 3 had many more social contacts than the rats in pens 1 and 4. In Calhoun's terminology, the ''velocity'' of the social contacts in the two middle pens was greatly increased.

Calhoun describes a series of consequences of this setup; significant for our study are the following phenomena:

1. The behavioral patterns of the males fell into three categories:

a. One group showed withdrawal behavior, feeding at times when no other males were around; they did not consort with females; they sat in a corner in a sort of daze.

b. A second group of males would form packs and pursue females. They often showed grossly deviant sexual and aggressive behavior; Calhoun calls them the *probers*.

c. A few relatively normal males established what Calhoun calls a *harem,* mostly in pens 1 and 4. Here a dominant male gathered around him a number of females who raised litters.

2. The females:

a. Harem females raised their litters almost normally.

b. Females who did not belong to the harem of a dominant male were not able to raise their litters appropriately. They would not build the nest pregnant rats usually build; many of them could not carry their pregnancy to term; those who did often failed to nurse their young; in the event of danger they would start to transport the young from one place to the other but would drop them on the road to safety and forget them.

In many of the males, particularly in the probers, cannibalism occurred. Furthermore, various homosexual behavior patterns developed in some of the rats; fighting and biting behavior, etc., in others.

A further striking consequence of the increased population density was that in Calhoun's first series 96 percent of the progeny of the rats perished.

A second experiment was set up: Calhoun selected the four healthiest males and the four healthiest females, in the prime of rat life, at the age of six months, from each of two overpopulated rat colonies. He permitted these four pairs to survive, to mate, and to raise their litters in spacious living quarters.

In spite of the fact that these eight rats no longer lived in overpopulated environments, they produced fewer litters in the course of the next six months than would have been expected normally. None of their offspring survived to maturity, an indication that for the parents to have lived for six months in the overpopulated environment had inflicted irreversible damage on the female's maternal behavior, leading to the extinction of this strain.

THEORETICAL DISCUSSION

I

What factor in Calhoun's experiments is responsible for the damage suffered by the rats? I believe that this factor consists in an overload of stimulation, and I shall examine what "overload" represents in the case of Calhoun's rats.

In the colonies where the density of population is twice the normal (and perhaps also optimal) rate, the rats were exposed to *at least double* the number of perceptual and affective stimuli deriving from encounters between individuals than they would be under normal circumstances in the wild. Indeed, it is far more likely that with the increasing number of individuals the number of encounters increases exponentially, creating a severe overload of action-triggering stimuli. Calhoun calls this greater frequency "an increase in velocity." Overloading the reactive system of Calhoun's rats appears to lead to two major classes of deviant behavior: (1) frenetic activity, (2) pathological withdrawal. There is a whole gamut of transitional forms between these two extremes.

Among these transitional forms, I have mentioned the conspicuous behavioral disturbances in the males, withdrawal, frenetic activity in the probers, homosexuality, cannibalism, aggressors who bite every subject in sight, etc. In the females the disturbances of pregnancy and nursing patterns lead to the rapid arrest of the survival of the species.

How can the single factor of stimulus overload lead to such a variety of consequences, and to as dissimilar ones? Surprisingly enough, the answer to this question can be provided by results of studies concerned with nonverbal communication between humans.

In a series of recent papers I have explored the communication patterns, the nonverbal action exchanges between the human baby and his mother. I called these exchanges a "dialogue" (Spitz, 1963a). As Emerson wrote: "Words are also actions and actions are a kind of words." It seems to me legitimate also to call the rats' obviously nonverbal action exchanges, the mutual stimulation and response that take place between rats in the course of their social or sexual activities a "dialogue." It is convenient to conceive of this dialogue as composed of smaller units, or elements, and I suggest calling them *action cycles*. Following Craig (1918), each action cycle consists of an anticipatory, an appetitive, and a consummatory portion.

By increasing the density of his population, Calhoun created a situation which interferes with the proper course of the dialogue.

It is my proposition that in this situation the stochastic[1] progression of the dialogue between the individual rats broke down; the dialogue was transformed into a pseudo dialogue, that is, into an exchange of meaningless actions and inappropriate reactions. This breakdown is, for instance, evident in the behavior of the probers toward the females on the one hand, and of the rat mothers toward their litters on the other.

From the perspective of *the progression of the dialogue* this is what happens: every social contact in Calhoun's rat colony triggers either an innate or a learned response in the dyadic contact between any two animals. Because of the greatly increased population density and corresponding enormous multi-

---

[1]Stochastic refers to a series of events bound to each other in causal dependence, but determined by probabilities only.

plication of actual contacts per unit of time, few of the responses are permitted to run their natural course—to progress to their completion. In other words, the responses are not consummated. This happens because hardly has a given animal begun to react to one contact stimulus, when another response is triggered, and a third, etc., all interfering with the completion of the first, the second, the third, etc., behavioral cycle. This is how total disorientation ensues as a result of overpopulation. This disorientation leads to an imbalance, a growing chaos of the psychological, sociological, and sexual action cycles and therefore of the whole adaptation of the animals.

It appears that iterative, continuously repeated interruption of successively triggered action cycles is damaging to the psychological functioning and eventually to the psychological organization of the rats.

Do we know anything about the consequences of interrupted action cycles in man? We remind the reader that an action cycle consists of anticipatory, appetitive, and consummatory phases. In the history of experimental psychology the interruption of action cycles between the appetitive and the consummatory phases has been extensively studied in artificial settings. For this discussion I will select three such experiments, well known and well explored by both experimental psychologists and psychoanalysts, although the experiments and observations were not designed to explore the interference with the natural action cycle.

The first is the well-known psychological study known as the Zeigarnik effect (1927). This study demonstrated that uncompleted tasks are better remembered than the completed ones. In this case pathology is not involved. What happens is that the failure to complete the task leaves a residue in the psychic memory system, which in turn gives rise to an urge to complete the task. No spectacular consequences are produced because the experiment involves only minimal amounts of affect.

The second example is much more spectacular. On the basis of clinical observation Freud postulated that habitual coitus interruptus is a determining factor in the etiology of *actual* neurosis. In this example, which in psychoanalytic theory has been spoken of as "the toxicological model," the assumption is that the regularly repeated interruption of coitus before its consummation causes tension to rise, dams up libido, and that this leads to severe psychological disturbances. Dammed-up libido thus was assumed to leave a residue with the effect of a toxin, and it was left open whether a biochemical basis would be found for this phenomenon. Freud (1895a) specifically states: "A sexual noxa like coitus interruptus comes into force through summation" (p. 106).

My third example is one which has lain more or less dormant in our psychoanalytic literature for nearly 60 years. I am referring to Freud's discovery of the role of the day residues in dream formation and his proposition regarding the function of the dream.

We can deal summarily with the role of day residues: they represent what I like to call the opening wedge to *unfinished business*. By unfinished business I mean the uncompleted tasks of the day, as well as the vast store of unsolved problems and unreconciled conflicts which each of us carries in his unconscious. Freud (1900) deals exhaustively and convincingly with this topic in the *Interpretation of Dreams;* his formulations come quite close to what Zeigarnik was to demonstrate experimentally in another area more than 30 years later.

The second part of Freud's thesis, the one referring to the function of the dream, is of far greater, indeed of decisive importance to our present topic. He quotes W. Robert, who stated in 1886 that the "Instigators of dreams [are] . . . things which are in our minds in an uncompleted shape"; and Freud continues the quotation, "Dreams serve as a safety valve for the overburdened brain. They possess the power to heal and relieve." And elsewhere: "A man deprived of the capacity of dreaming would in course of time become mentally deranged, because a great mass of uncompleted, unworked-out thoughts and superficial impressions would accumulate in his brain . . ." [Freud, 1900, p. 79].

Twenty years and many thousands of thoroughly analyzed dreams later (among them my own), Freud returned to this explanation of the function of dreams and added: "Is this the only function that can be assigned to dreams? I know of no other."

I believe that these quotations do not require any further commentary. All of us have realized that Freud speaks here of the dream as a psychological drive, to take a word quoted just now, as a *safety valve* to protect the psychic organization from the damaging consequences of unfinished action cycles, interrupted before their consummation. This is the exact parallel to the etiology of the damage which I postulated for the consequences of Calhoun's experiment on stimulus-overloaded rats.

It is hardly necessary to recall at this late date that Freud's statement on the function of dreams has been tested and retested literally in many hundreds of thousands of dreams analyzed by our colleagues. However, over and beyond this, an experimental confirmation has been added thanks to the imaginative work of Charles Fisher and William Dement (1962; Dement, 1960) on dream deprivation. I will use only a single category of the many important findings of Fisher and Dement's experiments; their study, done on a group of subjects, demonstrated the following:

1. To some individuals, dream deprivation lasting for five nights (the limit of the Fisher-Dement experiments) is intolerable. They interrupt the experiment after one to four days.

2. Individuals deprived of dreaming for five successive nights appear to make up the deprivation by dreaming massively during the following five successive nights, up to twice as much, after they are permitted to dream without interruption.

3. In a certain number of individuals, dream deprivation for a period of five to seven nights led to a variety of changes indicating the possibility of a beginning personality disruption. These changes disappeared when dream deprivation was stopped.

With these three examples, the Zeigarnik effect, Freud's toxicological theory, and the dream function–dream deprivation experiments, I feel entitled to offer a tentative reformulation of Freud's toxicological model.

Behavior patterns consist of an anticipatory, appetitive, and consummatory phase we call action cycles. Interrupting action cycles prior to consummation produces unpleasure in various forms, only one of which is anxiety. We frequently also speak of this unpleasure as frustration. Consistent interruption of action cycles leaves a residue which is cumulative.

After a critical quantity of such residues has been cumulated, one single discharge through the ordinary consummatory process will not suffice to reestablish normal equilibrium. The cumulation of interruptions seems to need compensation, as shown in the Fisher-Dement dream-deprivation experiments. There comes a point at which the compensation of the accumulated undischarged appetitive readiness cannot be carried through without seriously interfering with the normal functioning of the organism. A conflict arises now between the need to compensate and the requirements of normal everyday functioning. At this point a vicious circle begins, for the need to compensate conflicts with the consummation of normal function creates an increasing quantity of unconsummated action cycles. These now will cumulate in their turn and lead to the disorganization and disruption of the compensatory attempts. The culmination of this process is what I call *derailment of dialogue*.

It appears that a damaging influence, be it toxic, be it purely psychological, is exerted through the consistently repeated interruption of action cycles prior to their consummation. Its effects become evident in different ways in different sectors of the personality. The damage impairs the adaptive capacity of the individual, his capacity for mastering his environment, his understanding of his environment. This leads step by step to an increasing measure of breakdown in communication and dialogue.

To this breakdown man, and, as we have seen from Calhoun's experiments, also rats (and possibly other gregarious animals) reacts with a spectrum of disturbances ranging from increased effort or attention to frustration and ultimately anxiety. This anxiety arises from the general consequences of repetitive frustration of the consummatory act; it follows that Freud's toxicological theory of anxiety is incomplete, in so far as it describes only *one* particular aspect of the general consequences of repetitive frustration of the consummatory act.

Actually, these consequences are of far more encompassing significance. The Zeigarnik effect, the dream function, the dream-deprivation experiment, and, on a lower level of integration, Calhoun's rat experiments show that.

It appears to me that we are dealing here with a psychological principle of vast and perhaps universal scope in living organisms. In the living organism, at least on the mammalian level, there seems to exist a tendency, a need, perhaps even a compulsion, to carry action cycles to their consummation. We can speak of this tendency as a gradient; provisionally I will call it *completion gradient*. This gradient ranges from a mild tendency in the Zeigarnik subject to the powerful compulsion demonstrated by the severe social pathology of Calhoun's rats where consummation was consistently inhibited.[2]

II

Analogies between animal and human behavior and the reasons for it are always problematic. I have stressed this many times, even in the present article. Yet the consequences of overcrowding in rat colonies demonstrated by Calhoun have so many parallels in our urban overpopulation that we cannot simply ignore them. We must at least take a look at them and point out the *difference* between seemingly similar phenomena in man and animal, the "disanalogy" as Robert Oppenheimer (1956) called it with a felicitous term.

Thirty-five years ago Freud (1930) discussed at length the problems human civilization is facing, the antinomies inherent in the task of domesticating the

---

[2] The thoughtful reader will notice a relation between the compulsion implicit in the completion gradient and that postulated by Freud (1920) for the "compulsion to repeat" (mostly called "repetition compulsion"). He made the compulsion to repeat responsible for the demonic character of certain aspects of the mind (Freud, 1919). This "demonic character" might be the aspect under which he would have classified the spectacle of the frenzied, growing chaos of the psychological, sociological, and sexual action cycles of Calhoun's rats, leading to a total breakdown of these animals' adaptation.

Propositions which Freud abandoned (or which his followers did not pursue) may have been unsatisfactory to him in the larger context of his systematic view of the psyche. However, I have found that such supposedly obsolete ideas of Freud always contained rewarding insights, which only his masterly clinical observation and his unique genius were able to provide. In the framework of the compulsion to repeat, I am inclined to believe that the completion gradient may play the role of the quantitative expression, as it were, of the energy involved. To be sure, that is by no means the only role in which the completion gradient is manifested.

libidinal and the aggressive drives. The intervening years have not brought a solution to this dilemma, only added to it other and increasingly dangerous elements, urban overpopulation among them.

Looking back over my own lifetime, it seems to me that there has been a rapid increase in juvenile delinquency, ever more sadistic; teenage crime; widespread and at the same time socially ostracized homosexuality; severe neurosis and psychosis; strange forms of social groupings with, to say the least, peculiar mores; ever more inappropriate child-rearing practices. All this has happened despite extraordinary advances in our psychiatric therapy, in our preventive and curative measures in the area of social and psychiatric problems, in the field of infant care; all this in the face of a snowballing number of billions poured into these preventive and curative measures.

Can it be that we are facing a chronic derailment of dialogue in man? Yet man was able to cope, and indeed has coped, with problems of communication where rat and monkey broke down. The organ which permits him to perform this feat is the ego. Man as a species has manipulated communication and its breakdowns through new and inventive adaptive methods.

But that he can achieve only *after* he has developed an ego, and with it the ability to learn in new situations and to elaborate devices to cope with these. Freud has called the organ which enables man to achieve this the ego; it is developed, organized, and modified in the course of exchanges in the framework of mother-child relations.

In animals, on the whole, inherited behavior patterns play a much larger role than an acquired ego. The importance of the latter is proportionate to the amount of postnatal care required by the neonate, that is, the measure and duration of the newborn's initial helplessness. Accordingly we may expect the process of acquiring a central steering organization (or what would roughly correspond to the ego in man) to be of far greater importance in nidicolous (altricial) animals than in nidifugous (precocial) ones. It is of interest that both the rats investigated by Calhoun and the rhesus monkeys investigated by Harlow (1959; see also Spitz, 1962) are altricials. But the duration of their initial helplessness is incomparably shorter than man's. Accordingly, the consequences of maternal deprivation as well as those of the wrong kind of mother-child relations are much less serious than would be the case in the human infant. This is evident both in Harlow's and Calhoun's experiments, so that we may assume that for the human species consequences of a break-down of communication in infancy, before the establishment of the ego, may represent greater perils than those demonstrated in Calhoun's rat experiment.

This proposition entails a more specific discussion of two aspects of our problem. One is the question: When is the ego mature (that is, robust and resourceful) enough to deal with inadequate and inappropriate object relations and with the derailment of dialogue? The other is the question of the dynamics which make the atrophy of meaning in the dialogue so damaging psychologically. I will take up this question briefly later.

Regarding the first of these questions, the maturity of the ego, I have postulated (1958b) that after passing through several successive phases, the earliest ego consolidation begins around 8 months of life and concludes its first stage around 18 months of life. I find myself in good agreement on this point with Piaget's (1936b) findings.

Implicit in this view of ego development is the proposition that the ego's capacity to deal with harmful environmental conditions increases with age. Up to puberty that is pretty obvious; it is no less true of adolescence and early adulthood.

Of course, this capacity to deal with the harmful environmental experience has its limits at any time. As we know from our more recent deplorable historical experiences, anybody can be broken down if one tries hard enough. And we also know that the tensile strength of different individuals differs greatly.

A good example of the purposeful use of derailment of dialogue is the technique of brainwashing prisoners of war—one of the many dubious achievements of man's so-called moral progress.

The nosology of the consequences of derailment of the dialogue caused by inappropriate meaningless exchanges—and that includes overloading with exchanges—remains to be worked out.

There are a great many indications that also in the case of overloading of dialogue the level of ego organization and the measure of ego strength determine whether the personality will be damaged or not, and if damaged, how severely. To my knowledge, these questions have never been investigated specifically either experimentally or observationally.

Yet, man's inhumanity to man enables us, if we so will, to study certain extreme conditions. I am speaking of such modern phenomena as for instance the Hong Kong refugees.

However, in the present study, I am less concerned with adults and more with the breakdown of dialogue in infancy, at that developmental stage when man is still comparable to the animal, when the ego is not yet established or is still *in statu nascendi*.

It is of course obvious that we cannot make either early inappropriate object relations or the breakdown of dialogue in infancy responsible for all the present-day ills of our culture and our society. But when it happens that such conditions produce a serious distortion in the normal development of the infant's personality, this is apt to trigger progressive maladaptation.

Several years ago (Spitz, 1959), I advanced the proposition that the embryological principle of dependent development, the unfolding of the epigenetic landscape, applies as rigorously to the growth of man's psyche as it does to the development of the fertilized ovum. This breakdown of dialogue in infancy involves the nascent ego and its first layer, forming a deviant base for establishing the next phase. If uncorrected, the deviation will become evident in increasing measure from phase to phase, eventuating in a skewed personality.

I believe, therefore, that we should take the various factors which can lead to the breakdown of dialogue in infancy very seriously indeed, and in the following pages I shall take up some of the reasons why this should be so, particularly from the viewpoint of dynamics.

If we consider more specifically the dialogue between mother and child, the difference between meaningless exchange and meaningful dialogue becomes ever more important and certainly more sophisticated. In the nursing couple, the newborn cannot and does not empathize with the mother's inner processes. He responds to them; his behavior is influenced by them on the neurophysiological level.[3]

The mother is something else again. In the nursing couple, her role is to empathize all along the line with what she believes to understand from the behavior of her baby. This empathy, which is in part conscious, and probably to a much larger extent unconscious, is characteristic of what we call a good mother-child relation.

But what of the mothers who are not capable of empathy? The emotionally disturbed, the narcissistic, the insecure mothers? The mothers concerned with their own emotional needs? And what of the mothers who, to draw a frank analogy with Calhoun's population-density experiment, are bedeviled by the stimulus overload due to urban overpopulation? Each of these mothers, each for her own individual reason, can only interpret the behavior of her baby in terms of her need, her lack, her confusion, her guilt.

The exchanges between such mothers and their babies will be meaningless dialogue. For they initiate actions which do not apply to the child's need; they interrupt his response before completion. How can a consistent code of communication be established, how can reality adaptation be achieved under these circumstances?

---

[3] Even on that level the neonate is protected from stimuli assailing him from outside by the stimulus barrier. This protection decreases progressively in the months following birth, as a function of the development (in the framework of mother-child relations) of the ego which will take over the task of scanning, selecting, and processing incoming stimuli.

The child tries to respond to contradictory signals, fails, becomes agitated and restless. The mother throws up her hands in despair: she cannot understand why just *her* child should be so difficult.

In this state of confusion the child will develop along one or the other narcissistic line, which may or may not mirror the mother's problems. The child's gratifications and rewards are no longer those achieved in normal object relations, but much more archaic and therefore neither reality-adapted nor prospective; for instead of *progressive* adaptation to environmental conditions, adaptation remains fixated at or close to the level of the stimulus barrier.

Of course, this kind of breakdown of the dialogue can occur only as long as the individual is completely dependent on maternal care. That is the case during infancy, before the consolidation of the ego. We do not encounter this kind of breakdown in adults. Adults have at their disposal well-organized, carefully elaborated devices of adaptation, to deal with such situations. In those cases when they cannot deal with them the adult disposes of a host of defenses with the help of which he can protect himself against unmanageable stimuli. Therefore, we will look for the consequences of the meaningless dialogue, of action cycles interrupted before consummation, in infants. One example of many will illustrate this process in a nine-month-old:

Jerry, hospitalized at 8½ months, weighing 9 lbs., 3 ozs., was diagnosed as "failure to thrive." All lab tests were negative. Medication and a variety of diets failed to improve his weight. After two weeks of unsuccessful drug treatment the psychiatric department was called in. A syndrome of regurgitation and rumination, combined with two-finger sucking, reaching into the pharynx, was observed. Thereupon medication was completely stopped: the child was placed in the care of a single kindly nurse; his arms were temporarily splinted to stop the finger sucking.

After two weeks, Jerry had gained 1 lb. 5 ozs.; after three weeks, a further 12 ozs. He left the hospital a few days later with a total gain of 3 lbs.

Psychiatric exploration of Jerry's mother uncovered her severe oedipal conflict, her constant fights and her unconscious compliance with her tyrannical, sadistic, opinionated father. The peculiarities of the mother-child relations are suggestively illustrated by one observation of the attending psychiatrist: he noticed how deeply the mother was pushing the nipple of the bottle into Jerry's gullet; she did the same, even more impressively, with a hard biscuit which she fed him later. The psychiatrist questioned whether she was not feeding the child too rapidly, and too far down his throat. She answered: "I was always taught that eating is something to be got over as quickly as possible."

I showed a film of the child's finger sucking and feeding himself a hard biscuit. His fingers, which reach deeply into the pharynx, move visibly, titillating his epiglottis and provoking regurgitation. The comments of the medical audience to this part of the film are revealing; several persons in the audience remarked: "It makes me want to gag!" Gagging and vomiting are the result of the child's manipulation of his fingers or of the biscuit he pushes in: he regurgitates and then ruminates the vomit.

We may surmise that the mother's peculiar mode of feeding established a kind of conditioning. Gagging and vomiting were consistently rewarded by further maternal reciprocity and by further food. This is a purely anaclitic behavior pattern. The gratification of the drive leans onto the need for food. It lies in the nature of human development that the emotional need, the gratification of the drive, should become progressively more important than the actual need for survival. The development of Jerry's behavior illustrates this strikingly.

To Jerry, gagging, retching, and vomiting became part of the mother-child relation. They became messages directed to his mother. They were the response he had learned to her ministrations, and they became the means by which he could successfully appeal to her for what passes for fondling in this singular mother-child relation. For the mother would respond to Jerry's vomiting message by *her* interpretation of what he wanted: she would feed him again, and again, and again.

The mother's conflicts make her behavior understandable. The psychiatric exploration revealed that she felt deeply guilty because her father disapproved both of her marriage and of her having a child. This guilt found expression in the treatment of her baby. For instance, when she moved the baby in her lap, she did not give support, but let his head drop like a stone over her thigh.

On the other hand, she felt equally guilty that she could not get her child to thrive; in her misdirected zeal to overcompensate this guilt she pushed the food into him as quickly and as deeply as possible. The latter resulted in conditioning the gagging reflex to the gratification of *both* food *and* maternal "affection." Very quickly food became secondary for Jerry. Maternal attention was achieved by regurgitating and ruminating. Furthermore, maternal attention could be replaced at any time by the child's two fingers pushed deeply into his pharynx.

This is the point where the derailment of dialogue between mother and child becomes unmistakably evident. Oversimplifying, I would say that pushing the food into the gullet combines the anticipatory and the appetitive phase of the action cycle. The consummatory act, which corresponds to this appetitive phase, is the propulsion of the food into the stomach. As shown by

Tilney and Kubie (1931), in the feeding cycle the progressive filling of the stomach reduces the infant's appetitive activity.

In Jerry's case the interruption of the cycle takes place before the food has reached the stomach. X-ray motion pictures showed clearly the uncoordinated activity of the esophagus leading to regurgitation of the food before the goal, the stomach, is reached.

For Jerry, filling the stomach does not become the primary consummatory aim. It is replaced by the need for maternal attention, for the oral and pharyngeal stimulation, which for Jerry has become the equivalent of fondling. As a result of her own preoccupation with her emotional problems, the mother offers Jerry the wrong kind of action during the appetitive phase of this dialogue. The child's response to her peculiar performance, namely, pushing things in too fast and too deep, is physiologically understandable: he gags, vomits, and finally ruminates the vomit. Jerry's response is the correct answer to the mother's *action,* but a meaningless answer to what she *thought* she was doing.

The further steps in the cycle will be that the mother endlessly repeats her inappropriate action. She triggers the appetitive nursing response and in the same act interrupts it by eliciting the gagging reflex. Jerry responds appropriately to the stimulus, but frustratingly to the mother's wish: he chews and ruminates the food, but only after vomiting it. This cycle goes on repeating itself. Communication does not take place. The cycle is interrupted and begun anew again and again and would have led eventually to the death of the child. On the archaic level at which this process took place, it seems to me that we observe the repetition compulsion in action, primitive and undisguised.

This is not the occasion for a detailed discussion of the dynamics of this case. I believe that it has put clearly into focus my thesis about the derailment of the dialogue: the anticipatory response leads to the appetitive part of the cycle. In Jerry's case the latter is interrupted by a new, contradictory stimulus, and consummation does not take place.

Comparing this observation with what happened to the overpopulated rats, we realize that what Calhoun describes as *increased velocity* is the iterative triggering of the anticipatory part of a large variety of action cycles. The action itself is interrupted before its normal conclusion, before the curve has reached the highest point, namely, consummation—therefore its culminating point is missing, and also its descending part.

We may then conclude that iterative, consistent interruption of action cycles creates psychological conditions resulting in social pathology of the kind described by Calhoun. In the animal, where the adaptive mechanism consists largely of inherited, unlearned behavior, this pathology leads to the extinction of the overpopulated group. If such conditions of increased population density are not compensated in the course of the evolution of the species, they will lead to its extinction.

In man, as mentioned above, there is another alternative: man, whose adaptation is learned through communication, through transmission of the fruits of experience from the preceding generation, is able to develop adaptive compensations within ontogenesis, *within* the life span of the individual. He is able to do that with the help of his unique adaptive organ, the ego, which performs these adaptations by developing the appropriate mechanisms of defense. That, as I pointed out, presupposes an ego developed to the point where it is able to perform this task.

If we draw a parallel between the experiment of increased population density in Calhoun's experiment and the conditions which exist in the tenements of our major urban centers, we realize that the consequences of the two are not readily comparable. In the history of humanity conditions of overcrowding have existed at various times and in various geographical locations. We may assume that each case produced its own consequences and its own cure; the latter might be explosively violent; or it might be institutionalized (perhaps the *ver sacrum* is one such institution, where local overpopulation was a factor). Other historical examples in our Western civilization might be found in the Rome of the Emperors, in Elizabethan London, and in Paris before the French Revolution.

Here we are more concerned with present-day overcrowding of the cities in our Western civilization. A study of these will have to distinguish between the adaptive consequences of increased population density for the adult and the destructive consequences of the derailment of dialogue, of the cumulation of incompleted action cycles for the infant. Particularly in the case of the latter such a study will have to make a sharp separation between *physical* overcrowding as such and Calhoun's *increased velocity,* that is, psychological overloading.

It should also be remembered that inappropriate mother-child relations can arise for a variety of reasons, only one of which is overpopulation; at present, it still surely is not a major one. However, up to now it has not been described and we were unaware of the dangerous potentialities of overpopulation. In view of present demographic trends we will do well to keep these possibilities in mind.

I cannot discuss these possibilities in the present paper, but I may note that juvenile gangs have become a growing problem in practically every country on both sides of the Iron Curtain. That these gangs do not originate exclusively in the tenements is an overload problem of its own. But however farfetched the analogy, the activities of the juvenile gangs are strangely reminiscent of Calhoun's "probers." And in reading Calhoun's description of the "withdrawn rats," one gets the uneasy feeling that we have heard of something not too dissimilar in our own culture (and in older ones, too). One is reminded of the cultists, of the beatniks, of the strange little communities found on the so-called lunatic fringe.

It will be the task of future research to determine whether and how gang formation is connected with damage inflicted *prior* to ego formation; also whether some of the other deviant phenomena might be connected with adjustments to urban overpopulation made at a more advanced stage of individual development.

These are highly speculative analogies; nevertheless they strongly suggest that we may be witnessing an increasing measure of the derailment of dialogue in our society. I believe that man will be able to cope with this problem; that with the help of his ego he will create devices to deal with these difficulties. Where he will not succeed—unless he realizes what he is up against—is the problem of the derailment of dialogue in infancy.

For when the dialogue breaks down in infancy, ego formation is inhibited, ego functions are distorted and atrophied; ego apparatuses are crippled and the integrity of the ego, of the principal organ of adaptation, is in jeopardy. Compensatory functions will be developed, which have little or nothing to do with the givens of reality—witness the adaptive derailment in the case of Jerry. Such an ego, if it survives, will show monstrous deformations, and probably will never be able to achieve the capacity to develop into a well-integrated partner in any kind of dialogue.

It does not take a prophetic eye to perceive these disastrous consequences. The case of Jerry makes evident *one* possible consequence: that with the derailment of dialogue the appetitive branch of the action cycle comes to replace the consummatory one.

I need not tell our readers that man has hunted for the delights of appetitive paradises ever since our ancestor Noah (Gen., 9:20, 21), and after him the daughters of Lot (Gen., 9:34, 35), discovered the beneficial effects of fermented grape. I am well aware of the uses of opium, of hashish, of certain mushrooms and other drugs found in nature over the centuries and millennia. Much of the use of these pharmaca was institutionalized in one way or another; often they were a significant factor in whole cultures, nations, or religions. But what we are witnessing in the last 100 years and even more spectacularly in the last 30 to 50 is something else again. In the last 50 years we have progressed at an accelerating rate from tobacco and alcohol (and perhaps we should include opium and hashish) to morphine, to cocaine, to heroin. We have borrowed marijuana from some of our neighbors and recently have gone them one better in our headlong progression, to varnish, to benzedrine, to lysergic acid, and to glue sniffing.

I want to repeat that urban overpopulation is not the only reason for these increasingly difficult problems. It is one of the reasons—I myself have spoken of other ones in the past. But it certainly is one of the most easily reproduced experimentally and therefore most easily studied. At the same time, the problem of overpopulation is one of the most difficult to control and the most threatening at the present stage of our history.

It is deeply disturbing that in the discussion of the problems of urban overcrowding, of increasing population density, the accent is on water supply, on smog, on sewage disposal, on water pollution, on living space, on transportation, highways, freeways, and what not—all, no doubt, vitally important questions.

Indeed, we may well ask whether these material impediments, obstacles, and perils, which threaten urbanization, might not be nature's *safeguards* against overpopulation which threatens man's very essence and his survival. In this role these obstacles to overpopulation are strangely similar to what we can observe in animal and plant ecology. Animals and plants *have* to comply with the *safeguards* of nature. But our technology permits us to overcome such obstacles, and thus imperils man and his survival at a much more vulnerable point, in his organ of adaptation, in his ego.

I have yet to hear anyone raising his voice about the dangers of overpopulation to man himself—I would be inclined to say, to man's very essence—about the danger to the ego, the one agency in man which possesses the resources to cope with these hazards—but when damaged cannot cope with them. I think that it is time that we, as psychiatrists and psychoanalysts, study this problem, point out this danger, and voice our *caveant consules!*[4]

SUMMARY

Systematic inquiries into the origin of certain emotional disturbances of infants show that consistent maternal care is vital for the child's normal physical, psychic, and social development, indeed, for his survival. The most elementary precondition for consistent maternal care is the physical presence of the mother or her substitute.

It has, however, become increasingly apparent that children's development can also be stunted, and that they suffer damage of varying extent by the attention of, and close contact with, a mother who dispenses what seems to be the "wrong kind of mothering."

---

[4] *Caveant consules ne quid detrimenti res publica capiat!* [May the rulers take heed lest some harm befall the commonweal!]

A model of the mother-baby interaction is proposed to explicate the dynamics of the "wrong kind of mothering" and its consequences: my proposition is that the mutual exchanges between mother and baby consist in a give and take of action and reaction between the two partners, which requires from each of them both active and passive responses. These responses form series and chains, the single links of which consist in what I call "action cycles," each completed in itself and at the same time anticipating the next link. I designated these seriated response exchanges as the "precursor of dialogue," as a primal dialogue.

The dialogue acts as a vector of the baby's development, influencing its direction and stimulating it to adaptive efforts and psychic growth. It follows that inappropriate mothering (quantitatively as well as qualitatively) results in what is referred to at this time as the "derailment" of the primal dialogue.

Controlled experiments with animals, findings of experimental psychology, and, lastly, clinical findings illustrate the mechanics of the derailed dialogue and its sequelae.

In the cases under review a surfeit of stimulation, a psychic overloading, resulted in the derailment of dialogue. Overloading prevents its subject from completing actions or responses initiated by him. Long-lasting overload results in the cumulation of "incompleted action cycles." The sequelae of this cumulation are profound changes in the behavior of the individual. These changes are manifested in a departure from the norms of individual and social behavior patterns that are maladaptive for the individual and asyntonic with his society, that is, asocial.

The derailment of the dialogue is triggered, perhaps even caused, by the nature of the social setting. One setting, overpopulation, is extensively discussed in connection with an animal experiment, and the implications for the human community are examined.

The Evolution of Dialogue

This study started as an attempt to investigate how the child begins to distinguish living beings from things, the animate from the inanimate. Unexpectedly the work led us to an inquiry into the origins of language, for language is absent in inanimate "things," computers notwithstanding. Some of the findings resulting from this investigation were presented in "Life and the Dialogue" (Spitz, 1963a). Here I shall continue and elaborate on the thesis of that first paper and in so doing refer to it whenever necessary.

In the psychoanalytic literature Winnicott (1953) in his important paper "Transitional Objects and Transitional Phenomena" comes closest to the problem of the early stage of differentiation between the animate and the inanimate. I believe I interpret him correctly in stating that he considers the child's continued relationship to an inanimate "thing," cuddly toy or otherwise, as a device serving several functions. On the one hand, the child uses it to achieve autonomy from the libidinal object; on the other, the child masters conflicts and problems in his relations with the libidinal object with the help of fantasies enacted on a transitional, an inanimate, object.

Mahler (1958) approaches the problem from the opposite direction. She describes how ego regression in the schizophrenic child goes to a level of perceptual *de-differentiation* at which primal discrimination between living and inanimate is lost. Mahler thus posits that at a given point in infantile development such a discrimination is acquired.

It will be our task to explore the process by which discrimination between the living and the inanimate is achieved in infancy and how this process relates to the development of language. I shall begin with a brief review of our knowledge concerning the preliminary stages of visual differentiation between animate and inanimate in the human infant's first year of life.

Around the age of four weeks, the infant responds to the human face in motion by following it with his eyes. However, at the age of three months, there is still no difference between his smiling response to an inanimate artifact of the human face and his smile at a living human's face, as long as both are in motion. At the next stage, beginning around the sixth month of life, the

---

Reprinted from *Drives, Affects, Behavior*, Vol. 2, ed. Max Schur. New York: International Universities Press, 1965, pp. 170–190.

child no longer accepts the inanimate object in place of the living partner, however briefly. Endowing the inanimate with the privileged Gestalt and with movement is of no avail.

We offer the following proposition: a critical period of transformation is situated at this age level, during which an adaptation to the inanimate on the one hand, to the living on the other, takes place. This adaptation involves discriminatory processes. We came to this assumption because we observed in the human infant at this age (second half of the first year) a variety of unexpected and unpredictable responses both to the living and to the inanimate.

The most conspicuous evidence of the child's adaptation to the living at this stage is the phenomenon of the eight months anxiety (Spitz, 1950a), which is essentially the human infant's affective response, characteristic of that age, to the approach of a stranger. In subsequent publications (Spitz, 1954, 1957) I called this period a "critical period of development." The eight months anxiety represents a step forward in perceptive discrimination between stranger and friend.

Occasionally in some infants we observed similar reactions also to the *inanimate;* we could not readily find an explanation for these reactions. In the course of our work we observed the frequency of these reactions to the inanimate. We found them in about one-third of all the infants observed by us. These reactions do not appear with the same reliability as the eight months anxiety. They are more scattered, less predictable, but once attention has been drawn to them, we may perhaps find laws governing this response also.

We noticed this phenomenon for the first time when we offered a 12-inch doll to infants who had never before seen one. Some of them reacted to it with anxiety. This reaction varies of course from child to child, just as the eight months anxiety does. It ranges from awe and reluctance to touch the doll to dismay and screaming panic.

I was not successful in correlating the presence of doll anxiety with the history of the individual child or with the presence or absence of eight months anxiety. However, the phenomenon appeared to be reinforced in children who had undergone separation. We discovered further that, though the doll would provoke the most spectacular anxiety responses (at the same period, though not necessarily in the same children), such responses could also be elicited by other inanimate objects.

These observations led me to the conclusion that the children's unexpected reaction to inanimate objects in the second half of the first year should be considered as one of the behavioral changes which indicate the establishment of what I called the second organizer of the psyche.[1] As the result of this development, the infant becomes capable, among other achievements, of distinguishing his mother, the libidinal object, from strangers, the animate from inanimate things. This implies a momentous development in the infant's thinking processes. I believe that this is the inception of the concept of "alive," of life.

Like the capacity to distinguish the libidinal object from everybody else in the world, distinguishing animate from inanimate is an achievement of major importance and as such fraught with conflict, sometimes manifested by anxiety. I believe that in this conflict the aggressive drive plays a significant role (see below).

Child psychologists have not paid much attention to the infant's selective anxiety reactions in response to particular inanimate objects. In the last decade, however, psychoanalysts have become aware of such anxieties in certain clinical cases. Ethologists too have become alerted to these reactions to the inanimate. The reaction appears to be rather spectacular in primates, but has been observed also in other animal species. I had the opportunity to discuss this problem with Konrad Lorenz, with Eibl-Eibesfeldt, and with their associates, as well as with Donald Hebb and his staff. They all consider the phenomenon to be a reaction to strangeness of some specific kind.

Hebb (1946) discovered that the plaster model of a monkey's head produces similar reactions. Hebb offered monkeys a number of artifacts; the most anxiety-provoking were those which represented the head of an animal of the same species. Hebb remarks that some strange variation of something familiar, a familiar object in a new context, is particularly potent in provoking anxiety.

What has all this to do with the question of how the child learns to distinguish the animate from the inanimate? In the case of animals this distinction is of major importance for survival. Obviously they acquire this capacity in the course of phylogenesis. But the role of learning in acquiring it becomes increasingly important as we go higher on the evolutionary scale.

One major aspect of this role becomes evident from Harlow's large-scale investigation on what he called "The Nature of Love" (1958, 1962; Harlow and Zimmerman, 1959). In a paper on early sexual behavior patterns (Spitz, 1962) I also touched upon the present topic. I discussed extensively Harlow's experiment of raising rhesus monkeys on surrogate mothers, made of wire and terry cloth, inanimate, of course. More specifically I discussed the consequences of this procedure. In a nutshell, the consequences are that the

---

[1] Elsewhere (Spitz, 1954, 1959) I have suggested that major transformations leading to a higher level of developmental integration are marked by the establishment of organizers of the psyche; I described three such organizers.

surrogate-raised monkeys cannot develop play or social relations. They are subject to uncontrollable anxiety and to outbursts of violent agitation, hostility, and destructiveness. When grown up, they have no sexual relations and show no sexual behavior of any kind. Asking myself what factor, present or absent, in the inanimate terry-cloth surrogate mother exerts such a destructive influence on the baby monkey's development, I came to the conclusion that it is the lack of *reciprocity* between the surrogate mother and the rhesus baby.

Here I shall examine a specific sector of the reciprocity between mother and child which I have called *the dialogue*. It forms such a large part of the mother-child relations that it might practically be equated with object relations. Of course, this is not a verbal dialogue. It is a dialogue of action and response which goes on in the form of a circular process within the dyad, as a continuous, mutually stimulating feedback circuit. Actually, it is a *precursor* of the dialogue, an archaic form of conversation. In the human it leads eventually to the acquisition of verbal communication, of speech.

This thesis is less speculative or theoretical than it may sound; witness an experiment related to me by Konrad Lorenz. He constructed dummies or rather lures which would elicit the following response of ducklings *(Tadorna tadorna)*. He found that the following response could be elicited by various moving artifacts, but then quickly died out, whether the artifact was duck-shaped or not. Next he installed a speaker into the lure which would produce the call of the mother duck. This too was unsuccessful in establishing a consistent following response. Only when a human mind activated the speaker, only when the lure vocalized *in response* to the duckling's "lost" peeping, could the following response be established reliably, consistently, and durably.

When such a dialogue was offered, it did not matter whether the lure was duck-shaped or not—I tried the experiment at Lorenz's Institute using a square box made of bright red plastic. When I activated the built-in duck call in response to the duckling's "lost" peeping, they followed unfailingly.

Lorenz believes that the fidelity of the taped call is of minor importance. I share this opinion, for when in another experiment I imitated the mother-duck's call vocally, without lure or tape, the ducklings followed me for over half an hour. Yet my crude vocal imitation of the mother duck was certainly less faithful than the lure of the tape-recorded voice.

Even this barnyard example shows how the dialogue involves more than merely action and response. That the duckling's vocalization is called "lost" peeping underscores the dominant role of affect in the process. What the mother duck responds to is a call for help. And the ducklings follow her, irresistibly drawn by the seemingly tenuous thread of the dialogue, which in the course of development will replace the warm closeness, the primal security, provided by the mother duck brooding over the hatching eggs.

If the role of affect is so evident in birds, we can expect it to have an even more significant function, but also an infinitely more diversified one, in man. Affect and dialogue are not limited unilaterally to the child—in our barnyard example the very response of the adult mother duck is also an affective one. While completely different from that of the ducklings, it fits into the offspring's affect and the offspring's into hers. The two affects mesh in mutual interaction.

I have discussed this circular interaction of maternal and infantile attitudes in man elsewhere (Spitz, 1962) and in a clinical context spoken of the maternal attitude as *diatrophic* (1956a); it complements the infant's attitude, which Freud (1914) called *anaclitic*. The two operate in conjunction. The concept of the anaclitic attitude is familiar enough. The diatrophic attitude can best be described as a greatly increased capacity to perceive both consciously and unconsciously the child's anaclitic needs and an urge to provide for their gratification.

But that is still far too static a picture. We should indeed not be speaking only of a circular process, because that makes it sound two-dimensional. A progression takes place from one circular process to the next one; as Heraclitus remarked, you cannot go through the same river twice. This progression is not only a three-dimensional one, it also takes place on a time continuum. It is a stochastic process, in which the emotions involved in the dialogue play a highly significant role.

Elsewhere (Spitz, 1963b) I advanced the proposition that emotions have an anticipatory function. Therefore emotions fit readily into the stochastic process of the dialogue. Indeed, we are safe in assuming that emotions are the motive power which activates the dialogue and its progression. Action is invested with emotion and so, of course, is the response to it; the quantities involved vary and so do the proportions. The child's initiatives provoke reverberations in the mother; these are expressed in the form of behavior, which in turn evokes an answering behavior in the child and so on, producing ever new constellations of increasing complexity, with ever varied energy displacements. Each of these dispenses gratification or frustration, and the emotions so produced leave traces in the psyche and in the memory systems of both partners. It is here that one aspect of the stochastic network[2] which characterizes the dialogue becomes evident. Any single trace modifies, but

---

[2] Stochastic network—a system of events bound to each other in causal dependence; at each critical point the next event is not invariably determined (as in the classical concept of causation) but has a certain probability of occurrence (English and English, 1958).

does not necessarily determine, the next circular process as it arises, its form, its structure, its unrolling, or the way it moves toward its goal, and thus compounds the rapidly increasing complexity of the dialogue.

The time dimension enters into the evolution of dialogue from several sources. The most obvious one is the continuous and predetermined progress of maturation.

Quite different and much less predictable are the other sources. First, there are the results of cumulating the memory traces of life experience. Another aspect of the time dimension is the sequential storage of memory traces in the *mnem* systems. That is not only demonstrable through psychological (psychoanalytic) exploration, it is also a simple fact of everyday experience. Yet, we are ignorant of how and in what form a temporal sequence can be incorporated into our memory, but we also do not know in what form it could be retained over long periods and then reproduced.

In this respect the discussions of the Hickson Symposium are instructive. There Lashley (1951) states: "Nearly 40 years ago Becher wrote: 'There is no physiological hypothesis which can explain the origins and relationships of temporal form in mental life; indeed, there is no hypothesis which even foreshadows the possibility of such an explanation.' The situation is little better today."

In this stimulating article Lashley offers some suggestions which may lead to the possibility of constructing a model for the functioning of temporal forms in mental life: "It is now practically certain that all the cells of the cerebro-spinal axis are being continually bombarded by nervous impulses from various sources and are firing regularly, possibly even during sleep. . . . I am coming more and more to the conclusion that *the rudiments of every human behavioral mechanism will be found far down in the evolutionary scale* and also represented even in primitive activities of the nervous system." Lashley concludes: "Every bit of evidence available indicates a dynamic, constantly active system, or, rather a composite of many interacting systems which I have tried to illustrate at a primitive level by *rhythm* and the space coordinates" (italics mine).

In the discussion of Lashley's paper Paul Weiss elaborates his concept and states: ". . . the working of the central nervous system is a hierarchic affair. . . . The final output is then the outcome of this hierarchical passing down of distortions and modifications of intrinsically preformed patterns of excitation. . . . The structure of the input does not produce the structure of the output, but merely modifies intrinsic nervous activities that have a structural organization of their own. This has been proved by observation and experiment."

In my own opinion (and I believe also in Lashley's, who mentions him) von Holst's (von Holst & Mittelstaedt, 1950) experiments provided us with some of the rhythmic patterns mentioned above. Von Holst worked on fishes, gallinacea, and flies. These are animals equipped with a nervous system functioning on a relatively low level of psychological integration. That, I believe, is why von Holst was able to get information on the functioning of rhythms and space coordination at a primitive level; the same applies to Weiss, who also worked on such animals.

In early infancy we are also dealing with mental processes on a relatively low level of integration. They represent rudiments, prototypes or precursors of the subsequently developing human behavioral mechanisms and modes of function. Therefore, careful observation of the precursor of dialogue in infancy may shed light on the genesis, structure, and mode of operation of subsequent psychic function, including the temporal forms. However, at the present state of our knowledge of the psyche, or for that matter, of neurology, we have not yet formulated any rationally acceptable proposition of the way in which this could take place.

Still another aspect of the time dimension is a basic property of the dialogue, namely, its prospective character. To anticipate is in the very nature of dialogue. However, as I stated in the earlier paper (Spitz, 1963a), only the living can engage in dialogue, take the initiative or respond to it, and by the same token anticipate initiatives. The inanimate neither acts nor reacts, it merely exists, it is there. Any initiative aimed at it reveals its inanimateness, because such initiatives are not followed by a circular action-reaction response and thus do not lead to any exchanges. Thus, engaging in a dialogue becomes the child's criterion in distinguishing the animate from the inanimate.

The fact that the child prefers the living to the inanimate made us conclude that the feedback from the live partner is experienced as gratification, though this term has to be taken in a wider sense. Exchanges with a live partner carry both gratification *and* frustration, both libido *and* aggression. The dialogue, the circular exchange of action and response, serves the child to test whether something he sees is animate.

This testing is very impressively demonstrated in one of my films in which a 12-month-old child is confronted with a baby-sized doll, stares at it, puzzled, from all angles, then approaches it, butting the doll with her head, then moves back and continues to stare and, when the doll does not react, begins to cry and show anxiety.

Though brief, the scene is most instructive. The child, on beholding the doll, is puzzled by something which goes beyond her previous experience. It *looks* like a baby, it is *dressed* like a baby, it *stands* like a baby. But there is something strange. What is it? And now our little girl uses a test, a device, to find out. She tries to initiate a dialogue (or rather the precursor of a dialogue) and fails: for the strange thing does not *act* like a baby.

Our little girl shows herself to be a natural operationalist, in that she uses the scant tools at her disposal, the action-response sequence of the dialogue, for testing reality. Those among our readers who challenge our speaking of the dialogue or of its precursor as tools may recall that Aristotle called language an *organon,* a tool, and that Karl Bühler (1934) elaborated the *"organon theory"* of language as a tool.

At the same time the performance of our 12-month-old shows how the aggressive drive operates. Butting the doll with the head is somewhere halfway between touching, a tactile exploration, and hitting, a manifestation of the aggressive drive, and kissing, a manifestation of the libidinal drive. I shall return to another sequence of this film which will further clarify this proposition.

Animate and inanimate differ basically from each other in respect to the opportunities they offer for the management of the drives and for their discharge to the outside. The inanimate is eminently suitable for the discharge of large amounts of aggressive drive.

It should be clearly understood that when I speak of the aggressive drive or of aggression I do *not* mean hostility. Hostility is goal-directed and specific—not so aggression. Discharge of the aggressive drive requires no *specific* action, it frequently remains unspecific and random in its goal, even though the action as such is volitional and directed. Accordingly, we see the infant in the last part of his first year of life hitting, chewing, breaking, throwing inanimate things and, as these do not retaliate or respond, this activity continues until the thing is destroyed, or removed, or the energy available is spent. Exploration of the inanimate also belongs in this category and here again the unresponsive inanimate permits practically unlimited continuation of the activity.

It has been argued that these activities represent only tension reduction. I would prefer to reserve this term for that stage of the infant's life in which all activity is still random and not directed by a central steering organization. In contrast to this randomness, no one who observes a one-year-old child can fail to be impressed with the fact that a *functioning ego organization,* going far beyond the limits of the body ego, is governing the child's activities. Therefore I feel that it is inaccurate to designate these volitional activities only as tension reduction; they do, of course, reduce tension, but this is also true of all later ego-controlled activities.

Most of the activities which the infant performs on the inanimate remain on a very archaic level, because the inanimate does not respond; all the initiatives have to originate with the child. This will obviously narrow down and possibly even eliminate any potential for a stochastic network. The opportunities offered by the inanimate thus are exceedingly limited and ultimately unrewarding. Dialogue cannot originate from the child's relations with the inanimate. All that he can achieve with an inanimate thing is to discharge on it limited amounts of drive energy. For his handling of the inanimate is ultimately self-limiting; at best it stops with the inanimate thing's destruction or disappearance. When that comes about, the particular inanimate thing in question offers no further opportunity for the discharge of remaining amounts of drives or newly arising ones. The inanimate thus carries within itself the seeds of unpleasure, for when the aggressive drive can no longer be discharged on the outside, it will produce internal tension, which may range from the familiar symptoms of boredom, irritability, restlessness, to more serious symptoms.

How different from this are the relations with a live partner! Both drives, the aggressive and the libidinal, are engaged to the full. The living partner does not remain a passive target for discharge. When I previously stressed that the inanimate is an obvious target for the discharge of the aggressive drive, I also implied that it is relatively unfit for discharging the libidinal drive. This is so obvious that one does not even think of questioning it.

A major mental operation is required of the subject to endow the inanimate thing with a semblance of object attributes. When this happens, the inanimate becomes a transitional object (Winnicott, 1953). Yet it is very probable that in the genesis of transitional objects there is also another process at work, namely, an archaic conditioning mechanism. For the transitional object is indeed transitional in the sense that it partakes of both worlds, the archaic world of the conditioned reflex on the one hand, the ego-regulated world of object relations, of the psyche, on the other.

Among the inanimate things, the transitional object has a unique position—it is the one privileged thing in one individual child's world for a given period of time. By and large, however, inanimate things are not thus privileged. Large amounts of aggressive drive can be discharged on them, but no significant quantities of the libidinal drive. It seems that reciprocity is an unconditional prerequisite for the discharge of the libidinal drive, Saint Francis notwithstanding, who called fire his brother and water his sister. Not only does the living partner respond, positively or negatively, to the child's aggressive and libidinal initiatives; he does much more, he takes the initiative himself and makes the child its target. And by calling him a partner, we have indicated that he is the child's counterplayer in the dialogue. The stochastic network offers the child inexhaustible resources for ever new, stimulating avenues for discharge of both libidinal and aggressive energy, opportunities to elaborate these discharges, to make them manageable, to make them ego syntonic, and to modulate them so that he can reap rewards from the dialogue in the form of affective gratification.

The intricate and subtle interplay of the child's drives with the living partner's personality and drive structure, their gratification in the framework of the dialogue, permits and incites the child to discover devices for drive discharge which are often pleasurable.

The dialogue thus appears as one of the tools of which intrapsychic processes avail themselves for the management of the drives in the framework of object relations. When and where does it begin? There cannot be any doubt that the precursors of the dialogue originate in the nursing situation. In the human it is here that we will find the first events heralding the development of devices which eventuate in verbal communication and discussion, as I have attempted to show in *No and Yes* (Spitz, 1957). There I also presented evidence which supports my thesis that these devices are of phylogenetic origin.

It is then interesting and instructive to realize that the fitness of the inanimate for the discharge of the aggressive drive persists unmodified right into adulthood, when we are allegedly rational. True, man has acquired speech, which serves to replace action by discussion, a signal achievement. Have we not heard lately our leaders say of endlessly protracted negotiation, "As long as they talk, there is no shooting!" Is not this the meaning of the endless speeches of the Homeric heroes before they fall to with sword and lance? Of the self-glorifying, boastful tirades of the chiefs of primitive tribes, before battle begins?

Yes, we have achieved discussion instead of action. But when discussion gets heated, we pound the table at our adversary—and obviously we mean *him,* not the inanimate piece of wood. But what has this to do with phylogenesis? Well, ethologists have uncovered an embarrassingly similar behavior pattern in animals, which so far they have investigated primarily in the conflictual situation arising between the mating urge and the urge to attack. Two examples only, the most familiar ones: the male herring gull, when courting a female, turns away and with its beak tears out a bunch of grass; the heron, when courting, turns his head away and hacks at a stone. After this the approach to the female is made. The meaning of this behavior is quite obvious, the preliminaries to an intraspecies fight consist in certain specific behavior patterns called by Lorenz *Imponierverhalten.* It is a threatening, a bragging behavior, often called "display behavior," designed to impress the opponent with the subject's imposing size, strength, power, and intention to attack. This appears to be what the herring gull conveys by tearing out a bunch of grass as he would his opponent's feathers. This is what the heron demonstrates when he hacks at a stone instead of at his adversary. The survival value of such behavior is great, for as often as not one of the opponents will turn away and abandon the field to the other after such a face-saving maneuver.

These behavior patterns are species specific. They are triggered by the approach of another individual, male or female, of the same species; thus the threatening behavior also becomes part of the courting and mating patterns. As the ethologists put it, tearing out a bunch of grass instead of the enemy's feathers is a displacement behavior, which, in the sexual situation, has become ritualized. The conflict is between the attacking response against any other individual of the same species and the mating response toward the female of the same species.

The structure of this behavior shows a certain similarity to our pounding the table instead of hitting our adversary, when discussion gets heated. But the parallel is even more embarrassingly close when we hear that the male gorilla, enraged by an opponent, stands up and begins pounding his chest before attacking. The conflict here is not between the urge to attack and the mating urge, but between attacking and running away. Indeed, this is the very same conflict which makes us pound the table in a heated dispute; and the same conflict causes Homeric heroes to deliver bombastic threatening speeches while rattling their shields and shaking their lances—it is the conflict between the urge to attack and the fear of the adversary. As long as we rattle our shields, as long as we pound the table, as long as we talk, there is no shooting; there is dialogue—and we are safe.

One of my motion pictures of the 12-month-old previously mentioned contains a remarkable illustration of displacement behavior in a conflict situation. This little girl is one of a pair of identical twins, age 0;11 + 26. She is standing in a cot, her sister behind her and to the right. The large baby-sized doll is offered again, whereupon the sister starts to cry. Our little girl now goes through an extraordinarily expressive performance, nearly a pantomime. She looks searchingly at the big doll. Then she looks at her weeping twin. Her glance shifts back and forth between doll and sister. She seems to compare them. Now she bends forward and touches the doll with her lips. Then she turns her head over her left shoulder, looks at her sister, bends over and touches the sister with her lips in a kissing motion. She turns back to the doll, looks at it searchingly. Then she bends forward and touches the doll a second and a third time with her lips. Finally, she turns away from the doll to the other side, to the railing of her cot, touches it with her lips, and makes a few tentative biting movements on it.

I think that the conflict, the puzzlement, the trying out of a nonverbal dialogue, which shifts forward and backward between doll and sister and sister and doll is dramatically evident. The turning away and biting the railing in the end represent displacement behavior practically identical with that of the gulls and the herons.

There can be no doubt that in this very elementary dialogue precursor we witness an attempt to deal with the libidinal drive, with the aggressive drive, and with an anxiety potential. This, of course, is also what takes place in the dialogue, both precursor and verbal, in the exchanges with a libidinal object, with the mother. But the mother does not permit the unrestricted discharge of aggression; she insists on, and because she is an adult, she succeeds in keeping the child's aggression within acceptable bounds; and the same goes for the libidinal urge. She guides the child in evolving devices which facilitate a compromise—to have one's cake and to eat it too—to discharge the drive in a socially acceptable manner. She achieves this not only through enforcement, prohibition, and gratification, in other words, through the ongoing dialogue between her and her child; she also achieves it by helping the child to reduce his drive pressure, so that he learns to protect himself against anxiety-provoking situations. These latter arise when drive pressure threatens to disrupt the integrity of the ego. At this early stage the ego is still relatively helpless; the child strives to safeguard the new and gratifying achievement of maintaining his autonomy.

The dialogue thus becomes an increasingly effective tool. With its help, the child can achieve drive gratifications which cannot be achieved through action. But the dialogue also permits him to avoid frustration, helplessness, anxiety, which would arise in the wake of some forms of drive discharge.

The dialogue, of course, does not comprise the totality of object relations. It was not my purpose to coin a new term, dialogue, with which to replace the concept of object relations. The concept of object relations is difficult to describe and encompass. My use of the term dialogue has the purpose of making more tangible one part at least of this rather abstract concept, to make it as tangible as any of our everyday conversations, discussions, arguments, disputes. The dialogue is only one facet of object relations; it is their concrete and visible part and at the same time their instrument. Object relations are implemented in the dialogue.

I am not losing sight of the fact that the most important aspects of object relations are the intrapsychic processes, the mute surge, the ebb and flow of intersystemic investments, structuration, etc.

Where in this picture is the place of the 12- to 18-month-old's conversations with inanimate objects in the course of his first make-believe games? In these conversations the partner is imaginary. Conversations with imaginary partners cannot be conducted unless they are modeled on an original, and such an original can only be a dialogue which has taken place in reality with a living partner.

The precursor of the dialogue between the child and a live partner must precede all meaningful relations with the living. *A fortiori* it is indispensable for any imaginary exchange with the inanimate. This statement does not require proof; it goes without saying that the newborn has extensive relations with his mother long before he pays any attention to an inanimate object. As we have shown, these relations with the mother take the form of the precursor of the dialogue.

For this proposition we possess some confirmation of a quantitative nature. The late Katherine M. Wolf had always maintained that inadequate object relations tend to lower the development quotient in the *sector* of manipulative mastery, that is, the capacity to handle things (personal communication). We were able to confirm this proposition by direct observation and through the developmental tests of the children described in our paper on hospitalism (Spitz, 1945b, 1946b).

In the light of the propositions advanced in the present paper, one is led to conclude that during the first year of life the child's handling and manipulation of inanimate things is an attempt at a dialogue with them. It should be considered a continuation of the dialogue with the living, but on inappropriate objects. Something of the kind was already evident when we discussed how the child uses inanimate things for the discharge of aggression. That in itself does not suffice for the development of a dialogue with the inanimate, for the children suffering from hospitalism do not even achieve this stage of hitting, biting, throwing, or destroying inanimate objects. In other words, they achieve neither a dialogue with the living nor the counterpart of this dialogue with the inanimate. Furthermore, the observer familiar with the behavior patterns of these affect-deprived children is struck by the activity (such as it is) that replaces both relations with the living and play (aggressive or otherwise) with toys. We observed the frequency with which these children performed endless weaving movements with their hands, fingers, feet, and toes, staring at them as if spellbound.

Other infant observers also commented on this topic; e.g., Lebovici and McDougall (1960) mentioned it in the anamnesis of a schizophrenic boy they treated; in infancy he had undergone emotional deprivation. In the latter part of his first year of life and far into the second and third years this child never played with toys, but "stared fascinated at his extremities." One wonders whether such children replace the precursors of the dialogue, of which they had been deprived, by a dialogue which they conduct with their extremities, particularly with their hands and fingers, moving them in spooky, weaving patterns. This assumption is strikingly confirmed by a review of our films, which show the deprived children moving their lips while staring deeply absorbed at their finger movements.

This pattern (though with a quite different, benign character and not as extreme and exclusive) is a normal item in the behavioral inventory of the 3- to 4-month-old (C. Bühler, 1937a; Rheingold, 1956). But that which is a normal achievement at 4 months is not appropriate at the end of the first year, for it should have been left far behind. When this behavior becomes the only activity of the 8- to 15-month-old, it takes on a very different and sinister significance (David and Appel, 1961; Spitz, 1957).

Toward the end of the first year of life the average normal child becomes aggressively active with inanimate objects. He hits them, chews them, pounds them, throws them. Not so the children suffering from hospitalism; they lie in their cots, listless, without interest in any activity. Their inability to implement all outward manifestations of the aggressive drive has an interesting counterpart in the children who suffer from anaclitic depression, recover from it, and become overactive. After such recoveries, we could observe that the massive outward manifestations of their aggressive drive become unusually frequent and violent. They would direct their destructive activity both at things and at other infants. They would, for instance, tear their clothing and their bedsheets to shreds. When with other children, they would bite them, or tear their hair out by the fistfull. We observed one child pick at a playmate's instep until he had torn off a piece of skin. It seemed as if in their aggressive destructive action they made little, if any, distinction between animate and inanimate. That was to be expected; for these were children who had been separated from their mothers, and therefore deprived of the opportunities for the dialogue through which, as we have explained, they would normally have acquired the devices necessary for the domestication of the drives and for the discrimination between the living and the inanimate.

These observations support the validity of Katherine M. Wolf's proposition. They also support my thesis that the precursor of the dialogue with a living partner must precede any dialogue with the inanimate. This can be seen also in children's first make-believe games, which consist almost exclusively of gestures, both nonverbal and verbal, purloined from the adults. Quite frequently the gestures, the performance, are clearly intended as a directed communication.

We have, for instance, a charming film of a little girl, 15 months old, who takes a bundle of diapers on her arm and goes from child to child in the playroom and gives each a diaper, without speaking. But from time to time she produces a little bow and smiles. This is a most revealing performance; it is the purely nonverbal form of the dialogue, the initiating of a conversation with a gift and a gesture. It is obvious that here the identification is with the adult's gesture only; for the little girl bestows her diapers indiscriminately on the nurse and on me, as well as on the children. Or, in another of our films, the child dials his toy telephone and "speaks" gibberish into an upside-down-held receiver, looking up at the observer from time to time. It is self-evident that these are examples of a transition from the nonverbal to the verbal dialogue. Parts of the gesture have already become word; the flesh has become spirit.

It will be a short step (in our adult reckoning!) from here to the verbal dialogue—all of 3 months. For during the first quarter of the second year the child's verbal proficiency consists of a collection of "global" words, serving mainly for "expression" and for "appeal" in the sense in which K. Bühler (1934) used these terms.[3] In the following 3 months the global words are put together into two-word sentences. By the time the child is 18 months old, around 20 of these global words have accumulated; but their use is limited by lack of grammatical facilities. It is through grammatical facilities that spatial and temporal referents are introduced into language; as long as these are missing, communication remains sketchy indeed. But that, as Kipling remarked, is another story.

After the eighteenth month the child will develop, from the global words which have accumulated, both a grammar and a syntax of his own, and begin to introduce grammatico-syntactical categories into his speech. Communication gains immeasurably, the dialogue differentiates more clearly persons from states and feelings, persons from each other, and persons from things. Furthermore, the child adds to his dictionary words for persons, things, and states, often of his own creation.

Clara and Wilhelm Stern (1907) mention a characteristic conversation from this stage: Peter, toward the end of his second year, sees snow falling for the first time, gets very excited and shouts: "Kiok, Kiok!" His mother informs

---

[3] The step which terminates the global word period (the period during which the dialogue is initiated by the child mainly in the make-believe games) is equally significant. I refrained from introducing my concept of organizer of the psyche and of critical periods of development into the present discussion. The organizer concept belongs to a rather far-ranging universe of discourse. It refers to a comprehensive generalization which encompasses both evolution and development. The data we possess on the development of language are still relatively scanty. They are perhaps insufficient to relate the fairly narrow frame of reference of language development to the much vaster one of the sequence, structure, and function of organizers. Conversely, it is legitimate to relate the steps in language development to the stages of Piaget's (1936b) theory of reversibility, for the two belong to the same level of conceptualization.

I am convinced that a close relationship exists also between Piaget's stages of reversibility and the successive organizers of the psyche. One example of this relationship has been described above; at the stage at which the child uses global words and conducts a semiverbal dialogue, he has also reached Piaget's fifth stage of reversibility, that is, the stage at which the child is able to solve the test of the two concealments of the wrapped-up object. In the field of semantic development this is also the stage which is characterized by the achievement of the "no" gesture, which is the indicator of the third organizer of the psyche.

him that this is called "snow"; to which he replies in a peremptory tone, "Peter, Kiok!" indicating that he will call it *Kiok* and not snow.

This also exemplifies the inception of verbal discussion in a semi-grammatico-syntactical form. The point is that this achievement can be attained only through the instrumentality of controversial exchanges with a living partner. Conversely, the conversation conducted during the first half of the second year in the make-believe games with toys was obviously completely unilateral, and the controversy, if any, only imaginary. Such conversations represent identifications with the verbal *gesture* of the adult.

We now come to the key issue of language versus action and its bearing on the discrimination between the animate and the inanimate.

With the evidence now at our disposal, we believe that it is questionable whether any of the verbal communications of the child at this age—I am referring to the beginning of the second year—are much more than the make-believe conversations, even when actually directed to an adult. It is equally questionable at this stage whether the child in his own "conversation" has made a distinction between the category of word language and that of gestures. Accordingly, in his *verbal* behavior, he has hardly begun to distinguish the animate from the inanimate.

In contrast, it is beyond doubt that such a distinction has been made by the child much earlier in the realm of *action*. In this argument we distinguish action, a neuromuscular behavior with immediate alloplastic goals, from gesture, which has the immediate purpose of signifying, of a representation. From the viewpoint of verbal communication, this is still a transitional period. The word, the symbol, is just being established and is still unsuitable to serve and function adequately in all those sectors of life in which action has already been operating efficiently for some time.

To put it in chronological terms: the distinction between the animate and the inanimate in terms of action becomes evident between the ninth and the twelfth month (Spitz, 1963b). At that stage the precursor of the dialogue (in the form of actions and of expressions of emotions) is already so conspicuous that we were able to demonstrate it visually, notwithstanding the limitations of silent motion pictures.

Between 12 and 18 months the distinction between the animate and the inanimate is processed anew. It is included in a newly emerging dimension in reality testing. We will call this new dimension the *semiverbal conversation*. Due to this added dimension a far more searching test of the differences between animate and inanimate will be conducted by the child.

The data of my study do not yet allow me to draw a conclusion whether it is the ongoing dialogue with animate and inanimate that leads to concept formation and verbal facility, or, alternately, whether the achievement of verbal facility leads to a sharpened distinction between animate and inanimate. Probably there is an interplay between the two devices. I am inclined to believe that the first of the two devices is the more effective and the more important one, as is evident from the argumentation in my book *No and Yes* (Spitz, 1957). It is, however, obvious that at this stage we cannot study the dialogue outside of the framework of object relations.

In summary, our investigation of the precursor of the dialogue and of the progressive transformations it undergoes until it leads to verbal conversation has shown that the precursor already contains as prototypes many other elements of the later, verbal dialogue. But these prototypes do not serve only as models for later development, they also act as devices for the management of the drives, for their neutralization, for evolving the highly sophisticated psychological devices of the defense mechanisms. The precursor of the dialogue thus appears as the bridge across which the surround makes its influence felt, across which it becomes effective in developing and establishing all the major psychological devices and structures.

The present series of articles are thus only a first approach to the study of the dialogue and its precursors. It is evident that the major part of the work and investigation lies ahead. Freud began by focusing psychoanalytic attention on the verbal production of adults. Under the leadership of Anna Freud, this exploration was continued to the school child and preschool child. Through this intensive study of verbal behavior within the guidelines of psychoanalytic theory, a contribution, enormous in extent, extraordinary in its impact and importance, and unique in the history of science, was made over the years. The theoretical guidelines which made this achievement possible, through the study of verbal behavior, have equal validity for the study of infantile non-verbal behavior, as I have attempted to demonstrate with observations and experiments. There is every reason to apply the searchlight of psychoanalytic exploration to the infant's and toddler's preverbal productions, to the precursor of the dialogue.

The present article gives a few examples of this approach. Far more extensive material can be found in the pioneer study conducted by Dr. John Benjamin on these lines with an exacting scientific methodology; and we are beginning to reap the fruits of his tireless and dedicated work.

But the field is vast. One single research organization can cover only relatively small sectors. It is my hope that these articles will encourage others to approach the exploration of the embryology of thought processes in man through the investigation of dialogue and its precursor in the infant.

PART 3

THE EMERGENCE OF EGO

Editor's Introduction

The seven papers in this section are contributions to the psychoanalytic theory of ego formation. The first two, published a decade apart, deal with the organization of perception and the central role of affect in this process, a topic that only now appears to be coming into its own in psychology (see Zajonc, 1979; Emde, 1980a). These papers also highlight the central role of the face in both early perception and affective experience. Spitz's thinking about the face was not predicted by the prevailing psychoanalytic notions of the time, which emphasized the breast, and it undoubtedly helped to stimulate two decades of infancy research on the development of facial discrimination (see review in Haith and Campos, 1977). Today, our outlook is different. The face is central in one major theory of emotion (see Izard, 1977), it is the subject of a burgeoning area of research in emotional development (see Ekman and Oster, 1979; Emde 1980a), and it is a focus for much detailed research on the interaction between caregiver and infant (see D. Stern, 1977).

Spitz returned to the topic of the relationship of affect and perception in "Bridges," his last major published paper. There he pointed out that the young infant is biologically predisposed, by virtue of affective preferences, to select from a "barrage" of stimuli only those that have importance for survival. In this sense, affects endow the stimulus experience with meaning. But, he speculated, this is true in another sense. Affects also contribute to meaning by making memory registration more likely and by enhancing the development of anticipatory function. One is reminded of Piaget's largely untested speculations in this area (Piaget, 1973; see also Décarie, 1962; Bell, 1970). These discussions of Spitz's offer rich material for stimulating new hypotheses.

Other papers in this section deal with the biological origins of psychological defenses, with emotional regulation, with the emergence of self, and with the processes involved in the integration of early experience. Although interdisciplinary in his interests, Spitz uses the language and concepts of psychoanalytic metapsychology throughout these papers. Several of his concepts are particularly relevant for today's formulations.

In "Early Prototypes of Ego Defenses," "Ontogenesis," and "Further Prototypes of Ego Formation," Spitz discusses his concept of "prototypes" of defenses and coping behavior. Prototypes refer to early undifferentiated modes of function that "serve as the physiological *models* for the later establishment of psychological functions." As such, they may be considered innate physiological "structures" that require development—i.e., repeated interactions with the social environment—before they become transformed into psychological "structures." In his use of prototypical modes, Spitz offers a bridge concept for psychophysiology analogous to what Erikson proposes for psychosocial development in his discussion of "Zones, Modes and Modalities" (Erikson, 1950). Wolff (1967) has pointed out how this kind of concept of developmental modes also offers the potential for linking Piagetian schema theories of memory development with trace theories such as exist in classical psychoanalysis.

Spitz's discussions of emotional signaling in "Ontogenesis" and of the emergence of self in "Metapsychology and Direct Infant Observation" are especially relevant for today's theoreticians. According to Spitz, the anticipation of unpleasure begins to function as a signal some time between the ages of three and six months. Information may then be channeled in two directions: (1) A *centripetal,* internal signal results as mounting tension of the emotion announces an impending danger of overload. (2) A *centrifugal,* external signal results as the facial and behavioral expression of the emotion communicates the impending state (and action) to others. The process becomes crystallized during the third quarter of the first year when there is a "definitive link between felt emotion as a signal for the ego and the expression of emotion as a communication to the surround." Current research and thinking is now at the point of investigating hypotheses derived from these formulations and integrating them with advances in our understanding of cognitive development and of discrete emotions. (For reviews of recent research from the point of view of developmental psychology, see Sroufe, 1979; from the point of view of psychoanalysis, see Emde, 1980b.)

The excerpt from "Metapsychology and Direct Infant Observation" contains what is probably Spitz's most concise statement of his theory of self development. As he describes what he believes to be three stages of self formation in infancy and alludes to self transformation in adolescence and later, Spitz links his observations with the clinical theory of psychoanalysis. It is worth reviewing this thinking in the midst of today's renaissance of interest in the self in psychoanalysis (e.g., Kohut, 1971, 1977) and developmental psychology (Lewis & Brooks-Gunn, 1979).

Spitz's theory of psychic organizers in infancy was initially published in monograph form in *The Genetic Field Theory of Ego Formation* in 1959, but he further developed and clarified it in "Further Prototypes of Ego Formation" and "Bridges." Spitz states that the psychic organizer is to be thought of as equivalent to *"the development of a new modus operandi. . . . It introduces a better adapted way . . . on a higher level of complexity."* Such a mode of functioning will persist until increasing complexity results in the need for another modus operandi and regulation at a higher level; this will result in a more highly integrated reorganization with another organizer. As Spitz put it, "Every successive organizer in the further course of development introduces a new formula of regulation, successively more complex and better adapted." As a developmental theoretician, Spitz was intensely preoccupied with the dynamics of how such major reorganizations could take place. It seemed to him that over the course of infancy there was an increasing asymmetry between stimulus input and discharge or mastery. He theorized that at certain times there is such an increase in quantity that it reaches a critical point; at such times—perhaps also influenced by maturational timing mechanisms—this quantity switches to a new quality. Spitz was intrigued that these kinds of fundamental transformations were discussed not only in modern nuclear physics but also by Karl Marx.

Modern developmental psychology is now beginning to confront the mysteries of developmental transformation. Partly this is because we have not seen the continuities that we expected in infancy and early childhood. Looking prospectively we have not been able to predict outcomes, even though we reached understandability about lines of development when we looked retrospectively aided by our clinical theories. But this is also because our psychology now has methods for looking directly at developmental transformations; these include multivariate approaches and statistical approaches that can look at individuals developing over time (instead of group behavior, which can become "averaged out" over time). Spitz's theory of organizers provides a background for today's interest in developmental transformation. Not only has it led to some specific research programs (see, for example, Emde, Gaensbauer, and Harmon, 1976), but it also has been the forerunner of many lively theoretical discussions that continue today (see Kagan, Kearsley, and Zelazo, 1978; McCall, 1979; Sameroff and Harris, 1979).

Diacritic and Coenesthetic Organizations: The Psychiatric Significance of a Functional Division of the Nervous System into a Sensory and Emotive Part

As with everything pertaining to the psyche, the bane of psychiatric problems has been that they present not only a psychic, but also a somatic aspect. Psychiatry has therefore tried to approach its problems from first one aspect and then the other. Up to a comparatively recent date the approach was a purely empirical one, following the lines of trial and error.

In the course of time the need of a theoretical basis became pressing. Psychiatrists first tried to meet this need with the help of anatomical criteria. The organicists in particular endeavored to find the cause of mental disease with the help of histological investigation of the central nervous system. However, the result of these investigations was unsatisfactory.

The approach from the psychological side came later. It was made by Freud at the end of the last century. His concept, psychoanalytic psychiatry, followed the lines of a functional division of the personality and provided several entities within the psyche. These entities differ in their structure, in their content, in their dynamics, and above all, in their function. Notwithstanding this, they are not only interactive, but are parts of one system of which they can and do alternately assume control. Furthermore, their limits are considered to be variable, so that any of these systems could, under certain circumstances, replace parts of any of the other.

The idea of a functional approach has also appealed to neurologists. Its first great exponent was probably Sir Charles Bell (1806) in the eighteenth century, in his book *The Anatomy and Philosophy of Expression*.[1] This same question of functional division has been taken up again and again in the course of the nineteenth century. The most recent literature on the subject has been

---

Reprinted from *The Psychoanalytic Review*, 32:146–160, 1945.

greatly influenced by the work of Cannon (1934) in the physiological field on the one hand, and on the other by the work done on encephalitis lethargica in the twenties of our century.

From the psychiatric standpoint the interest of this approach lies in the fact that it divides the neural system into two organizations which differ functionally from each other, but which at the same time can influence each other widely. A duality within the nervous system and the interaction of the two organizations supplies us with a more flexible explanation of the multiple phenomena presented by the human organism than does the monistic concept.

Such a functional approach also has advantages from the psychiatric point of view, which make it desirable to apply it to a larger area of the phenomena of psychiatry, psychology and neurology. It seems to me that the functional aspect is the common ground on which both the psychiatric and the neurological manifestations of a phenomenon can be visualized and perhaps understood.

This points the road to a possible solution of the ancient problem of finding a connection between psyche and soma and to correlate the manifestations of the one to those of the other. This is an extremely tempting goal. It is the object of this paper to bring us somewhat nearer to it. The approach which we have chosen lies along the lines of a functional differentiation of neurophysiological units within the totality of the nervous system.

Sir Henry Head (1908) made experimental attempts to differentiate two systems of perception. Little remains nowadays of his original concepts except the name, which is being more and more widely used in a sense different from the one which he had defined. The recent authors working in that field of neurophysiology on which this paper is based are too numerous to be

---

[1] Sir Charles Bell was the first to state clearly the existence of two functionally opposed nervous organizations within the central nervous system. He calls them ideomotoric and cardiomotoric. This corresponds to a very ancient division, so ancient and reappearing so constantly in ever modified forms, that this division must either correspond to a strong need of human thinking, or to convincing observable facts. We have no reason to repudiate the first or to neglect the second.

For the benefit of convinced opponents of any dichotomy when applied to biological problems, I wish to give, both as a justification and as a contribution to our conceptual framework, a short outline of the origin of our classification. The outline is schematic and therefore a number of details are omitted—but it is not the history so much as the genesis of an antithesis between emotional and cognitive energy within the psyche which we wish to describe. The genesis shows five periods.

A. *The metaphysical antithesis* in Greek philosophy speaks in terms of sensuality and cognition. The first traces of this assumption are to be found in the writing of Herakleitos and Empedokles. It is clearly expressed by Plato in the metaphor of the "Charioteer." In this metaphor the runaway black horse (lust) is contrasted with the docile white horse (courage). Aristoteles brought the contrast into a scientifically applicable form. In ancient philosophy the difference between vegetative and animal souls found its final expression in the teaching of Plotinus.

quoted. The work of many of them, like that of Kurt Goldstein (1936) and of Grinker (1937, 1939), is familiar to all and has inspired much of what will follow in the present paper. Less well known but equally significant is that of Kueppers (1923, 1931) and Papez (1937, 1939). On the psychoanalytic side Schilder (1928), Kubie (1934, 1941a,b), Hartmann (1939), Hendrick (1942), Kardiner (1932, 1941), and others should be mentioned.

In what follows I shall frequently refer to the work of the French neurologist Wallon, who not only uses a psychological approach in his physiological methods, but who also subordinates his whole concept to a functional point of view.

Henry Wallon (1925) succeeded in dividing the human nervous system into two organizations which are widely divergent as to their anatomy, their physiology, their manifestations, etc. On the other hand there is the closest interdependence imaginable in regard to the way in which they function. He has called these two organizations the sensory system and the emotive system. Following Head's (1908) terminology in the division of perception, he attributes to the sensory system "epicritic perception" and to the emotive system "protopathic perception." Wallon's work has expanded considerably the original definition of protopathic perception, while maintaining the definition of epicritic perception as introduced by Head.

The viewpoint of a functional division is maintained by Wallon throughout his book, without his succeeding, however, in elaborating it in a systematic manner. This I propose to do in what follows by expanding Wallon's viewpoint in order to achieve a system covering the whole neural organization. At the same time we will abandon the terms protopathic and epicritic which have

B. *The ethical antithesis* of passion and will is already preformed in the teaching of the Cynics and the Stoics. It becomes a central problem in the Middle Ages, filling the pages of Saint Augustinus' "Confessions" and of Thomas of Aquino's "Summae."

C. *The epistomological antithesis* of "clear knowledge" and "confused knowledge" appears in the philosophies of Descartes and Spinoza. "Clear knowledge" is defined as the device for discriminating between the single elements of experience and also for analyzing the single factors within these elements. This definition makes the transition to a psychological classification easy.

D. *The psychological antithesis* of perception and apperception is stated by Leibniz. In a purely descriptive manner Leibniz has anticipated the distinction between conscious and unconscious. This differentiation of Leibniz is of decisive significance for the whole psychology of the nineteenth century (Wundt, Lotze, Fechner, Helmholtz, and others) and of the twentieth century (Freud, Piaget, Wallon, Bühler).

E. *The neurophysiological antithesis* of vegetative (autonomous) and animal system in the work of Bell. This contrast has been expanded, modified, and elaborated with the aid of detailed investigation of the central nervous system. (Function of the Thalamus: Déjérine and Roussy, 1906; Head, 1908; Gelb and Goldstein, 1920; Dusser de Barenne, 1937. Hypothalamus: Economo and Poetzel, 1929; Economo, 1931; Cushing, 1932; Bailey, 1933; Davison and Selby, 1935; Fulton and Bailey, 1935. Extrapyramidal System: Sherrington, 1906; Vogt and Vogt, 1920; Denny-Brown, 1929; Foerster, 1936.)

been preempted by Head and instead will call the two systems the emotive or coenesthetic[2] and the sensory or diacritic[3] system.

The sensory or diacritic system centers in the cortex. Among its functions are conscious thinking as well as intentional and volitional acts. Its perception takes place through the sensory organs. These sensory perceptions are able to distinguish intensity in an approximately quantifiable manner; furthermore, they are localized and circumscribed. The executive organs of the sensory system are the striated long skeletal muscles of the limbs. These muscles function in a phasic manner with sudden contractions and relaxations according to volitional impulses.

The emotive or coenesthetic system, on the other hand, has its centers in the striopallidate region, the thalamic region, and the hypothalamus. Its psychic manifestations are to be found in the emotions, the affects, and in certain attributes of dreams. Its somatic manifestations are visceral and postural. Its perceptive function is better qualified by the adjective "sensitive" than "sensory," since its manifestations are perceived as vague, extended, diffuse sensations such as gastrointestinal, sexual, precordial, or dizziness sensations, etc.

The executive organs of this system are the smooth muscle fibers and the so-called postural muscles. The postural function[4] is one of the most important in expressing affects and emotions. The mimic musculature also belongs in the postural category, since it serves to express emotions. The difference between the functioning of the long skeletal muscles and that of the short muscles of the trunk which insure the postural function is the following: While

---

[2] Coenesthetic from Greek *koenos:* common—*eisthesis:* sensibility (Hinsie & Schatzky, *Psychiatric Dictionary*).

[3] Diacritic from Greek *diacrinein:* to separate, distinguish; *dia:* through—*krinein:* to separate (*Webster's International Dictionary*).

[4] The importance of the *postural function* has only recently begun to be appreciated by the medical world at large. Teachers of calisthenics are better informed on this subject than most physicians. The importance of the osseous structures of the pelvic and the shoulder girdles is generally understood. What is less clearly realized, is the significance of the intricate and powerful muscular structures which support, connect, and interlace the system of spinal column and thorax with that of the pelvis. Absolutely and relatively, the mass of the muscles in the trunk, particularly along the spinal column, surpasses that of all the rest of the body. The reason for our inattention to the significance of this powerful and complicated musculature lies in the fact that most of its activities take place without the intervention of our consciousness. In its massivity it forms a basis for the rapid movement of our limbs. At the same time, it constantly changes the tonus of its constituent smaller parts, relaxing or contracting smaller muscles or muscle groups for the purpose of maintaining the general equilibrium of the body. It is noteworthy that these contractions take place at a slower rhythm than those of the muscles of the limbs and seem to come close to the tonic contractions of smooth musculature. Our unawareness of this large part of our body has a result which is important for the psychiatrist. Not even the mimic expression of our face gives such a reliable account of our mood as does our body posture. The slumping attitude of depression, the rigidity of the obsessional, the easy relaxation of the normal mood, speak volumes to eyes which are able to see.

the skeletal muscles with their long, sudden contractions function in a phasic manner, both the smooth and the postural muscles function in a "tonic" manner, that is, in a much slower rhythm. Actually the postural muscles serve to maintain a certain tonus of the body which is indispensable as a base from which the sudden volitional movements of the limbs and their phasic muscles can start.

Our justification in thus dividing the nervous system into an emotive and a sensory organization is that they represent functional units operating along entirely different lines. At the same time, within each of these organizations the mode of functioning displays a certain uniformity.

Thus, for example, within the sensory organization, perception is localized and circumscribed, the thinking process is cognitive, and activity is volitional. These three functions operate according to the "intentional"[5] mode.

Intentionality is such a general characteristic of all sectors of the sensory organization that, if we want to give this organization as a whole a designation deriving from its way of functioning, we would seem to be justified in calling it the "intentional organization."

We have already mentioned that one of the attributes of the intentional organization is consciousness. We will have to add that it operates in a time-space continuum. Within this continuum it has to isolate and differentiate from each other perceptions, representations, and actions. Furthermore the mental processes of the intentional organization are the means by which we can connect with each other any of these perceptions and ideas. This is what we call association. These connections can be severed at will. If such were not the case, that is, if the connections became indissoluble, choice of action would become impossible. This would preclude judgment and decision.

Assuming a division within the whole of the human neuromuscular organization, of what will that part, which we have called the intentional system, consist? It consists of sensory perception, plus cortical areas, plus pyramidal tracts, plus endorgans in the voluntary muscles.

Now, let us look at the other organization, the emotive or coenesthetic. Nothing is localized or circumscribed here. Our emotions, be they fear, rage, or love, cannot be localized. Neither can we localize vertigo or visceral functions; the latter take place without even becoming conscious. In fact, the attribute of consciousness does not describe emotive experience adequately. Details are indistinguishable within the emotive experience, even degrees of

---

[5] Intentional, is a term introduced by Franz Brentano (1874). Here it is used in the sense of describing the mode of functioning of a system which establishes objects that remain identical to themselves, which adapts itself to them, and manipulates them. In this definition all the functions of the sensory system are described; for to establish objects identical to themselves is to perceive; to adapt to them means to consign them to memory or to imitate them; and lastly, the manipulation of objects takes place by means of volition and of thought processes.

intensity hardly exist. If we become conscious of the emotive experience at all it is in the form of a total phenomenon.

This is a form of perception which differs fundamentally from sensory perception. Properly it should not be called perception at all, but *reception*. As we will see later, the executive aspect, the motility of the emotive system, also differs fundamentally from that of the intentional system. If we ask the neurophysiologists what organization within the nervous system of the human being they consider adequate for the production of such experiences, they offer us only tentative answers. Kempf (1921), for instance, has made an attempt in this direction. Others, like Grinker (1939), have been unavoidably compelled through their work on the hypothalamus to conclusions closely related to our own. Wallon (1925) was the one who came closest to describing the details of such an organization of the nervous system. We have enumerated its components above, the thalamus, the hypothalamus, the autonomic and the striopallidate.

However, we have to find the functional mode with which satisfactorily to describe the operations of the emotive system. In the first place, from the point of view of perception, it does not distinguish details, but perceives only totalities. The same applies to its motricity, to its executive aspect. This operates according to the all-or-none law.

Perceiving only totalities means that not only will no details be distinguished, but that *two* elements of a given environmental situation will be perceived as *one* perception. If, at the receptive end of the system, only totalities can be perceived; if, at the executive end, on the other hand, the reaction to a totality takes place according to the all-or-none law, then it is obvious that it is sufficient for *one* of the several elements of the totality to reach the perceptive threshold to set into motion a trigger release which activates the all-or-none reaction.

Since, however, details are not perceived, but only a given threshold, it is immaterial *which* part of the original experience acts as a repeat stimulus, as long as it reaches the threshold.

This is a sequence of events which diverges strangely from the one to which we are used in our sensory world, where the stimulus-response pattern prevails and the response is proportionate to the stimulus. But there are some familiar exceptions within the stimulus-response pattern which parallel the sequence described above. Those exceptions are to be found in the field of the conditioned reflex. We may say therefore that the emotive system functions according to the laws of the conditioned reflex and if we wanted to designate it according to its mode of functioning, we would call it the "conditional organization," as contrasted with the "intentional organization."

The following chart of the properties and functions of the two systems will be helpful. (See Table 1.)

TABLE 1.

	Emotive Organization	Sensory Organization
Quality	Coenesthetic	Diacritic
Perception	Sensitive (visceral sensitivity)	Sense organs
Sensation	Vague Diffuse Extensive	Localized Circumscribed Intensive
Centers	Striopallidate Extrapyramidal Hypothalamus Autonomic Thalamus	Cortex
Executive organs	Smooth muscles Postural muscles Mimic muscles Viscera Glands	Striated skeletal muscles
Muscle function	Tonic Nonvolitional	Phasic and volitional
Psychic manifestations	Emotions Dreams	Conscious Thinking
Mode	Conditional	Intentional

Let us apply our concepts to one of the examples chosen by Pavlov (1927, 1928). A buzzer is pressed and food offered to a hungry animal, whereupon salivation sets in. According to our assumption, the emotive reception will perceive the two elements, buzzer and food, as belonging to the same situation. Once this is established, once the buzzer reaches the threshold necessary to elicit salivation, it will become irrelevant whether one offers the animal the buzzer or whether one offers it food. It will salivate in both instances, the all-or-none reaction will take place. In this example the association between the two elements of the total situation cannot be severed by *intentional* processes. The drawback of our example is that its emotional content is of a very low intensity. As we will see later, situations with an emotional content of really high intensity influence the emotive system in a much more decisive manner. When high-intensity emotion characterizes the experience, the linkage between the elements of the situation becomes practically indissoluble by *any means* whatsoever.

A peculiarity of the emotive organization which Wallon (1925) also mentions in his book, is worth noting at this point—namely, that in the emotive system one single experience of high emotional valency suffices to establish a conditioned reaction which will be extremely difficult to destroy. Wallon based this statement on the case histories of 214 feeble-minded children which he published in his book and which were observed during a period of 20 years.

This finding is in accord with the examples of conditioning through emotive experience which are to be found in the traumatic neuroses.

Kardiner (1941), in his beautiful report on case histories of traumatic neuroses, describes those cases in which attacks are provoked by external stimuli resembling those which occasioned the original loss of consciousness. A gassed patient is thrown into an attack when perceiving volatile oils. Another patient whose initial trauma took place during a heavy downpour in the trenches, has a seizure when his feet become wet. No other stimulus produces his attacks and, as Kardiner puts it: "These cases behave as if their attacks were finely conditioned reflexes."

Actually, these attacks *are* delicately conditioned reflexes. Our reluctance to call them by this name stems from the fact that we have been accustomed to Pavlov's concept of the "conditioned reflex." Pavlov creates conditioned reflexes by offering the animal sensory stimuli which provoke reactions in the emotive organization. The connection between the sensory stimulus, as offered by Pavlov, and the emotive visceral reactions is an extremely loose one; but, more important, the emotional content connected with the emotive reaction achieves only a comparatively low degree of intensity. As a consequence, the animal has to be exposed to numerous repetitions of the sensory stimulation before the emotive conditioned response is established, and even then the reaction is an extremely precarious one and apt to be lost with the greatest ease.

If we are to understand this contrast between Pavlov's concept of conditioning and that which obtains in traumatic neurosis,[6] we have to realize that under average circumstances the emotive system is not exposed to the direct interference of the environment. Environmental stimuli have to pass through

---

[6] The lack of space makes it impractical to bring out in its whole detail and in its whole significance the contrast between Pavlov's concept of the conditioned reflex and our view of the conditioned reaction which takes place in the emotive system. A detailed discussion of this problem will be published in a separate article. [See "Ontogenesis: The Proleptic Function of Emotion," this volume. Ed.]

the selective apparatus of the sensory system. This selective system provides for the discharge of a very large part of these stimuli in the form of action, perception, etc., and permits only a very small number of stimuli to reach the emotive system. These residual stimuli can therefore achieve only a comparatively low threshold of intensity.

In the traumatic neuroses the order of magnitude of the environmental stimuli is such as to overwhelm and put out of function the selective apparatus of the sensory system, thus exposing the emotive system to direct stimulation. Therefore an emotive stimulation of a very high degree of intensity results—witness the enormous amount of emotional reaction which takes place in consequence of the experience.

This irruption into the emotive system therefore appears to be dependent on quantitative and also on affective factors.

The direct stimulation of the emotive system results in the complete predominance of its perceptive organization over that of the sensory system during the traumatic episode. This predominance in turn implies a perception, or rather a "reception" which takes place in terms of total experience. As shown previously, such total experience is the prerequisite for the immediate establishment of a conditioned reflex.

Here is the explanation why conditioned reflexes thus created required only *one* experience to become established instead of many, and why they show such extraordinary stability that they can hardly be destroyed by our most energetic intervention. Actually, they become a part of the personality, mold the rest of the personality according to their own pattern and result in a structural change of the rest of the psyche. This change has to be abolished piecemeal before we can cure such cases.

However, the traumatic neuroses are states occurring in the fully developed personality, where a long process of maturation and development has created a complex psychic structure. Such a complication is undesirable for the purposes of investigation; too many factors obscure the picture, too many structural elements can be made responsible for the resulting condition. It seems desirable therefore to examine the phenomena of such traumata at an earlier age, when the picture is more clearcut. Wallon's observations also were made on children.

A striking peculiarity of the relationship between the emotive and the sensory system encourages us to do so. This peculiarity lies in the fact that in the perceptive field, at least, the two systems are to a large extent mutually exclusive—another is that they develop at different periods in the individual and in a different rhythm.

Experiments on infants made by Ripin (Hetzer & Ripin, 1930), Gesell (Gesell & Ilg, 1937), Wislitzky (Hetzer & Wislitzky, 1930), and Wolf (Hetzer

& Wolf, 1928) have proved that at birth the sensory system is practically nonexistent; that is, though anatomically it is more or less present, its function has not yet been established. The inception of its functioning, as proved by other experiments on infants by Ripin, Rubinow and Frankl (1934), and many others, takes approximately four months and its full development, according to our definition of this term, is achieved somewhere around the second year, as shown by Piaget (1936a).

But the emotive system is already functioning in the first four months. This also has been proved by experiments made on infants by Ripin, by Marquis (1931), and by Wildernberg-Kantrow (1937).

It is with this phenomenon in mind, namely, the difference in the time of the development of the two systems, that an observation made by Margaret Ribble (1938, 1939) on sucking frustration becomes significant for our thesis. Certain infants, when making their first attempts to suck, encounter difficulties in getting hold of the nipple. After two or three failures they become stuporous. These babies give the appearance of having abandoned cerebral function, they fall into a comatose sleep, with Cheyne-Stokes respiration, extreme pallor, and diminished sensitivity. They appear to have regressed to a fetal, quasi-vegetative, mode of functioning.

The condition is rarely relieved simply by introducing food into the stomach. The infants must be treated with the remedies one applies to states of shock, such as saline clysis, intravenous glucose and blood transfusion. After recovery they have to be taught to suck by stimulation of the mouth. If the condition is not dealt with immediately, it threatens the life of the neonate.

The mouth is the organ which forms the first link or transition from an emotive vegetative mode of life to that of sensory orientation. Although the trauma suffered by these infants occurs in the sphere of sensory stimulation, it is perceived by the emotive system of the infant's organism. This is because, as we previously indicated, the neonate has no means other than the emotive system for dealing with any stimulus. Therefore this trauma will represent a negative conditioning in the emotive sphere. This negative conditioning makes the infant refractory to any further sensory stimulation.

Another well known condition is that of hospitalism. We are referring to those infants who, after a prolonged stay in welfare institutions during their first year, develop a psychiatric picture ranging from psychopathy to feeble-mindedness. Experiments by Durfee and Wolf (1933) have shown that infants younger than four months do not develop these lesions, nor do those babies who entered institutions after their second year, as observed by Lowrey (1940) and Bakwin (1942).

It is significant that this span of time (from the fourth month to the second year) exactly corresponds to the period in the infant's life in which an integrated sensory organization is acquired. Experimental investigation has proved that the trauma suffered by infants in public welfare institutions was due to the lack of stimuli. This lack of stimuli made it impossible for a normally integrated sensory perceptive organization to develop. Consequently, the adaptation of these infants to their environment was handicapped by inadequate sensory perception and equally inadequate motor reactions. They reacted therefore with the only organization at their disposal, that is with the already established emotive organization. But there the emotive organization is confronted with a task to which it is not equal. The living organism has developed in the course of evolution, a succession of more and more highly integrated systems of orientation. The lowest, the trial-and-error method of the protozoa, is approximately on the level of an orientation such as could be achieved by the emotive system. Such an orientation can only be effective when the survival of the individual is immaterial, because spendthrift production of individuals insures the survival of the species. From this kind of orientation, successive stages of evolution have finally produced our diacritic method of orientation, based on a highly differentiated diacritic perception of the environment. This differentiated diacritic perception has a high survival value for the individual. When the individual has to fall back on the primitive emotive organization, the orientation to the environment will become completely insufficient for an adequate response. The emotive organization reacts to all and any stimuli only in an emotive manner, either with fear or rage or with such well-known visceral reactions as enuresis, loss of sphincter control, etc.

It is evident that a retardation of development of the sensory system produces an imbalance in the relation between this system and the better developed emotive system.

This discrepancy increases with age. During the early, exclusively emotive stages, during the first few weeks, we insulate and protect our infants from environmental stimuli; the older they become, the more we expose them to violent stimulation. The emotive system can only react to this stimulation with the cataclysmic manifestation with which we are familiar in psychiatric pathology.

It is interesting to note that the methods described by Ribble (1941) for reestablishing the disturbed functions of the infants—namely saline clysis and intravenous glucose—stimulate the emotive centers, besides involving chemical stimulation and the reestablishment of circulation in the central nervous system. In the case of traumatic neuroses it is significant that the most successful cures were those which, in one way or another, attempted emotive conditioning.

The reason for this is obvious. In all these cases the sensory system has failed and is useless for the awareness of security. Yet the awareness of security is a sensation of which we only become conscious when it is in jeopardy. It is the result of the adequate functioning of our sensory organization. But the sensory organization, a late acquisition in the course of embryological development is a superficially situated, very delicate, and easily injured apparatus. In contrast to this, the emotive system is difficult to put out of action as long as the subject is alive. It may be used therefore as an avenue of approach in reconditioning the organism and, eventually, in reestablishing a sense of security. This system lends itself to this process all the better because of its peculiar readiness to accept conditioning.

This point of view enables us to achieve a better understanding of the etiology and of the treatment of psychosis and of neurotic imbalance. We have only to remember the recent advances in the treatment of psychosis. Without wishing to give a theory of the shock therapies, I think it is safe to state that all these modern methods attack the emotive system. The mildest of them is the malaria therapy, which, with its shaking chills creates a marked revulsion of autonomic balance. But the others, insulin, electric shock, metrazol, are increasingly severe interventions into the coenesthetic system, shaking it to its foundations. What they seem to lack is a specific coordination with the psychiatric condition to which they are applied and a specific connection with the causes of these conditions.

However, psychoanalysis, which does not attack the emotive system in this violent manner, also has proved its curative value in psychiatric conditions. Can it be that there exists a connection between the psychoanalytic method and a neurophysiological sector of the human body, such as the coenesthetic organization?

While the shock therapies attack the somatic components of the emotive system, we have to remember that this system is the bridge between the somatic and the psychic. One of its aspects comprises the autonomic, the visceral, and the postural functions, but the other aspect (as stressed by its name, the emotive system), manifests itself as affects and emotions, in other words, falls into what we consider to be the province of the unconscious.

The aim of a well-conducted analysis is to get into contact with the unconscious. The experienced analyst knows that the patient's intellectual understanding of the cause of a symptom will not cure him, that it has to be "affectively reexperienced." This means that the patient's understanding has to reach the emotive system *via* his affect. A proof of this fact is the frequency of emotive manifestations which accompany such insight.

During the early days of cathartic analysis Freud aimed solely at the emotive affective reaction. The introduction of transference analysis enabled us to find the coordination of symptoms and affects. The recent development of ego analysis and our understanding of defense mechanisms have further introduced into our treatment the possibility of combining the attack on the emotive system (that is on the id), with a conditioning and deconditioning process directed toward the ego. Thus we may formulate the aim of analytic treatment as the deconditioning of the emotive system, in so far as it has wrested autonomy from the control of the ego and functions as an intruder in the ego-sphere. Simultaneously with this deconditioning and with the help of the emotive system's dynamic leverage a reconditioning of the ego takes place. As Freud put it in the New Introductory Lectures: "Ego shall be where Id was."

We have made a series of assumptions which may seem hazardous. They will prove themselves if they are able to suggest new ways of approach for the treatment of psychiatric conditions. Should this be the case, our assumptions would offer the possibility of diversifying treatment according to the additional etiological factors we have introduced.

When we will be able to distinguish within the actual clinical picture the factors of environmental retardation from those of emotive etiology; when we will be able to gauge the lesion inflicted on the emotive system and the amount of reaction formation to this evoked in the sensory system—then the age-old controversy between the somatic and the psychic approach will have resolved itself to the benefit of the patient.

Summary

A division has been made within the whole of the human nervous system.

The central nervous system is divided into two parts called respectively the diacritic sensory organization and the coenesthetic emotive organization. The significance of this division for the approach to traumatic neuroses, to modern psychiatric therapy and to psychoanalytic theory is elaborated with the help of pathological phenomena observed in early infancy.

The Primal Cavity:
A Contribution to the Genesis of
Perception and Its Role for
Psychoanalytic Theory

In recent years, two forms of psychoanalytic approach to the phenomenon of sleep have claimed our interest. I am referring to Lewin's (1946, 1948) interpretative and reconstructive work on the dream screen, on one hand, and to Isakower's (1938) clinical observations on the psychopathology of going to sleep, on the other. It is my belief that these two studies cover two aspects, and, beyond this, two stages of a regressive phenomenon, which has its counterpart in ontogenetic development. The regressive phenomena described by Lewin and by Isakower fall into the area of "normal" psychological functioning. The developmental data which I shall present in what follows, will serve to retrace the same process in the opposite, in the progressive direction. I hope to show that the dream screen hypothesis of Lewin and the clinical observation of Isakower have their parallel in the independent findings of direct infant observation and in the neurophysiology of perception. The convergence of the three lines of research, Isakower's, Lewin's, and my own, is noteworthy. Each started from a different point and, using different approaches, yields findings which are mutually explanatory. I have first spoken of such convergences in a communication on "Experimental Design" (Spitz, 1950c) and stated that in psychoanalysis such a convergence can occupy the place which validation has in experimental psychology.

THE DREAM SCREEN AND THE ISAKOWER PHENOMENON

Lewin's hypothesis takes as its starting point Freud's statement that the dream is the guardian of sleep. The fundamental wish-fulfilling nature of the dream ensures the continuation of sleep. In this function the dream is the manifestation of a regression to the emotional state of the infant when it goes to sleep at the mother's breast after having drunk his fill. Certain of his patients' dreams appeared as if projected onto a screen which, Lewin holds,

Reprinted from *The Psychoanalytic Study of the Child*, Vol. 10. New York: International Universities Press, 1955, pp. 215–240.

is the visual memory of the breast. He further assumes that this dream-screen-breast is always present in dreaming; that in the "blank dream" it actually is the dream content. He connects these findings with his other proposition, that of the oral triad of the wish to eat, to be eaten, to sleep (to die).

Isakower's contribution is the clinical observation that some of his patients, when in the reclining position, particularly when subject to elevation of temperature, or in the predormescent state, have certain sensations which partake of the mouth, of the skin surface, and of the hand sensitivity. The somewhat vague sensations are of something wrinkled, or perhaps gritty and dry, soft, filling the mouth, being felt at the same time on the skin surface of the body and being manipulated with the fingers. Visually the sensation is perceived as shadowy, indefinite, mostly round, approaching and growing enormous and then shrinking to practically nothing.

Lewin's and Isakower's observations have proved extraordinarily fertile both clinically and theoretically. The clinical observations of numerous analysts, including myself, have confirmed their findings.

When, however, I confronted Lewin's hypothesis with the findings of my own research on perceptive development, a difficulty arose. Lewin's description of the dream screen has a perceptive aspect and an affect aspect. We will begin with the discussion of the perceptive aspect, for since Freud's earliest writings perception has been rarely explored by psychoanalysts.

THE BEGINNINGS OF PERCEPTION

Both Lewin and Isakower state that the phenomena described by them are based on the memory of what they consider to be the first visual percept, namely, the mother's breast. My own work on the earliest stages of perception, conducted by the method of direct observation on infants, led me to experimental findings which at first appear to contradict their conclusion. In agreement with the statements of the academic psychologists Volkelt (1929), Hetzer and Ripin (1930), Rubinow and Frankl (1934), and Kaila (1932), I came to the conclusion that the first visual percept is the human face; to be more exact, it is a Gestalt configuration *within* the human face.

This first visual percept cannot be achieved at birth. It is progressively developed in the course of the first three months and is reliably perceived, and reacted to as such, in the course of the third month of life. I have elaborated these findings in my experimental study "The Smiling Response" (1946d and the 1948 film), in which I have also shown experimentally that at this period no other visual percept is recognized or reacted to in the same reliable manner as the human face.

This is a decisive turning point in the development of the psyche during the first year of life. It is the turning from passive reception to active perception, and accordingly I have called it, in analogy to an embryological concept, an "organizer" of psychological development. We will come back later to some of the details of this phenomenon.

The period prior to the crystallization of this first visual percept has been described by Hartmann (1939) and Anna Freud (1952a) as the period of *undifferentiation*, by myself as that of *nondifferentiation*. The term nondifferentiation should be understood in a global, total sense: on one hand, the infant does not distinguish what is "I" from what is "non-I," the self from the nonself, let alone the constituent elements of his environment. On the other hand, his own faculties, be they modalities of feeling, of sensation, of emotion, are not differentiated from one another; finally, no differentiation within the psychic system or even between the psyche and soma can be demonstrated. A case in point is the phenomenon of the so-called "overflow" in the newborn.

The subsequent differentiation is a progressive one, maturational on one hand, developmental on the other. It is in the course of the first three months, more or less beginning after the sixth week, that we can detect experimentally certain areas in which the infant begins to distinguish visual percepts. The first such percept to which it reacts is the human face. Toward the middle of the second month of life, the infant begins to follow the movement and displacement of the human face. Later, after about ten weeks, he responds to the human face with a differentiated manifestation of emotion, that of smiling.

With these observational facts in mind, let us now imagine the perceptual world of the infant before differentiation has begun; to achieve this, it is well to project ourselves backward to the memories of our own childhood and to realize how gigantic every remembered street, house, garden, piece of furniture appears in our memory; and how, if we happen to see it again 20 years later, it seems, surprisingly, to have shrunk.

This shrinkage of remembered impressions is due to the increase of our own size, for man is the measure of all things. Considering that the infant's face is one-third the size of the adult's face, and that the infant's whole length at birth is little more than one-quarter that of the adult, one begins to realize how gigantic the adult appears to the infant.

Swift illustrates this in *Gulliver's Travels,* a point mentioned by Freud (1900, p. 30); Lewin (1953a) refers again and again to this distortion of the infant's perception. The distortion is even more accentuated through the fact that the perceptive angle of the infant's vision, when approached by an adult, has to be an extremely wide one—we do not usually see people as close as the infant sees them. Lewin did not overlook this; he speaks of the "diplopic, amblyopic baby, with its weak powers of accommodation and its confused depth and color perceptions'' (1953b, p. 183). (See also Margolin, 1953.)

We can assume that the baby, if indeed it perceives anything, perceives moving, shifting, gigantic, vaguely colored and even more vaguely contoured inchoate masses. In the midst of this chaos certain of these shifting masses reappear periodically and are associated with certain recurrent sensations, feelings, emotions. They become associated, in short, with need satisfaction.

It is at this point that my observations on infants appear to contradict both Lewin's and Isakower's assumptions. The reason for this divergence is a twofold one; one has already been mentioned: namely, that the fiirst percept to be crystallized out of the shifting nebular masses in the world of the baby is the human face. The second is an easily demonstrable fact which can be checked by anyone who takes the trouble to observe a nursing baby. The nursing baby does not look at the *breast*. He does not look at the breast when the mother is approaching him, nor when she is offering him the breast, nor when he is nursing. He stares unwaveringly, from the beginning of the feeding to the end of it, at the mother's face.

Therefore, I offer the proposition that the Isakower phenomenon does not represent the approaching breast—at least not from the visual point of view. In my opinion it represents the visually perceived human face. All the phenomena, all the details described in Isakower's and Lewin's examples, as well as in those provided by other analysts, are to be found in the human face. The cracks, the wrinkles, the roses, the spots—but let Gulliver in Brobdingnag speak: "Their skins appeared so coarse and uneven, so variously colored when I saw them near, with a mole here and there as broad as a trencher, and hairs hanging from it thicker than pack threads, to say nothing further concerning the rest of their persons'' (Swift).

It would seem that the facts of perceptive development cannot be reconciled with either Isakower's or Lewin's assumptions. Such is not my opinion; on the contrary, I believe that my findings, and the observable data of perceptive development, actually form the bridge between the Isakower phenomenon and the Lewin propositions, and round them off in certain aspects. The real point of juncture is to be found in the observation that the infant, while nursing at the breast, is at the same time staring at the mother's face; thus breast and face are experienced as one and indivisible.

It should be remembered that at birth the newborn perceives only sensations originating *within* his body. He is protected from outside perceptions by the stimulus barrier. How, then, does the turning from inner stimuli to outer perception, be it even of the inchoate kind described earlier, come about? It seems to me that the present state of our knowledge permits the following proposition:

We possess one localized perceptual zone which includes in itself both the characteristics of interior and exterior perception. From birth on and even before (Minkowski, 1924-1925, 1928; Hooker, 1942, 1943), a readiness for response to stimulation can be demonstrated in and around the mouth. This behavior is of an aim-directed nature. We may, with Konrad Lorenz (1950), call the readiness underlying this response an *innate releasing mechanism, an IRM*. Like all IRM's, it has survival value.[1] The resulting behavior consists in the following: The whole outside part of the mouth region, of the "snout" (nose, cheeks, chin, and lips), responds to stimulation by a turning of the head toward the stimulus, combined with a snapping movement of the mouth. The function of this response is to take the nipple into the mouth.

We call this behavior the sucking reflex. Though it can be elicited by appropriate stimulation in the fetus and even in the embryo, at birth it is unreliable like all innate behavior in man. In reflexological terms, it is neither stimulus-specific nor response-specific; that means that it does not *always* take place in response to the stimulation of the snout, nor does it *only* take place in response to the stimulation of the snout.

But despite this comparative unreliability it is one of the most reliable responses at birth. Its reliability is second only to that of the clutch reflex, which is the closing of the hand on palmar stimulation; in the same order of reliability as the clutch reflex is its antagonist, described by me under the name of the *digital stretch reflex* (Spitz, 1950b) which consists in the stretching of the fingers on dorsal stimulation of the phalanges. It is noteworthy that sucking and clutching—the two archaic responses which show directed behavior and which are far and away more reliable than all others at this period—are to be found in connection with the hand and the mouth; and, moreover, that they are both directed to an action of "taking into," as it were. It is surely significant that the regression in the Isakower phenomenon concerns the selfsame organs, the hand and the mouth.

One may speculate on the question of whether the unreliability of these responses may have its cause in the fact that they are provoked by stimuli originating on the outside of the body, so that they impinge on the sensorium, which at this stage is not yet cathected. But, as we have stressed before,

[1] IRM (innate releasing mechanism) is a concept introduced by animal ethologists (Uexküll, Lorenz). The concept has hardly ever been defined in the literature, except in terms of the releasing stimulus. An exception to this is an attempt made by Tinbergen (1950, p. 309). The approximate definition given by Tinbergen elsewhere (1951) will suffice: "There must be a special neurosensory mechanism that releases the reaction and is responsible for this selective susceptibility to a very special combination of sign stimuli. This mechanism we will call the Innate Releasing Mechanism (IRM)" (p. 42). We may complete it by a definition given by Baerends (1950): "The mechanism beginning at the sense organs, ending at the center released and including the sensitivity for characteristics of the object, we will call the releasing mechanism" (p. 338).

reception of inner stimuli is already present at this stage. Accordingly, we have next considered a stimulation which involves simultaneously both the outside and the inside. Such a stimulation takes place when the nipple is placed *inside* the newborn's mouth. In view of what we have said above, it is not surprising that this stimulation elicits a much more reliable response at this period; the response consists in sucking and in the concomitant process of deglutition.

What appears to me significant in this phenomenon is that the *inside* of the mouth, *the oral cavity,* fulfills the conditions of partaking for perceptive purposes both of the inside and of the outside. It is simultaneously an interoceptor and exteroceptor. It is here that all perception will begin; in this role the oral cavity fulfills the function of a bridge from internal reception to external perception.

Both Isakower and Lewin have included some of these ideas into their reconstructive approach to the problem. Isakower has assumed that the combination of the oral cavity with the hand corresponds to the model of what he defines as the earliest postnatal ego structure, and that the sensations of the oral cavity are probably unified with those of the external cutaneous covering.

Lewin (1953b) in his "Reconsideration of the Dream Screen," quotes Dr. Rogawsky to the effect "that the original cavity might well be the inside of the mouth, as discovered and perceived by the suckling's finger. Accordingly, the earliest impression of the mouth would serve as a prototype of all later ideas of body cavities."

I would agree with this formulation, but would make it more specific. It is misleading, in my opinion, to speak of the suckling's finger discovering or perceiving anything. At this early stage (the first weeks of life) the organ in which precursors of perceptions are received is the oral cavity and not the finger. We have, therefore, to consider rather what the oral cavity perceives when something—in the case suggested by Dr. Rogawsky, the finger—is introduced into it. Even earlier than this, the nipple, and the jet of milk coming from it, have acted as the earliest postnatal liberators from thirst. How enduring the memory of the unpleasure of thirst is can be seen from the repetitive mentioning of the gritty, sandy sensation in Isakower's examples.

To me this finding is not surprising. I have stressed again and again in the last 20 years that speaking of hunger in the newborn and infant is a misnomer. The sufferings of hunger are not comparable to thirst, nor do they occur in response to as brief a deprivation as those of thirst. We are all too prone to forget that at birth the infant shifts from the life of a water dweller to that of a land animal. During the intrauterine period his mouth cavity, larynx, etc., were constantly bathed in the amniotic liquid. After delivery a continuous stream of air will dry out the mucosa with great rapidity, particularly since the salivary glands begin to function only many weeks later. This drying out of the mucosa will cause all the discomfort sensations of a dry mouth, throat, nasal passages, etc., connected with thirst; and not with hunger. Thirst, or rather dryness of this area, will therefore be one of the first experiences of discomfort in the infant.

But the experience of relief from unpleasure through the nipple which fills the newborn's mouth (remember the disparity of sizes!), and the milk streaming from it, is only one part of the picture, a passive experience. The act of sucking and of deglutition is the infant's first active coordinated muscular action. The organs involved are the tongue, the lips and the cheeks. Accordingly, these are also the muscles which are the first ones to be brought under control, a fact which makes the later smiling response possible.

Similarly these will be the first surfaces used in tactile perception and exploration. They are particularly well suited for this purpose because in this single organ, the mouth cavity, are assembled the representatives of several of the senses in one and the same area. These senses are the sense of touch, of taste, of temperature, of smell, of pain, but also the deep sensibility involved in the act of deglutition. Indeed, the oral cavity lends itself as no other region of the body to bridge the gap between inner and outer perception.

True, the quality of this perception is a contact perception, not a distance perception like the visual one. Hence, a further transition has to occur from tactile to visual perception.

I have already mentioned one factor in this transition: the fact that the nursing infant stares unwaveringly at the mother's face as soon as his eyes are open. We have to add to this a second factor, namely, the maturational and developmental level of the infant's sensory equipment, including the central nervous system on one hand, the psychological development on the other, during the first weeks and months of life, previously characterized as the stage of nondifferentiation. Stimulation occurring in one system of the body is responded to in others. Overflow is the rule of the hour. We may again advance a hypothesis: when the infant nurses and has sensations in the oral cavity while staring at the mother's face, he unites the tactile and the visual perceptions, the perceptions of the total situation, into one undifferentiated unity, a situation Gestalt, in which any one part of the experience comes to stand for the total experience.

The Modality of Primal Perception and Its Three Subsidiary Organs

It has become evident in the course of this discussion that this first experience of the baby is not a simple one. We had to expand our approach to the genesis of perception by including in it emotional qualities, those of pleasure and unpleasure, as well as dynamic qualities, namely activity and passivity. That, however, is inevitable in all developmental research, as I have shown elsewhere (Spitz, 1946d), because affects are the initiators of all perception, emotional development its trailbreaker, indeed the trailbreaker of development in all sectors, hence also dynamic development.

Obviously the source of these affects of the infant is a physiological one, a need. As Freud (1915a) stated, the drives originate at the dividing line between the soma and the psyche. It is the need which produces the tension that is expressed by the affective manifestations of unpleasure. It is the need gratification which leads to tension reduction and quiescence. This dynamic process activates the first intraoral perceptions, which take place on a dividing line again, that between inside and outside.

The site of the origin of perception and of psychological experience has far-reaching consequences. For it is here that the task of distinguishing between inside and outside has its inception; this discrimination becomes established much later and will lead in an unbroken development to the separation of the self from the nonself, of the self from the objects, and in the course of this road to what is accepted and what is rejected (Freud, 1925a). I might mention in passing that the time necessarily elapsing between the arising of the need and the reduction of tension introduces a further element into our picture, that of the capacity to wait, the capacity to tolerate tension or, in a term recently become fashionable, that of frustration tolerance.

The particular anatomical location and physiological function of the oral cavity enables it to distinguish the outside from the inside. This leads us to a qualification of a generally accepted psychoanalytic proposition stressed by both Isakower and Lewin. It is correct that the breast is the first object; it is probable that the breast, or rather the nipple, forms a part of the first percept; but direct observation proves that the breast definitely is not the first *visual* percept.[2] This is because at this earliest stage of life *distance* perception is not operative, but only *contact* perception. It is of special interest to our discussion to examine what organs besides the oral cavity are involved in the contact perceptions of the nursing situation. Three such organs are in evidence from birth.

1. Of the three, the most evident is the hand. Its participation in the nursing act is obvious to every observer. At birth this participation is in the nature of overflow; the sensorium of the hand is not cathected as yet, as shown by Halverson's experiments (1937). He found that the clutch reflex on palmar

---

[2] *Percept,* the thing perceived, should be clearly distinguished from *object* (libidinal); the latter originates through the focusing of a constellation of drives onto a percept. Perception of the percept is the prerequisite of object formation.

stimulation is reliably elicited when tendons in the palm are stimulated—a stimulation of deep sensibility—and was unreliable on cutaneous stimulation. The activity of the hands during nursing, when both hands find their support on the breast, consists in a continuous movement of the fingers which clutch, stroke, claw, and scratch on the breast. This activity will accompany the nursing process consistently during the subsequent months. It will become more and more organized, probably as a function of the progressive cathexis of the hand's sensorium. We can imagine the development as beginning with an activity of the mouth, overflowing into the hand; at a somewhat later stage this is proprioceptively perceived and, when the sensorium is cathected, also exteroceptively. This early coordination of mouth and hand function and its progressive development is in agreement with the embryological and neurobiological finding that maturation proceeds in a cephalocaudal direction.[3]

2. The second organ which participates in the nursing situation is less evident. It is the labyrinth. Both Isakower and Lewin speak of the frequent presence of dizziness, murmur and noise in the phenomena they describe. This finding is supported by direct observation on the newborn. It has been shown experimentally that the stimulus which leads to the earliest conditioned response in the newborn is a change of equilibrium. The experiment consists in the following: If, after about eight days of life, the breast-fed infant is lifted from his cot and placed in the nursing position, he will turn his head toward the person holding him and will open his mouth. It is immaterial whether the person in question is male or female. What does this experiment show, what is the sensory organ involved in this reaction of the newborn?

When we lift the newborn from his cot and place him in the nursing position, we set in motion in the labyrinth a neurophysiological process of a very special nature. This process is a gravity-induced shift of the endolymph within the labyrinth, resulting in two sensory stimulations of a completely different nature in two spatially separate parts of one and the same organ. The pressure of the endolymph on the lining of the semicircular canals results in changes of the equilibrium sensation; the same pressure will simultaneously provoke auditory sensations in the organ of Corti in the cochlea. The morphological difference between the lining of the semicircular canals and that of the cochlea is responsible for the difference between the two resulting sensations. The sensations connected with the stimulation of the semicircular canals will be

---

[3] Hoffer discusses the relationship between hand and mouth in two articles. In the first (1949) he investigates the function of the hand in ego integration and in the development of early ego functions. His conclusions are in accordance with the above statements; but they deal with a later stage than the cavity perception described by me. In his second article (1950), he introduces a new concept, that of the "mouth-self" which is progressively extended to the "body-self" through the activity of the hand which libidinizes various parts of the body. This process also occurs at a later stage than the one discussed in my present article.

dizziness and vertigo, those connected with the stimulation of the Corti organ will be auditory, probably vague, rushing, murmuring, roaring noises which may be similar to the sensations described by Isakower and Lewin (see also French, 1929; Scott, 1948; Rycroft, 1953). We can then envisage that the newborn experiences the being lifted into the nursing position as an interoceptively[4] perceived experience with all the vagueness, diffuseness and absence of localization that is characteristic of prothopathic sensation.

3. The third organ involved is the outer skin surface. Isakower's as well as Lewin's descriptions emphasize the vagueness of the localization. Isakower speaks of the big and then again small "something," gritty, sandy, dry, which is experienced both in the mouth and on the skin surface, simultaneously or alternately; it is experienced like a blurring of widely separated zones of the body. I believe that we do not have to postulate intrauterine memories here. It seems to me rather that this is the echo of an experience that is analogous to that of thirst in the mouth—only that it involves the skin surface instead. Up to delivery the skin surface had been in the least irritating and most sheltering environment imaginable. It was surrounded by liquid and protected even against this by vernix caseosa. After delivery it is exposed to the roughness, unevenness, dryness of the textiles into which we wrap babies. It is inevitable that the stimulation due to these textiles will be infinitely sharper than we adults can imagine; that it will take quite a long time, weeks and months, until the newborn's skin has adjusted to these stimuli and toughened sufficiently to relegate them to the normal environmental background.[5]

It might be assumed that to the newborn the sensations of skin discomfort are indistinguishable from discomfort in the passages of mouth, nose, larynx, and pharynx. From our knowledge of the nondifferentiation in the perceptive sectors (and all others) this must indeed be so.

The sensations of the three organs of perception—hand, labyrinth, and skin cover—combine and unite with the intraoral sensations to a unified situational experience in which no part is distinguishable from the other. This perceptive experience is inseparable from that of the need gratification occurring si-

---

[4] In the following I will speak of interoceptors and interoceptive systems, using the definition given by Fulton (1938) and Sherrington (1906): "The interoceptors are divided into two groups: (1) the proprioceptors (muscles and labyrinth) and (2) the visceroceptors (gut, heart, blood vessels, bladder, etc.)."

[5] Two highly pertinent papers of M. F. Ashley Montagu (1950, 1953) came to my attention too late to incorporate his findings into the present paper. Basing himself on some theoretical considerations, and on a series of observations on nonhuman animals (Hammett, 1922; Reyniers, 1946, 1949), he concludes that the skin as an organ has a hitherto unsuspected functional significance for physiological and psychological development. Laboratory evidence indicates that in the nonhuman mammals the licking of the young by the mother activates the genitourinary, the gastrointestinal, and the respiratory systems. Some evidence is offered that matters may be, if not similar, at least analogous in man (Drillien, 1948; Lorand and Asbot, 1952).

multaneously and leading through extensive tension reduction from a state of excitement with the quality of unpleasure to quiescence without unpleasure. We do not postulate any memory traces, be they even unconscious, of this situational percept of the newborn. Whether engrams are laid down at this stage also remain unanswerable.[6] But this selfsame situational experience, repeated again and again, will many weeks later eventually merge with the first visual percept and be present simultaneously with it, remaining attached to it in first unconscious and later conscious visual imagery.

The cluster of factors which go into the nursing experience of the newborn therefore can be enumerated as follows:

1. The psychophysiological factors of unpleasurable tension and its reduction through nursing.

2. A factor which in due time will become a psychological one, that of activity.

3. The neurophysiological perceptive factors of the oral experience of sucking and deglutition involving a number of proprioceptive sense organs situated within the mouth.

4. Simultaneous sensory experiences of the hand and of the outer skin.

5. Simultaneous interoceptive experiences in the labyrinth.

THE ACHIEVEMENT OF DISTANCE PERCEPTION

On reflection it must be evident that the majority of these factors—with the one exception of skin discomfort—belong to, or at least are very close to, perceptions of changes going on in the inside of the neonate, that is, proprioceptive perceptions. Even in regard to the hand we may assume that the movements do not represent a response to a tactile sensation, but an overflow into the hand musculature of the innervation of the nursing and deglutition activity. As for the labyrinth sensations, these belong patently to the coenesthetic (protopathic) system and share with this the diffuseness, vagueness, and lack of localization.

We have to stress again that the whole experience with all its percepts and sensations is centered inside or linked up with the oral cavity and belongs to the modality of contact perception. That modality must also be postulated for the perceptions of the labyrinth which originate on the inside of the body. This contact perception, taking place *inside* of the body, is the crystallization

---

[6] It is perhaps useful to remind ourselves in this context (and also in reference to the dream screen and to the Isakower phenomenon) that from the beginning Freud (1900) stated that the first mnemonic traces could only be established in function of an experience of satisfaction which interrupts the excitation arising from an internal need. This experience of satisfaction puts an end to the internal stimulus (p. 565).

point for the first modality of the perceptive process and is secured with the help of the endlessly repetitive experience of the unpleasure-pleasure cycle.

In the course of maturation, a second modality appears—distance perception in the form of the first visual percepts. Through the baby's unwavering stare at the mother's face during nursing the visual experience is merged into the total experience. The infant still does not distinguish inside from outside, what he sees with his eyes from what he feels with his mouth.

A large number of disappointing experiences—namely, waiting periods intruding between the perception of mother's face and the lowering of need tension through food in the mouth—are required before a differentiation between the two can take place. Until that occurs, mother's face—not the visual percept of mother's breast!—will mean "food in the mouth" and relief from unpleasure. It can be experimentally proved that at this stage—the third month of life—the visual percept of the maternal breast produces no change whatever in the hungry baby's behavior.

That much of this applies to the hand and its sensations, is obvious. After all, the simultaneous activity of the baby's hand during nursing is familiar to every mother. We may assume that also in the hand it is not so much the tactile percept which is connected with the intraoral experience, but rather a proprioceptive percept, that of the contraction and relaxation of the hand muscles which is perceived in the same manner as the contractions of the oral muscles in sucking. That something of the kind must be taking place can be shown in motion pictures, where it is amply evident that in the nursing baby the closure of the hand is performed in the same rhythm as the sucking movement of the mouth. The "taking into" quality of these hand movements appears to me to justify the proposition that they are experienced by the infant as belonging to the sucking movements of the mouth. Perhaps we are justified in expanding this proposition to the child's coenesthetic sensations. When the child is lifted and cradled in the mother's arms, pressed against her body and held securely during the act of nursing, it comes near to the blissful intrauterine state in which need tension never arose and the insecurity of our modern baby cot with its lack of support was unknown.

An excellent illustration of all that I have discussed above has been provided to me through the courtesy of a colleague from Havana, Dr. Carlos Acosta (personal communication, 1955). In the course of the analysis of an adult patient, Dr. Acosta noted a number of unusual dreams, hallucinatoryform visions and similar manifestations, of which I will quote a few.

Case O. V. Twenty-one-year-old white male. He came into treatment because of overt homosexuality. He is an extremely infantile individual, given to day-dreaming which borders on the hallucinatory, with an I.Q. of 74. Both the testing psychologist and Dr. Acosta agree that the patient's I.Q. actually is higher and that the test situation is distorted through the patient's emotional difficulties. It was not possible to determine whether he is a case of arrested development or whether his symptomatology is the consequence of a regression; I would lean toward the former.

Four communications of the patient which bear on our discussion follow:

1. The patient visits his girl. Sitting next to her he falls asleep and on awakening he peeks into her décolleté and sees "the breast cloudy, with spots, like a glass from which milk was poured out, the glass remaining covered with a film of milk, forming spots," which he compares to *"manchas en mujeres embarazadas"* ("chloasmata in pregnant women").

2. Lying on the couch during treatment he hallucinates as follows: "There is a piece of white bread, shaped like a pear, with its point toward me, approaching me, coming closer and getting bigger. . . . Funny, now it has jumped suddenly to my thumb and is much smaller."

3. The patient reports on another day that the previous morning the chore of boiling the breakfast milk filled him with resentment because while the milk was on the fire, he was masturbating and indulging in fantasies, but worried that the milk would boil over. In his masturbatory fantasy he imagined that he was having intercourse with his girl and was sucking her breast. He associated the milk boiling over in the pot with that coming out of the girl's breast and with the sperm spurting out of his penis. In this fantasy part of the sperm was going into the vagina (and spurting out of the breasts), another part was splashing onto the floor.

4. When confronted with maternal-looking women, he gets a peculiar sensation when they look at him. He feels the inside of his mouth contracting [Analyst's note: like a contraction of the buccal and labial musculature], and he associates to this a "displeasure" in the stomach, like heat or emptiness. He had the same feeling in his mouth when he hallucinated the "clouded breast" vision of his fantasy. The contraction of his mouth muscles forces him to turn away and hide his face from such a maternal woman, because he does not want her to see him making faces. He remembers that he had this feeling as a very small child when mother carried him in her arms at her breast from one room to another; he also remembers the feeling of dizziness and nausea. This he has also at present when riding on a bus and "the air rushes into his mouth." The circumstances leading to his mouth sensations often also provoke similar sensations in the inside of the belly, which then contracts in the way the inside of the mouth contracted.

CONSIDERATIONS SUGGESTED BY THE CASE MATERIAL

In the various dreams and observations reported by Lewin and Isakower as well as by an ever-increasing number of analysts who in the meantime have written on the subject, a large number of the constituent elements of the picture we are concerned with can be found in one place or another. Some of these elements belong to dreams and normal states, others are found in pathological conditions. The case described by Dr. Acosta seems to bring together in one and the same individual all these elements. I feel, therefore, that it makes further examples repetitive because it is sufficiently representative of the large body of observations published on the subject.

Communications No. 1 and 2 describe phenomena which are strikingly similar to and in some particulars even more vivid than those reported by Isakower. That the patient brings together the breast-shaped object with his thumb, has particular significance for our further remarks. It impresses me as an example of the mode of operation of what, for want of a better term, we have to call the ''psyche'' in early infancy; this ''psyche'' causes different percepts with similar functions to be merged into one another; this merging is the result of a lack of differentiation. In the example quoted above thumb sucking and nursing have the same function, namely to release tension. The percepts are different, but the function is identical.

But Communication No. 4 suggests conclusions which are more far-reaching. Here sensations in the oral cavity, which refer to subliminal mnemic traces of the nursing situation, are brought into relation by the patient with sensations within the abdomen, on the one hand, envelopment in the mother's arms and body, on the other.[7]

In the case of Dr. Acosta's patient, the hand and simultaneously the equilibrium sensation (both in the ''being carried'' memory) as well as the intra-abdominal sensation are combined with the intraoral experience (French, 1929; Rycroft, 1953). It is this summative aspect of the nursing experience which has motivated me to speak of the inside of the mouth as the primal cavity. I believe that the data provided by the reports of Dr. Acosta's patient rather convincingly substantiate the opinion held by Isakower, Lewin, and myself: intrauterine fantasies at a later age are based on a regressive imagery of early intraoral experience.

The patient's description bears out what I had postulated earlier: the oral

---

[7] Two points are worth mentioning, although they do not belong into the framework of the present article. One is O. V.'s sensations of muscular contractions of his mouth region, which he associates with fantasies connected with the breast, with breast-feeding and with seeing ''maternal-looking women.'' He is so intensely conscious of these contractions that he has to avert his head for fear that ''the woman may notice that he is making faces.'' This suggests that the *Schnauzkrampf* symptom in the schizophrenic may be connected with wishful fantasies of breast-feeding and with the mnemic traces of the proprioceptive percept of mouth activity during nursing.

The other point is that, when the patient travels on a bus and ''the air rushes into his mouth,'' he has a feeling of dizziness and nausea. He says that this feeling is like the feeling he had as a very small child when his mother carried him in her arms at her breast from one room to another. We may well add this finding to Freud's assumptions on the origin of flying in dreams (1900, pp. 271 ff.; 393 ff.) on one hand, on the other to his hypotheses on the production of sexual excitation (1905b, p. 201). In the latter he specifically states that the stimulus of rhythmic mechanical agitation of the body operates in three different ways: on the sensory apparatus of the vestibular nerves, on the skin, and on the muscles and articular structures. He even mentions the impact of moving air on the genitals. He connects these childhood experiences with later developing train phobias. The contribution of Dr. Acosta's patient appears not only to confirm fully Freud's findings, but to add to them the information that the origin of the multiform traveling phobias may reach back to the nursing period of the infant in the first year of life.

cavity, in which the interoceptive and exteroceptive perceptive systems are united, forms the basis of a perceptive mode (we might call it "perception according to the cavity mode"), in which inside and outside is interchangeable and in which furthermore a variety of other sensations and perceptions find their focus.

It may be added here that this early intraoral experience consists of taking into oneself the breast while being enveloped by the mother's arms and breasts. The grown-up conceives of this as two separate experiences. But for the child they are one experience, single and inseparable, without differences between the constituting parts, and each constituting part being able to stand for the whole of the experience. This is essentially the paradigma of Lewin's formulation: "to eat and to be eaten." It is a most vivid example of the mode of functioning of the primary process.

PERCEPTION OF ENVIRONMENT VERSUS PERCEPTION OF SOMATIC EXPERIENCE

There are certain aspects in the preceding discussion which are reminiscent of the brilliant, but in part erroneous, speculations of Silberer. Lewin has referred to them, and stressed how misleading many of his concepts were. In one of Silberer's articles, "Symbolik des Erwachens und Schwellensymbolik überhaupt" (1911), he states the symbolic imagery can express two things, content and the state or the functioning of the psyche. I believe that in my foregoing discussion it has become evident that his assumption has to be revised and that the infant's as well as Dr. Acosta's patient's experience can be separated into two perceptual aspects:

1. The aspect of perception mediated to us by our sensorium. This is the perception of the outside, the perception of things and events.

2. The second aspect is that of the perception of states and of functions; not, however, the states and functions of the psychic apparatus of which Silberer speaks, but rather the states and functions of the musculature, of joints, of position—in other words, an interoceptive perception. Dr. Acosta's patient describes a few of these perceptions of states and functions; I postulate their existence in the first period of nursing and probably, in a progressively decreasing measure, throughout the first year of life.

These two perceptive aspects, however, do not encompass the totality of the experience. We have already stressed several times that an instinctual gratification is connected with it. This implies the presence of affects and emotions of some kind, which provide the percept with its valency and with the quality of an experience. In the adult, affects may evoke visual imagery or, vice versa, visual imagery may evoke affects; but the two, affect and visual imagery, originate at two different stages in the infant's development. One may speculate whether the percept activates also the arousal function of the reticular system which, according to Linn (1953), is capable of mobilizing further affects.

LEVELS OF INTEGRATION AND PERCEPTUAL FUNCTION

We can now examine the degrees of regression attained in the dream screen described by Lewin and in the Isakower phenomenon. In dreaming, we relinquish the level of the verbal symbolic function and regress to the level of symbolic imagery (Freud, 1917a).

In the infant, the level of imagery is presumably reached after the third month; that of verbal symbolic function, approximately around 18 months. According to our experimental observations, we may assume that somewhere from 3 to 18 months the infant perceives mainly in images and operates mentally with the memory traces laid down by visual percepts. It is around 18 months that verbal proficiency becomes sufficiently established, enabling the infant to begin to replace in his mental operations an increasing number of visual percepts by verbal symbols.

We believe that the infant passes in the course of his first two years through three stages, or, as we can call them also, through three levels of integration of increasing complexity.

1. The first level is that of the coenesthetic organization, when perception takes place in terms of totalities, because it is mediated mainly through the coenesthetic system on one hand, through interoceptive- and tango-receptors on the other.

2. The second level is that of diacritic perception, when distance receptors come into play, when visual images become available, but when the mnemic traces of these images are still impermanent, at least in the beginning. This is due to the fact that they are in the process of acquiring what Freud (1915b) calls in his article on the unconscious in a specific context *"topisch gesonderte Niederschriften"* ("topographically separated records").

3. The acquisition of language marks the inception of the third level of integration. This presupposes an ego development, the development of the abstractive capacity, called by Kubie (1953) the symbolic function.

In waking life adults operate on the last of the three, on the level of symbolic function. In dreams they normally regress to the level of visual perception and imagery. This is the level at which Lewin's dream screen can become perceivable.

In his paper "The Forgetting of Dreams," Lewin (1953a) with the help of a reconstructive procedure arrives at formulations closely resembling mine. He deduces logically that if a regression occurs from the visual imagery level at which the dream functions, then there should be memory traces older than these pictures. Thus, as I do, he sees these memory traces "more like pure emotion," made up of deeper tactile, thermal, and dimly protopathic qualities which are in their way "memory traces" of early dim consciousness of the breast or of the half-asleep state. And, if I read him correctly, he believes that it is to this level of integration that the subject regresses in the so-called blank dream.

It follows that the level of regression involved in the Isakower phenomenon harks back to an earlier period, that which precedes the reliable laying down of visual mnemic traces or at least to a period at which a significant number of visual mnemic traces has not yet been accumulated. I would be inclined to say that while the regression of the dream screen goes to the level of the mnemic traces laid down somewhere between the ages toward the end of the first half year and reaching to the end of the first year, in the Isakower phenomenon the regression reaches to the traces of experiences preceding this period. Obviously, these age ranges represent extremely wide approximations.

We may now examine the dream screen in the light of our assumptions. Following Freud, Lewin has pointed out that the dream itself already marks a disturbance of sleep. The function of the dream is to act as the guardian of sleep. The dream screen, which represents the breast, is derived from the infant's experience of going to sleep after nursing at the breast. This is exemplified by Dr. Acosta's patient who, when describing and reliving his hallucinatory experiences, frequently becomes drowsy and falls asleep on the couch. We might say that the dream screen described by Lewin is the achievement of a wish fulfillment, the gratification of a need, the symbolically used mnemic trace of satiated quiescence. The visual dream, on the other hand, is the symptom of the ego having become alerted to an extent sufficient to abolish the complete regression into dreamless sleep and to enforce a reversal of the regression to the level of visual perception, the level of three to eighteen months. The quality of satiated quiescence in the dream screen places the regression into the earlier part of this period.

It is not likely, however, that the dream screen is the visual image of the breast. It is much more probable that it is the result of a composite experience, which in the visual field represents the approaching face of the mother, but in the field of the other percepts involves the sensations within the oral cavity. This is perhaps also an explanation of the fact that in so many of the dream-screen reports the dream screen appears dark, at other times colorless, amorphous. Lewin actually speaks of the dream screen being like a composite Galtonian photograph in certain dreams—only he conceived this as a blending of different images of the breast. I would rather call it a synesthesia of many different senses, the visual constituent of which is derived from the percept of the face.

What, then, is the relationship between the blank dream discussed by Lewin and the Isakower phenomenon? Perhaps it replaces in the sleeping state what the Isakower phenomenon is in the predormescent and pathological states. The level of regression in the two phenomena is comparable. Lewin considers the regression a topographical one in the blank dream. In the light of our findings on infant development we may add that it is also a genetic regression (in the terms of Freud, 1917a, "a temporal or developmental regression"). It goes to a level which is earlier than the regression to the visual mnemic traces. It goes to the level at which mnemic traces were laid down in sensory modalities other than the visual ones.

This may provide the explanation of why the blank dream is devoid of visual content. We know from Freud and from our daily experience with patients that the dream operates primarily with visual images. It operates much more infrequently on the higher level of verbal symbols; Lewin mentions this and Isakower (1954) in particular has commented on the phenomenon in his paper "Spoken Words in Dreams." But the dream also has difficulties in representing emotional content as well as the mnemic traces which belong to the period in which they were not associated to imagery as yet. At that early period in life, emotional content of a very primitive nature and the mnemic traces of bodily functions were associated to the traces of coenesthetic functioning. It is in good accordance with this that when reporting blank dreams, the subjects comment on the tone of affect which accompanies it, whether that be an affect of happiness or one of terror. And the coenesthetic mnemic association is confirmed by the fact that in some cases the blank dream is accompanied by orgasm—in the case of one of my patients orgasm could only be achieved in a blank dream.

We now may follow Isakower in his careful discussion of the processes which take place in the ego when a regression to the phenomenon observed by him occurs. He postulated two such consequences: (1) A disintegration of the various parts of the ego and its functions. (2) A dedifferentiation of the ego.

Isakower describes, within the many-faceted process of going to sleep, one specific consequence of the disintegration of the ego. This is the change which takes place through the withdrawal of cathexis from the outward-directed sensorium and a concomitant increase of the cathexis of the body ego. This formulation of the going-to-sleep process (in the adult) has an exact counterpart in our observations on the way in which the newborn functions. The newborn is incapable of perceiving the outer world. This has been shown in numerous findings of experimental psychologists as well as in our own. The sensorium is not yet functioning because, in terms of the dynamic viewpoint, the newborn has not yet cathected it.

THE STIMULUS BARRIER AND THE DISTRIBUTION OF LIBIDINAL CATHEXIS

This experimental finding enables us to understand Freud's concept of the stimulus barrier from the economic and the dynamic viewpoint, from that of the distribution of cathexis. The stimulus barrier is not to be understood as an obstacle in the path of the reception of stimulation originating in the environment. It is to be understood as consisting in the *uncathected condition of the sensorium*. In other words, the receiving stations are not energized as yet.

Conversely, the totality of the available cathexis of the newborn is directed toward his own body, a state of which we speak as the primary narcissistic stage. Isakower assumes an overcathexis of the body ego in the sleeping adult. Whether in the newborn one can speak of an *absolute* overcathexis of his own body, is questionable. There can be no question, however, about the disproportion between the infinitesimal amount of cathexis directed by the newborn toward the sensorium as against the enormous amount of cathexis allotted to his own body. We may speculate on this disparity in the distribution of cathexis. In a way, this condition is a continuation of the intrauterine situation. During the intrauterine period the mother has two roles: first, that of protecting the foetus from danger. In this role she carries out all the sensory and action functions needed for the purposes of adaptation to the conditions of living. Her second role could be described as that of assimilation because she also performs all the embryo's metabolic and catabolic functions. But after birth, these two roles are redistributed. The protective role against outside stimulation which the mother had during the period of gestation will be continued, for she still has the task of performing for the newborn the function of the sensorium as well as those of the action system. However, she can no longer perform the newborn's metabolic functions as she did during pregnancy. To survive, the organism of the newborn has to take over these functions and has to cathect the interoceptive system for the purposes of metabolic functions. Accordingly, toward the own body there will be no stimulus barrier. Therefore the responses of the newborn are a function of the messages transmitted by the interoceptive system; but as there is no localization within the interoceptive system's reception, these messages will be undifferentiated. They will operate in terms of the economic viewpoint, that is, of the pleasure principle. Such perceptions of himself as the newborn receives are of a total or global nature and cannot be assigned to specific systems; therefore the motor apparatus will respond to them by diffuse, undirected excitation and overflow.

In the adult's falling asleep as described by Isakower we have the withdrawal of cathexis from the sensorium and the increased cathexis of the body ego. We may add to this that the motor pattern of the sleeping adult also approximates that of the newborn in its undirected responses. The basic difference between the adult and the newborn lies in the fact that while the adult cathects a body ego, an organized structure of body representations in the psyche, there is no such thing in the newborn. The newborn has still to develop the body ego, and what we witness in the newborn is not a withdrawal of cathexis but a nonexistence of cathexis.[8]

CATHEXIS AND PERCEPTUAL EGO FUNCTIONS

The falling apart of the ego functions in the adult as described by Isakower might be spoken of metaphorically as a consequence of a weakening of the cohesive forces of the ego, which is a result of the process of falling asleep. In the newborn these cohesive forces have still to come into being and are only developed as a function of the constitution of the ego. It is an attractive hypothesis to assume that when the ego is weakened, be it by the process of falling asleep or by pathological processes, one of the first attributes of the ego, its cohesive force, will be diminished and the cooperation of the ego constituents ceases; or, in terms of present-day communication theory, "intracommunication" becomes impossible (Cobliner, 1955).

The second consequence of the regression in the Isakower phenomenon is spoken of by him as a dedifferentiation of the ego. He believes that the dedifferentiation takes place somewhat later in the process of going to sleep than the dissociation of the ego components; therefore, when the body ego has arrived at this stage, when it is overcathected, it has reactivated an archaic developmental level. He stresses that on this archaic level perception is directed toward the process of the subject's own body, toward the changes in intracorporal tensions, and not toward the external stimuli which may provoke them. He mentions that in the waking adult this mode of perception remains in function in one organ only, the vestibular organ. There it is the perception of intracorporal changes informing us (and frequently in a very disagreeable

[8] It will be seen from this discussion that when I speak of the phase of nondifferentiation, I am referring to something much more inclusive and general than what Hartmann, Kris, and Loewenstein have described in "Comments on the Formation of Psychic Structure" (1946, p. 19). They refer specifically only to the absence of differentiation between the ego and the id, and the undifferentiated phase is the one in which both the id and the ego are gradually formed. My concept is much more closely allied to Hartmann's (1939) discussion of the same concept in *Ego Psychology and the Problem of Adaptation*.

manner, indeed!) of changes taking place in our surroundings. We have nothing to add to these propositions of Isakower. By and large, they have been paralleled by our preceding discussion of the new born's progressive development which corroborate his conclusions.

Freud (1915b) stated that affects and emotions represent our awareness of discharge processes. The intracorporal sensations of which we have spoken actually are discharge processes. This may be the reason for their close connection with affects and in particular with anxiety.

SUMMARY AND CONCLUDING REMARKS

We may summarize by saying that adults, who operate on the level of the symbolic function, will regress normally to the level of visual perception and imagery in the dream; it is at this level that Lewin's dream screen becomes perceivable. When a disturbance of going to sleep occurs, as in febrile disease, or when a dissociation of the ego in waking states takes place, then a further regression to the level of the coenesthetic perception may occur in which the Isakower phenomenon becomes available.

The level of coenesthetic perception belongs to what I would call the experiential world of the primal cavity. It is the world of the deepest security which man ever experiences after birth, in which he rests encompassed and quiescent. It is to this world that man escapes when he feels threatened by pathological conditions in febrile states; also when in the waking state the ego becomes helpless through dissociation, as in toxic conditions. The method of escape has a double mechanism: the withdrawal of cathexis from the sensorium, on one hand, the hypercathexis of the body ego, on the other. The particular sector of the body ego representation which seems most highly cathected is the representation of the primal cavity. This distribution of cathexis makes the experience of the Isakower phenomenon possible.

From the point of view of therapy these considerations underscore the necessity of understanding the patient in terms of earliest orality, as has been stressed repeatedly by Lewin. When we deal with the adult, however, the approach to earliest orality is not a direct one, for the mnemic traces of earliest primal cavity experiences as such are not available to the patient and cannot be communicated to him by the therapist in terms of these experiences—the terms for them do not exist in language, they can only be paraphrased. Many, but certainly not all mnemic traces of the primal cavity experiences are attached in the course of development to memory traces in the nature of images, acquired and mediated by the visual and by the auditive senses. Later still, in the course of the elaboration of the symbolic function, word representations will be attached to these images. This is the linkage between the memory traces of object representations and the memory traces of word representations. The therapist, in his therapeutic endeavor, has to travel this road in the inverse direction, from the abstractive word to the concrete representation that evoked the original affect.

A better understanding of the intraoral experience and of its ramifications into experiences of hand and skin surface suggests nonanalytical therapies in the case of the deeply regressed psychoses. Up to now such therapies have scarcely been attempted.[9]

The world of the primal cavity is a strange one: indistinct, vague, pleasurable and unpleasurable at the same time, it bridges the chasm between inside and outside, between passivity and action. The earliest sensory experiences of events taking place in the primal cavity are dealt with on the level of the primary process, yet they lead to the development of the secondary process.

In its nondifferentiation this world is the matrix of both introjection and projection, which therefore appear primarily normal phenomena, though we become really aware of their proliferation in pathological processes.

The perceptive modality of the primal cavity will also form the matrix for later developmental stages of perception in sensory organs with a very different function. The specific morphology of the particular organ will determine the mode of function—yet it will hark back to the inside-outside mode established by the intraoral experience, as for instance in the distinction between the "I" and the "non-I," the self and the nonself.

We may say in conclusion that the mouth as the primal cavity is the bridge between inner reception and outer perception; it is the cradle of all external perception and its basic model; it is the place of transition for the development of intentional activity, for the emergence of volition from passivity.

When, however, the body relaxes diurnally in the passivity of sleep, the

---

[9] This communication was already in the hands of the editor when Louis Linn's paper "Some Developmental Aspects of the Body Image" (1955) was published.

His remarks parallel in many aspects the views expressed in my present paper. He reports on M. Bender's recent experiments in simultaneous sensory stimulation of adults. Bender's findings (1952) corroborate our direct observations on perceptual development and function in infants and their psychological concomitants.

Bender investigated two simultaneous stimulations of the *same* sensory modality. Our own propositions refer to simultaneous experience of stimulation in *different* sensory modalities. Linn's own work also deals with the fusion of two sensory modalities into a single perceptual event. We are referring to the patient who, when touched simultaneously on face and hand, reported this as "the hand of my face." The reader will note the similarity between Linn's observation and the conclusions drawn by me on the blending into a single event of the contact percept and the visual distance percept in earliest infancy. I am inclined to assume that the body ego originates from the sensations experienced in the oral cavity. The latter are vastly predominant in earliest infancy. This is in agreement with Linn's ingenious hypothesis on hand-mouth identity and with his explanation of the scotomization of the hand in adult perception.

activity of the mind will retrace its way toward the primal process, and the primal cavity then becomes the cavernous home of the dreams.

Some Early Prototypes of Ego Defenses

Conflict and defense are among the most fundamental and important concepts introduced by Freud in his earliest psychoanalytic publications. He mentioned them already in the letters to Fliess; they remain the focus of our attention to this day. Freud continued refining these concepts and, speaking of the instinct being turned back on the ego and of the instinct undergoing reversal from activity to passivity, he remarked: "Perhaps they represent attempts at defense which, at higher stages of the development of the ego, are effected by other means" (1915a, p. 132).

Here a development of the defenses from a more primitive to a more organized stage is clearly suggested. Subsequently this suggestion was taken up by other authors, beginning with Anna Freud's (1936) discussion of the chronological sequence of defense mechanisms. In 1939, Hartmann started exploring some of the early physiological prototypes for later psychological defenses, a question taken up more recently by Menninger (1954) and Greenacre (1958).

It is the purpose of this paper to apply the genetic principle to some of the defense mechanisms of the ego in an attempt to uncover some of their physiological prototypes. In this attempt I will consider phenomena of neonate behavior and functioning, both perceptual and neurophysiological. I have selected them because their mode of functioning seems to present sufficient analogies with the mode of functioning of specific later defense mechanisms to warrant investigation. In some cases, I will be able to point out certain transitional features. It will remain for the future to develop a genetic sequence stringent enough to justify the assumption that ontogenetic development has led to the use of physiological prototypes as patterns for psychological mechanisms. My purpose, then, will be to emphasize certain primitive ways of functioning, mainly in the neonate. The modes of functioning refer to (1) the field of perception; (2) the processing of stimuli both in the afferent sector of the central nervous system and in its efferent sector; (3) the accumulation of tensions and the ways in which these are discharged.

To preclude any possible misinterpretation of my theoretical position, I must stress that when I speak of perceptual and neurophysiological prototypes of defense mechanisms, I am not implying in any way that any of the defense

Reprinted from *Journal of the American Psychoanalytic Association*, 9:626–651, 1961.

mechanisms of the ego are innate. What *is* innate is the variable capacity for learning and the variable modes of adaptation (Benjamin, 1959), for making use of neurophysiological and morphological givens for the purpose of coping with environmental conditions. In the course of this process, devices on a higher level of complexity are elaborated, among them the defense mechanisms of the ego. What goes into these are therefore certain properties of innate neurophysiological function, which will serve as prototypes of the adaptive devices elaborated as the result of interactions with the environment. It is hardly necessary to stress that in these interactions the mother is the exclusive representative of the environment in the beginning and that in this role she remains the most important figure during the first two years and one of the most important subsequently. What I am saying, then, is that not only are the defense mechanisms created, or at least decisively influenced, as a result of the mother-child relations, but also that these mechanisms make use for this purpose of certain properties, of modes of functioning, either actually or potentially present at birth.

Hartmann and Greenacre have limited their considerations of such prototypes to physiological functions which appear to them to serve a *defensive* function already in the neonate. The neonatal physiological defense which these authors select is mostly analogous in its defensive function in some way to the one which the psychological defense mechanism will also serve eventually. In the case of Hartmann (1939) this limitation is rather surprising, for he specifically and repeatedly has stressed that at their origin all the psychological defense mechanisms of the ego serve the purpose of adaptation and only later that of defense.

My assumption is that in the course of development, physiological functions are psychologically processed and give rise to adaptive mechanisms of defense. It seems to be an unnecessary limitation to restrict the role of these defense mechanisms to the same function which their original physiological prototype had. In my opinion, in the course of this process, the defense mechanism which eventually develops may acquire a function quite different from that of its original physiological prototype.

In parallel with Hartmann, and independently of him, I developed the idea of physiological prototypes of defense as an amplification of Freud's (1895b) proposition, according to which the defenses become pathological only when used in exaggeration. I do not, of course, exclude that some of the prototypes of defense mechanisms also may have adaptive or other functions and need not serve for defense only.

Greenacre's (1958) highly original approach is different in its fundamental concepts. She also considers only those processes which serve defense functions physiologically. But her considerations are centered predominantly on physiological defensive functions which do not have a counterpart in those defense mechanisms of the ego with which we are usually concerned. An instance in point is what she calls "watery defense." By this novel concept Greenacre means the system's use of water in different locations of the body and for different regulative and protective functions, viz., as a mechanical pad, as a solvent, as a cooling agent, as a factor in hydrodynamic and in chemical balance. She connects these purely physical, adaptive, homeostatic, regulative, and protective reactions with a variety of phenomena: (1) with the mechanism of displacement; (2) with the allergies in widely separated organ systems; (3) with somatic symbolization and somatization. It seems to me that her approach shows great promise as a heuristic principle for future psychosomatic investigations. Whether it is more than an analogy in the field of the prototypes of ego defenses, as we commonly classify them, remains to be seen.

Karl Menninger's (1954) approach to the defense mechanisms is on a broad and comprehensive front. He attempts to place them in the framework of a unitary theory of organic life and its manifestations, but provides also an unbroken transition to the inorganic. He develops a theoretical system of the adaptive processes which comprises four hierarchical classes of regulatory devices. From the viewpoint of the defense mechanisms, as described by Sigmund Freud and Anna Freud, that involves a major reorganization of our thinking in several respects. As my presentation is organized on the lines of our traditional concept of defenses, I will have to forego the discussion of the new approach introduced by Menninger.

Early neurophysiological prototypes do not necessarily follow the same defensive pattern as the later ego defenses. Some of these prototypes are givens of embryological development, and as such impress one as being predominantly somatic. Others again are phylogenetically inherited, as anlage which will mature after the individual is born and therefore, although the somatic still plays the larger part, they may be open to the forces of ontogenetic development and modified by them. Finally, there may be certain prototypes which appear well after birth and will unfold and become established after a number of ontogenetic patterns are already present or developing. In these the participation of phylogenetic somatic factors is of lesser significance and environmental forces predominate.

The most conspicuous among these environmental forces is, of course, the influence of the mother, which makes itself felt in the mother-child relation. Psychoanalysts need hardly be reminded that the nature of the mother-child relations, the vicissitudes of their unfolding, and their ultimate fate determine the selection of the particular set of defense mechanisms which the child will elaborate and from which he will mold his individual character structure. We can confidently say that the prototypes represent simply what is *available* to the child during his first year of life or two. It will be the nature of the mother-child relations as they unfold in the course of development which governs the choice of the particular prototypes suitable for the given situation. Actually, the term "choice" implies a freedom of selection, which at this age is non-existent. We would do better to speak of the individual mother-child relations forming a gradient which impels the psychological development of the child toward the preferential usage of one prototype rather than any other in the service of defense. It is not the purpose of our present study to discuss the selective processes going on between the mother-child relations and the early prototypes of defense mechanisms. It should be mentioned, however, that under normal circumstances certain defense mechanisms will emerge at given points of the child's development.

I have attempted the investigation of the emergence of one such defense mechanism in the course of normal development, namely, that of identification with the aggressor (Spitz, 1957). It would seem desirable to undertake other such investigations for the purposes of ascertaining at what point of normal development the physiological prototypes of defense mechanisms are transformed into the beginnings of defense mechanisms proper. We would thus acquire what might be called an inventory of the age-adequate appearance of defense mechanisms. This knowledge would make a more systematic approach to the question of the influence of mother-child relations on the formation of defenses possible.

Beginnings have been made in this respect. Greenacre (1958) and Bergman and Escalona (1949) formulated propositions in regard to excessive and untimely amounts of stimulation leading to premature ego formation. I would rather speak of such untimely stimulation as leading to premature activation of defenses on the somatic level and resulting in deviant ego formation. Let us recall that during the months following birth, the mother acts as the child's protector against incoming stimuli. If she fails in this role, she may prematurely become an overstimulator instead of a protector, and perhaps activate prototypes of defense mechanisms, or even defense mechanisms proper.

Our present purpose is to discuss some of the neurophysiological givens at birth and in the first year, which may serve as prototypes of later defense mechanisms of the ego. What the fate of these prototypes can be in the individual case will have to provide the subject of other investigations.

The basic defense mechanisms of the ego, as discussed by Freud on various occasions, and particularly as described by Anna Freud in the introductory chapter of *The Ego and the Mechanisms of Defense* (1936) comprise the following: (1) repression, (2) regression, (3) reaction formation, (4) isolation, (5) undoing, (6) turning into the opposite, (7) turning against the self, (8) projection, (9) introjection, (10) sublimation.

To these should be added denial, displacement, and intellectualization. For a variety of reasons, the latter do not figure in every enumeration of the defense mechanisms. For instance, the concept of denial was worked out specifically by Anna Freud in several chapters of her book and distinguished from negation. In simplest terms we might say that, while denial is an unconscious mechanism, the same cannot be said of negation. As regards displacement, it appears to be counted by some authors (Greenacre, for instance) among the defenses. Most of us will consider it not so much as a defense mechanism, but rather as a basic mode of functioning of the unconscious.[1]

Let me begin with what to me seems to be the most familiar mechanism of defense, namely, repression. It is the one which has been described earliest, together with the concept of defense, in the *Studies on Hysteria* (Breuer & Freud, 1895) in Freud's correspondence with Fliess and in his various drafts for the "Project for a Scientific Psychology" (1895b). It also gives me the opportunity to present right from the start an illustration of some differences between my concept of prototypes of defense mechanisms and that of other authors.

On the one hand I share with them, and particularly with Hartmann, the opinion that the prototype for repression lies in the infantile phenomenon of the *stimulus barrier*. The latter was first described by Freud in 1914 in the article "On Narcissism" and extensively discussed in 1920 in *Beyond the Pleasure Principle*. Freud elaborates here, and later in greater detail (1925b), that the *external covering* serves as a barrier against incoming stimuli, while the next layer has been differentiated as an organ for the perception of stimuli. However, even this second layer processes only minimal quantities, samples, as it were, of the incoming stimuli.

This state of affairs is extraordinarily striking in the newborn. Here the threshold of the stimulus barrier is so high that the incoming stimuli simply do not penetrate unless they literally break through the protective layer,

---

[1] As for intellectualization, there can be no doubt that this device plays a major role as a defense mechanism, particularly in certain developmental stages like puberty. It would be an interesting task to delimit it from sublimation; for the moment we might say that while sublimation remains fully in the realm of desirable normal development, intellectualization, to a very significant extent, serves a pathological function.

It becomes obvious that restricting our investigation to the earliest prototypes of defense mechanisms within the first and part of the second year of life will eliminate from our considerations some of those enumerated above, like sublimation, reaction formation, and intellectualization. We do not believe that all of these have *somatic* prototypes. They appear to belong to a series of psychological devices developed at a higher level of complexity and based on previously established *psychological* devices.

The formation of sublimation is obviously predicated upon the presence of the superego. The same probably holds true of reaction formation. Intellectualization has, we believe, its prototype just at the transition line between the age level with which we are concerned, that is, between the first 12 to 18 months and the stage which follows.

swamping the organism with unmanageable quantities of excitation. This breakthrough actually does occur during the birth process and was described by Freud as the "trauma of birth."

Freud's theory of the trauma of birth as the prototype for later anxiety is the outstanding model for our approach to physiological processes and physiological phenomena as prototypes of later defense mechanisms. Freud (1926) said:

> The foetus can be aware of nothing beyond a gross disturbance in the economy of his narcissistic libido. Large amounts of excitation press upon it, giving rise to novel sensations of unpleasure: numerous organs enforce increased cathexis in their behalf. . . .
>
> The process of birth constitutes the first danger situation, the economic upheaval which birth entails becomes the prototype of the anxiety reaction. . . .
>
> To anxiety in later life were thus attributed two modes of origin: the one involuntary, automatic, economically justified, whenever there arose a situation of danger analogous to birth, the other produced by the ego when such a situation merely threatened, in order to procure its avoidance.[2]

Immediately after birth the system gets rid of the excitation caused by the breakthrough of the protective layer. In normal cases it is a matter of less than ten seconds until quiescence returns, and the stimulus barrier is reestablished. I do not share Hartmann's and Greenacre's opinion, according to which the stimulus barrier is created by a *withdrawal* of cathexis from the sensorium. While that would also result in a protection from incoming stimuli, such an explanation introduces dynamics into a process in which they do not yet play a role.

I do not believe that a cathexis of the sensorium, or, to be more exact, of sensorial psychic representation, exists at birth, at least not in the sense in which psychoanalysts use the term "cathexis." Neither Hartmann nor Greenacre have tried to postulate that the sensorium had been cathected already *in utero* and the cathexis withdrawn in the course of the birth process, although Greenacre practically implies this. In my opinion, at birth neurophysiological maturation has not yet proceeded to the point at which the sensorium *could* be "cathected" in the current sense of the term (Spitz, 1957, 1958a).

I do think, however, that not only *maximal* stimulation leading to a breakthrough of the protective barrier become effective in the neonate; *minimal* stimuli also provoke a response, even though quite irregularly and unreliably. If this were not the case, we would not be able to elicit reflexes in the

---

[2] [Spitz is quoting from the version entitled *The Problem of Anxiety*, New York: Norton, 1926. This quote appears in slightly different translation in the *Standard Edition*, Vol. 20, on pp. 135, 150–162. Ed.]

newborn, let alone that slow postural turning toward warmth repeatedly mentioned by observers.

Let me offer a hunch as to the nature of the dynamics involved in the neonate's responses to minimal stimuli. A psychic representation existing at birth or a cathectic displacement to such a representation cannot be postulated; we do not even believe that one can speak of precursors of psychic representation or cathexis. What the irregularity and unreliability of the responses to minimal stimuli do suggest is that excitation is generalized, and will flow now into one or another neural pathway. When it happens to hit the sensorium of the particular sector being stimulated, a response will be obtained in that sector, but the next time such a response may not occur.

This also readily explains the turning toward warmth (probably a phylogenetically inherited innate releaser mechanism and key stimulus), for the stimulus of warmth is present during lengthy periods and will therefore act as a continuity in time and not as a discrete single event, where the chances of generalization of the excitation are obviously much smaller than in the case of a continuous stimulus. A stimulus present during lengthy periods makes it possible for some part of the random excitation to overflow into the pathways which will provoke the thermal responses.

This proposition also permits the explanation of the possibility of establishing a conditioned reflex after one or two weeks of life. If one and the same sensory sector is repeatedly stimulated, some of this stimulation will get through and lead to a reaction from time to time. If this process is repeated sufficiently often, the repetition will contribute to the channelization of this particular pathway, as the repetition is reinforced through the reward offered by the discharge of excitation made possible. Still, at our present stage of knowledge, I feel doubtful whether such channelization is possible in other than emotionally reinforced situations, like that of feeding, on the positive side; or in situations involving pain, on the negative side.

A comparison will serve to clarify what I mean when I state that the maturation of the neurophysiological apparatus at birth has not yet reached the point at which the sensorium *could* be cathected. Take, for instance, a burglar alarm which was installed in one's home. One can switch it off; then it does not respond to anybody entering the premises. Conversely, take the case that the house is a new one and the central power station of the city is not yet delivering current to it; then the burglar alarm will not function either, whether the switch is off or on. The state of the neonate's perceptual system is that of the house which has not yet been connected with the central power station. The receiving stations, that is to say, the representations of the sensorium, are not yet energized and a maturational process has to take place before they are.

In Freud's proposition (1925a) the external covering serves as a *barrier* against incoming stimuli, while the next layer has been differentiated as an organ for the *perception* of stimuli. The first layer will continue to function as a protective barrier, unchanged throughout life. The second layer is destined to mediate perception and will eventually be modified to do just that; but it does not yet function in this manner at birth, because its psychic representation has not yet been cathected. Thus, at birth, the still uncathected second layer is added to the first protective layer and represents an additional protection against incoming stimuli. This explains the high threshold of the neonate. This is the difference between neonatal perception and perception at later stages of development; at this later stage, the second, the perceptual layer's psychic representation has been progressively cathected as the result of interaction between development and maturation.

The stimulus barrier is an extremely elementary form of prototype for the very complicated mechanism of repression. The only element repression and stimulus barrier have in common is the lack of cathexis. But while in the case of the stimulus barrier at birth the receiving station has not yet been cathected, in the case of repression proper cathexis has not only been withdrawn, but a countercathexis is established. This is particularly striking in that special case of repression which Laforgue (1926) has called scotomization.

This last consideration suggests that there may exist intermediary steps between repression and its most archaic prototype. Hartmann (1950) has postulated that the closing of the eyelids represents a transitional step, a forestage of later defense both against within and against without. But closing the eyelids is not the specific prototype for repression; it rather seems to me that the particular form of defense for which the closing of the eyelids might be considered a prototype is the mechanism of denial. If you will recall the comparison with the burglar alarm, the closing of the eyelids would be like switching off our burglar alarm, because we are too terrified of the burglar and hope he won't notice us. Both denial and scotomization fulfill exactly this purpose.

Of course, closing of the eyelids in the first hours of life is still very inadequately organized. One can, though quite rarely, observe children at that age sleeping with one eye open and one eye closed, or even with both eyes open. The closing of the eyelids will become progressively organized and function in proportion to the measure in which the threshold of the stimulus barrier decreases. This taking over the function of the stimulus barrier in one particular sector of the sensorium illustrates well the transitions of which we are speaking. We may speculate whether the closing of the eyelids should be considered as the prototype for the *withdrawal* of cathexis in denial and repression, while the stimulus barrier would be the prototype for the phenomenon of absence of cathexis.

We should, however, remain aware that closing the eyelids is not the same as withdrawing cathexis; it is not its homologue (and even less the homologue of denial). There exist, nevertheless, sufficient similarities between the two to consider the withdrawal of cathexis in denial the *analogue* of closing the eyelids. In the first place, the *result,* both in closing the eyelids and in withdrawing cathexis, is identical: perception of an external impression is warded off. The means of achieving this are different in the two cases.

In denial the cathexis of the painful impression is withdrawn and subsequently canceled (A. Freud, 1936). Closing the eyelids, however, is a muscular activity, a physical avoidance that is initiated by a sensation which is homologous to the one which initiates denial: the sensation of a painful impression which the ego wishes to cancel. Thus the two end points of the process, the painful impression at the *beginning* and its warding off as the *outcome,* are identical. It is the middle, the process leading to the end result, which differs.

In postulating that denial is an analogue of the infantile closing of the eyelids we have to consider not only in what respect they are identical but also in what aspect they differ.[3] Let us consider first the events leading to the physical action of avoidance involved in closing the eyelids, e.g., when the infant is bothered by the sun shining in his eyes. This painful external impression provokes the need to end the unpleasure. The steps which are taken to achieve this goal then involve cathectic shifts which result in activating the muscular apparatus and will eventuate in the closure of the eyelids, thus ending the painful external impression.

An example will clarify in what respect denial differs from the above. A patient comes into the analyst's office on the first of the month to find his bill lying, as usual, white on the dark couch, next to the pillow. He ignores it throughout the whole hour, although as a result of his threshing around he audibly crumples the paper of the bill with his shoulder. He continues ignoring it on getting up and his attention has to be called to it as he is leaving.

The difference between this performance and closing the eyelids consists in the fact that the activation of the muscular apparatus through cathectic shifts is eliminated from the process of avoidance. The cathexis of the painful external impression is identical; but the perception is warded off centrally, presumably by withdrawing cathexis from it, instead of peripherally with the help of the musculature. This incidentally represents a saving of energy, according to Freud's definition of the thought process. In the case of denial the trial action of the thought process alone is sufficient to achieve the goal.

---

[3] In the words of Robert Oppenheimer (1956), "One has to widen the framework a little and find the disanalogy, which enables one to preserve what was right about the analogy."

It appears probable that denial in this form is an integral part of our psychic functioning. We are well aware that perception is a selective process. Not only psychoanalysts, but more recently experimental psychologists, have rather generally accepted the idea that perception takes place selectively as a function of the affect involved. It was implicit in this hypothesis that the affect in question would be a positive one. I believe that one should consider the possibility of the existence of a large number of possible perceptions which do not take place under normal circumstances also as a result of their negative affective quality, much in the manner of the negative hallucination. Fenichel (1945) came rather close to this idea.

We are not postulating that our selective perception is based exclusively on the pleasure affect for the perceived and the painful affect for the non-perceived. Our proposition is that the economic point of view has to be applied to perception as we have been used to applying it to other phenomena. If we do that, we become aware that the term "painful external impression" becomes a relative one. That was to be expected, for the economic viewpoint is regulated by the pleasure-unpleasure principle. In other words, perception is regulated by a gradient which goes from more pleasurable to less pleasurable. The pleasurable is more readily perceived than the less pleasurable; that this gradient involves extremely fine distinctions becomes evident in the well-known fact that the meaningful is more readily perceived than the meaningless.

These considerations belong in a psychoanalytic theory of perception and probably also of learning. For our present purpose it serves to make us realize that the precursor of the mechanism of denial is to be found in the archaic, physical avoidance of unpleasure expressed in the closing of the eyelids, which appears prior to the development of thought process and conscious perception. After these are acquired, a model for the inhibition of perception at the subjective source of perception is given by the selective nature of perceiving.

The ultimate establishment of the mechanism of denial as a pathological process would then appear to be not much more than placing this normal way of functioning of the psychic apparatus in the service of the neurotic goal. The patient who ignored the bill on the couch inhibited its perception because the transference situation of the moment demanded this scotomization of reality. In other circumstances he might have equally overlooked a piece of paper lying on the dinner table because the plate of soup was more meaningful and pleasurable. In the case of the bill, an active withdrawal of cathexis took place; in the case of the soup, cathexis was fully engaged and nothing remained for the paper.

If we go on from the dynamics of denial to those of repression, we are faced with a further complication. We have to explain in what way countercathexis enters the process described above when repression occurs. One possible explanation has been discussed by Freud in *Beyond the Pleasure Principle* (1920). When speaking of the specific unpleasure of physical pain, Freud states that "cathectic energy is summoned from all sides to provide sufficiently high cathexis of energy in the environs of the breach. An 'anti-cathexis' on a grand scale is set up."

The search for physiological prototypes of defense mechanisms thus leads us to investigate phenomena very different from each other in their nature and significance for the organism as a whole, phenomena as different from each other as the neurophysiological threshold of the stimulus barrier at birth is from the neuromuscular action of closing the eyelids against too much light, with the reaction to pain thrown in for good measure. Later still another possible prototype for the withdrawal of cathexis will be discovered.

The first two, threshold and lid closure, are observable phenomena. They occur at different levels of organization and both of them are similar in their functional "purpose." The third, the reaction to pain, is of a different dignity. It is a proposition belonging in the context of the libido theory, though a well-substantiated one. The functional principle of each of these three will have to serve as prototype for a psychological operation performed at a much later stage of development. At that stage the organism has already achieved psychic structure, that is, at the very least, the differentiation between the ego and the id. At that level the functional principle operating in the phenomena of the threshold, in that of lid closure, and in cathectic operations in response to pain, will be integrated into the process we call the mechanism of repression.

Whether a genetic continuity can be demonstrated between these prototypic phenomena and the ultimate development of the mechanism of repression must be left to the findings of future investigators. Our proposition regarding these prototypes is modeled on Freud's application of the genetic principle in connection with embryological and neurophysiological data. The extraordinary heuristic value of this method encourages us to risk its application also in the field of defenses.

There would be very little purpose in indulging in such speculative exercises, were it not for the fact that the defense mechanisms are man's armamentarium for adaptation and mastery, for survival, and ultimately for further evolution. Defense mechanisms are at the very origin of man's capacity to think, to speak, to perform mental operations (Spitz, 1957). It must be our concern to discover how they originate and what may lead to disturbances in their formation. Therefore, even if at present the investigation of their prototypes may appear to be a bootless errand, it belongs to what I would call fundamental research in the field of psychoanalysis. As in all fundamental research, we cannot say at present where it will lead us.

I have dealt overlong with one single defense mechanism with the purpose of making you aware of the complexities of the problem. I will try to deal more briefly with the others which I have mentioned, beginning with projection and introjection. In *Beyond the Pleasure Principle,* Freud offered a suggestion regarding the origin of projection. He stated that when inner excitation provokes too great an increase in unpleasure, then there is the tendency to treat it as if it came from outside; because, if the unpleasure-causing stimulus is outside, then the defense of the stimulus barrier can be used against it.

To this proposition can be added information gained from the observation of perceptual development. During the first weeks of life, up to the second month, there is no difference in the infant's reaction to stimuli coming from the inside or from the outside. The first observable behavior which suggests that the infant distinguishes the "I" from the "non-I" appears in the second month of life.

The lack of a boundary line between the "I" and the "non-I" forms the necessary prerequisite not only for projection but also for introjection. The boundary will be progressively consolidated in the course of the third to the sixth month of life through actions performed in the course of the infant's relations with the "non-I." In the course of these actions the "I" is increasingly identified with what one feels inside. The "non-I" becomes more and more what one can see outside only, *after having lost it.* Before that, one felt it inside because at that stage it still belonged to the undifferentiated totality. I have spoken advisedly in oral terms, because of the tendency to equate introjection with incorporation with food intake. It is also along these lines that I discussed elsewhere (Spitz, 1957) the establishment of the boundaries between the "I" and the "non-I."

As regards projection, Abraham (1924) advanced the proposition that at the beginning of life projection can be related to anal and urinal elimination which, in my opinion, is an extrapolation derived from the analysis of adult patients. I have come to conclude from direct observation that under normal circumstances, during the first four to five months of life, the infant is not much aware of what goes on in the anal region. He becomes increasingly aware of this toward the end of the first year of life. This is also in good agreement with the findings of neural development. In contrast to Abraham, we believe that the prototype available for projection at the three-month level is regurgitation and vomiting. This is a conviction which forces itself on the observer when he watches certain infants who refuse food. It is difficult to resist the impression that what has been incorporated, that is to say, *intro*-jected through the mouth, is *re*-jected and then *pro*-jected through this identical route. This is also in line with the distinction set up by Freud (1925a) in his article on negation where he writes: " . . . what is bad is to be outside me."

It is not only in repression, denial, projection, and introjection that we can see the analogues to the modes of functioning of infantile perception and its inhibitions. For instance, it would be easy to visualize as one of the prototypes for the mechanism of isolation the steps which lead from the infant's totality perception to the distinction of the "I" from the "non-I," and from there to the diacritic detail perception of the surround.

Burness Moore, (1958), investigating the origins of isolation, claimed separation experiences as one of its precursors. He suggested that the earliest of these is the birth experience, followed by the vicissitudes of the mother-child relations in the framework of child care, to the differentiation of the self from the nonself, and culminating in the anal experiences of bowel movement and sphincter control. Moore specifically states that he does not consider separation as the only source of the defense mechanism of isolation.

As in so many other defense mechanisms, perceptive modalities and the dynamic shifts connected with them are probably the earliest prototypes of isolation. Specifically, the transition from diffuse, undifferentiated perception to the segregation of Gestalten from the chaotic surround and then the circumscription of the essential elements of these Gestalten appear to provide prototypes for isolation. However, the progressive segregation of the essential elements of a Gestalt takes place within the framework of unfolding object relations also. Moore's assumption that separation becomes operative as a prototype of isolation is correct. But we must add that the experience of separation will be selectively screened and molded according to the modalities of perceptive development prevailing at the time of the experience.

As stated elsewhere (Spitz, 1957), the perception of the difference between the "I" and the "non-I" comes about through the endlessly repeated experience of the loss of the need-gratifying preobject in the feeding situation; in Moore's terms, through the separation from the preobject. The two, the perceptive experience and the separation, are in close interaction, one facilitating and directing the other, and we cannot say which is first.

Another instance of an inhibition of perception as prototype of an ego defense is sleep. The effectiveness of sleep as a defense in infancy, discussed elsewhere (Spitz, 1957), was illustrated by the case of Monica (Engel and Reichsman, 1956). The infant withdraws from an unpleasurable percept by going to sleep and by regressing in fantasy to the archaic sleep of satiation after nursing. Thus sleep may be considered as the prototype of all defense. Perhaps sleep can be referred to as an ideal defense, or even better, as the earliest defense. It is an anaclitic defense, for *as a defense* it leans onto the physiological function of sleep.

In sleep cathexis is withdrawn from the sensorium. That is a dynamic process which will serve as the prototype for the withdrawal of cathexis in regression. This does not invalidate the proposition that the closing of the eyelids plays a role as one of the prototypes for both repression and denial. After all, the first step in composing oneself for sleep is the closing of the eyes. It is well to remember, however, that in earliest infancy "sleep" can occur without closing of the eyes, though that is rare. This seeming paradox shows that no single physiological phenomenon fulfills all the prototypic conditions for the later defense mechanisms. Can we then postulate that sleep as such is the prototype for regression?

The answer to this question has to be qualified in two directions. In the first place, according to psychoanalytic theory, sleep itself involves a regression. We therefore have to ask ourselves, "*To* what does the neonate regress, and *from* what does he regress?" This question imposes on us the second consideration, namely, the realization that "sleep" is too general a term and that there may be different kinds of sleep at different stages of life.

An extensive investigation on the problems of sleeping and waking has been conducted by Kleitmann (1939) and his associates on infants beginning with the third week of life. This work, as well as that of others, has recently been psychoanalytically discussed by Sanford Gifford (1960) in a scholarly paper in which the significance of the sleep-wakefulness pattern and its evolution is shown to be a useful indicator of the unfolding of early ego development. Gifford concludes, as I have, that the three-month level is a nodal point in this process. He speaks of the exchanges between mother and child for this development and calls these preobjectal relations. I agree with Gifford that this does not contradict my proposition that the preobject, the human face, is established only in the third month. The preobject is necessarily the product of preobjectal relations. It is within the framework of the preobjectal relations that the physiological prototypes are situated. In the course of the preobjectal relations the diurnal rhythm of sleep and wakefulness, the adrenocortical activity, the temperature curve, the establishment of the occipital alpha rhythm, etc., are progressively achieved. But at present, we do not yet know enough about the sleep-wakefulness pattern in the first three weeks of life.

With the aforementioned observational facts in mind, let us reconsider our concept of sleep. Analytically we postulate that in sleep cathexis is withdrawn from the sensorium (or rather from its psychological representation). Looking at the neonate, remembering what we have postulated regarding the neonatal stimulus barrier, we may ask ourselves: What cathexis is withdrawn? And from what representation? With the picture of the neonate as I see it, there is no cathexis of the sensorium yet, and therefore none can be withdrawn. Nor is there a psychological level from which a regression could be performed, even if we speak of this regression only in terms of the memory and perception systems. All these will exist only in the future.

I am therefore inclined to think of "sleep" in the neonate as something very different from sleep at a later age. I am somewhat hesitant to say this, but I have the idea that even physiologically neonatal "sleep" will prove to be different from sleep as we know it, after the ego has been established. There are hints of this in the subsequent synthesis of the various physiological functions presented by Gifford. After all, we have only to go back a few hours or days in time before the delivery to realize that the terms "sleep" and "wakefulness" have become meaningless. The fetus's activity *in utero* certainly does not imply anything comparable to being "awake," be that activity performed by the skeletal musculature or by the smooth involuntary musculature as in the case of singultus, peristalsis, etc. (Benjamin, 1960). Why must we postulate that sleep is acquired ready made at birth? *Natura non fecit saltum.*

I am rather inclined to assume that what we call sleep in the neonate is a phenomenon *sui generis* from which sleep, as we adults know it, will develop later. This is the reason why I have always spoken of the neonate as *quiescent,* and not as sleeping. Sleep and wakefulness will be segregated out of this state of "neonatal sleep" as a result of interaction between maturation and development. The chapter on this development and its details still remains to be written. On the other hand we have accumulated some information on the establishment of the perceptual and the memory systems. To establish them, the infant needs time and experience, and it is interesting to note that, as time progresses, as the infant accumulates experience, as memory traces are laid down, the infant's sleeping pattern changes. The half-sleeping, half-waking periods tend to disappear more and more, and sleep becomes organized into larger time units, coordinated with the alternation of day and night on the one hand, with the feeding pattern on the other.

You will understand that, with such views, I have little inclination to indulge in speculations as to whether sleep represents the wish to return to the intrauterine situation. My inclination, as expressed elsewhere (Spitz, 1955c), is to follow Lewin's (1946) and Isakower's (1938) propositions and to consider *real* sleep as a regression to the satiation at the breast. This distinguishes real sleep from the sleep of the neonate. Real sleep, the kind of sleep which is a product of development and which can be observed after the third month of life, is endowed with meaning, with psychological content. Its prototype, however, the physiological sleep of the neonate, is devoid of psychological content.

This discussion of regression and sleep shows that it is quite difficult to distinguish which is the cart and which is the horse. One gets the definite impression that regression and sleep come into being simultaneously in the course of the first few months of life. Sleep, as stated, must be considered, at least at its origin, as a physiological pattern; whereas in the sense in which we use the term, regression unquestionably is a psychological one.

Permit me to repeat: (1) sleep in the proper sense of the term appears to develop from the stimulus barrier; (2) this takes place as a function of the increasing accumulation of memory traces and experience; (3) in sleep, in contradistinction to the stimulus barrier at birth, cathexis is withdrawn from the sensorium; (4) regression begins to operate *pari passu*. We may therefore conclude that we probably have here before us a close linkage in time of a physiological prototype, neonatal sleep, and of a psychological defense mechanism, namely, regression.

Of course, the linkage is not only in time. Inevitably the sleep mechanism in some way influences regression and regression influences the sleep mechanism. One must therefore speak of an interaction of the two. One may further assume that the early preobjectal relations in their turn will make their influence felt with the help of the regression mechanism in the development of the eventual sleep pattern.

One would probably be justified in stating that in this sense regression rather than sleep proper is the first of the defense mechanisms to appear. But then one immediately realizes that at this early stage one cannot yet postulate the existence of an ego. Therefore, what we seem to have before us here is a defense mechanism without the ego. Actually we should say that this earliest regression is the prototype of the later ego defense mechanism of regression. With this the physiological function, sleep, becomes the *physiological* prototype of a *psychological* prototype.

For, make no mistake: the regression which we postulate in the baby's first few months during the process of sleep will be vastly modified when it becomes a defense mechanism which the ego can use for its purposes. And even this is still very different from what Kris (1944) has described as regression in the service of the ego.

Sleep can equally be considered the prototype of denial; this logically follows from my previous linkage of denial with the stimulus barrier.

One may further speculate whether sleep might also be the prototype of undoing. Somewhere one senses a relationship between the two. On further reflection, one realizes that undoing is involved in a special phenomenon connected with sleep, namely, in the dream. That is probably most vividly illustrated in the deservedly famous "dream of the strawberries" (Freud, 1900).

It appears licit to assume that the dream is an extremely archaic mental phenomenon. Freud assumed that the infant resorts to hallucinatory wish fulfillment when gratification of the drive is not available. This refers to a form of psychic activity which at a later stage probably will be elaborated and subdivided into a number of psychological phenomena, such as the dream itself, daydreams, hallucinations, and delusions. I believe that hallucinatory wish fulfillment in infancy is probably the earliest mental activity and comes into being at the period at which neonatal sleep turns into regular sleep, which is differentiated from clearly distinguished waking, that is, sleep proper. How much later actual dreams appear we have no way of knowing, though changes in facial expression and mouth movements of sleeping infants are suggestive and would indicate that it must be very early. We may then assume that that function of the dream which is present at this archaic stage, namely, the changing of unsatisfactory reality through a mental operation into gratifying fantasy, is available from the beginning. This corresponds to the proposition on infantile omnipotence introduced by Freud (1900, 1909, 1911) and elaborated by Ferenczi (1913).

It is clear that neither the function of wish fulfillment of the dream, or its function as guardian of sleep, nor that of transforming unpalatable reality into desired imaginary gratification are the same as the mechanism of undoing. In the latter, the id wish is permitted to find its conscious expression in the form of a derivative on the condition that, in the same act, it is immediately turned into its opposite and annulled. In Fenichel's (1945) terms, undoing is made up of two actions, the second of which is a direct reversion of the first.

There is a kinship between this way of dealing with the drive and the dream's dealing with reality and with conscious or unconscious wishes. This becomes particularly evident in the trigger action of day residues which initiate dreams, in which then the attempt is made to resolve problems we were unable to deal with while awake. I like therefore to speak of the dream as "unfinished business." One aspect of the dream process, namely, that of dealing with the id wish, appears to have been selected and organized in the defense mechanism of "undoing," in which the prohibited intention of the drive is manifested and, in the same act, nullified. It can be concluded that the stage of the physiological and psychological phenomenon of sleep which serves as a prototype for undoing is that at which the dream becomes possible. The prototype for undoing is not the physiological process of sleep, nor its psychological aspect, namely, regression, but a psychological concomitant, namely, the dream.

Undoing can be connected also with another archaic prototype, with the repetition compulsion. The prerequisite for the discussion of such a proposition would be a thorough investigation and clarification of the whole controversy centering around the concept of repetition compulsion.

I presume that in following the train of thoughts I have presented, you may have found it confusing that in some cases *one* defense mechanism could be led back to *several* different prototypes and that, on the other hand, I described physiological prototypes which appeared to be responsible for several different defense mechanisms; and finally, that at certain points combinations of both became visible. That is a confusion which I cannot deny and which, furthermore, is quite characteristic of the stage of development with which we are dealing and which I called the stage of nondifferentiation for good reasons. The physiological functions and systems are not clearly differentiated from each other at this stage; and even less so are the psychological ones which derive from them.

I probably should not employ the term "derivation" to describe the use of physiological prototypes in the evolution of ego defenses. What appears to take place is that the modalities of a given archaic and mainly physiological way of function will be applied on a higher and more complex level of function, on the psychological one. On this higher level the archaic *functional* modalities become integrated into a new entity, into the defense mechanism—and this without regard for their previous role and function.

Space will not permit here a more thorough examination of the remaining defense mechanisms. I will try to deal with them briefly. Freud and Anna Freud have stressed that "turning into the opposite" and "turning against the self" are not so much derived from the functioning of the ego but rather are characteristic of the drive itself. As regards "turning into the opposite," I am inclined to see its prototype in archaic ambivalence. I mean by this term a phenomenon which I am inclined to consider the precursor of psychological ambivalence. This phenomenon has to do with the nondifferentiation in every sector of the neonate's personality, which for the observer manifests itself impressively in the infant's behavior, starting with birth and throughout the first year of life (Spitz, 1957). Random functioning and behavior in every sector of the personality will be coordinated into clear-cut patterns only step by step. The adult observer is mostly unable to predict what direction an act initiated by the infant will take. It is even difficult to tell from facial expression whether the infant is starting to cry or to laugh. Some of this nondifferentiation still persists at the end of the first year and later, though in an ever-decreasing measure. The differentiation of the drives throughout the first six months is also still incomplete, thus facilitating and even favoring, the "turning into the opposite."

That probably holds also for the "turning against the self." Only here the incomplete differentiation of the drives combines with the incomplete differentiation between the "I" and the "non-I." One sees for instance infants in the first year of life inflicting pain on themselves in response to frustration. An impressive example is the case of an eight-month-old boy I observed in an orphanage. Whenever something caused him unpleasure he would begin to cry, and at the same time hit the left side of his face with his clenched right fist, with such violence that it could be heard several rooms away, until the unpleasure stimulus was removed. Such unpleasure stimuli could be completely impersonal; I filmed this child when he was performing this self-chastisement because the sun was shining into his eyes.

CONCLUSION

In the course of this discussion of the defense mechanisms I have not presented much new factual material. I have simply indicated a road along which research should be undertaken and might be elaborated. For it is unquestionable that the prototypes of the ego defenses will be processed through the mother-child relation in the course of development. It should prove worth while to investigate the following questions:

1. What kind of mother-child relations favor and facilitate what kind of defense mechanisms?

2. At what point do the mother-child relations transform the physiological prototype into the beginning of a defense mechanism?

3. It would seem desirable to verify Greenacre's (1958) and Bergman and Escalona's (1949) propositions according to which premature ego formation (or, as I would put it, what amounts of stimulation leading to premature activation of defenses) results in faulty ego formation. I may remind you that Greenacre's proposition refers to traumata experienced by the infant in the course of the birth process.

This is a proposition which might be expanded to include, during the months following birth, the mother's role as the child's protector against incoming stimuli. If she fails in this role, instead of the protector she may become the overstimulator. Will she not then prematurely activate prototypes of defense mechanisms, or even actual defense mechanisms proper?

The majority of our prototypes—I refer to the stimulus barrier, to the closing of the eyes, to the sleep-wakefulness cycle, to the process of differentiation between the ''I'' and the ''non-I,'' etc.—are situated in the undifferentiated stage and belong to what later will form the conflict-free sphere of the ego. They contribute, with the help of object relations, to the process of ego formation. It is to be expected that their premature activation in the direction of defense will lead to faulty ego development, to what I have described elsewhere (Spitz, 1959) as *asymmetric* ego development. Therefore, the investigation of the role of the prototypes of defense mechanisms and of the role of earliest defense mechanisms themselves in the formation of psychological structure would seem appropriate and desirable.

Many more questions could be asked. For instance, it would be desirable to investigate which of the prototypes is likely to lead to defense against the outside, such as denial, and which to defense against the inside, such as projection. Obviously, this paper cannot deal with the numerous problems which it raises and their exploration will have to remain for the future.

Ontogenesis: The Proleptic Function of Emotion

When in 1872 Charles Darwin reviewed the spectrum of the expression of emotions in man and animal, he found it necessary to write a book of more than 360 pages. He found that he had to consider the development of emotions both phylogenetically and ontogenetically. In the space at my disposal I will have to omit emotions in animals and consequently phylogenesis. I will limit myself to the ontogenesis of emotion in man. Even then I will not be able to do more than to examine its earliest phase, beginning with birth, to what we can observe in the first few months and to what we can conclude from these observations.

The numerous and mostly unclear definitions of emotion that have been attempted since Darwin's times are not relevant to this study, for which I will choose as my point of departure the following two statements by Freud: "It is surely the essence of an emotion that we should be aware of it, i.e. that it should become known to consciousness" (1915b, p. 177).

In other terms, Freud considers emotion to be something which has a *conscious* component. The second statement of Freud's reads: "Affects[1] and emotions correspond with processes of discharge, the final expression of which is expressed as feeling" (1915b, p. 178).

Freud consistently refuses to assume the existence at birth of a division of the psychic apparatus into conscious and unconscious; neither does he assume the presence of an ego, of memory, in one word, of psychic functioning *as such*, or of emotion, in the neonate. From personal observations conducted on a large number of neonates and from experiments performed on them, I can fully confirm Freud's thesis. I believe that one cannot speak of emotions in the neonate in the sense in which we speak of them in the adult. At birth one can only speak of excitation.

In the neonate this excitation appears to be preponderantly of a negative nature. For the sake of brevity, I will speak of this as unpleasure. I will not use this term in its popular meaning, but to connote an increase of tension,

Reprinted from *Expression of the Emotions in Man,* ed. Peter H. Knapp. New York: International Universities Press, 1963, pp. 36–60.

[1] In this paper the term "affect" will be used interchangeably with the terms "emotion" and "feeling." The literature does not distinguish clearly between them.

according to Freud's usage. Its counterpart, pleasure, will be used to connote decrease of tension. Neither of the two terms, as used here, will assert or deny any of the feeling connotations implied in the everyday usage of these words.

If in the neonate the negative manifestations seem preponderant, this is perhaps because their counterpart, the positive manifestations, are so inconspicuous and because they do not conform to the popular use of the term "pleasure." The positive side in the newborn's behavior is manifested primarily as quiescence, that is, as inactivity. The only active counterpart to unpleasure manifestations in the neonate is the "turning-toward" in response to certain key stimuli.

We would probably be well advised to speak of negative excitation and of its counterpart, of quiescence, as prototypes or precursors of emotions in the neonate. At this early stage, they are mainly manifested in the infant's facial expressions, in his random movements, and in his vocalization.

The concept of psychological prototypes was present in Freud's thinking already at a very early stage of his work and found its definitive formulation in his book *Inhibitions, Symptoms and Anxiety* (1926). He suggests that the physiological changes in the infant during delivery (i.e., in the birth situation), the excessive degree of excitation, the physiological consequences of the breakthrough of the stimulus barrier (i.e., the protective shield against stimuli in the neonate), are the somatic prototypes for the expression of the affect of anxiety. Thus the manifest part of the affective state of anxiety is modeled after an archaic mnemic image, which is the precipitate of neonatal traumatic experience. Freud furthermore advanced the proposition that the ontogenesis of affects generally tends to follow this pattern. This statement of Freud's will form one of the main arguments of my presentation.

In previous publications I have spoken both of prototypes and of precursors.[2] In the following, when I use the term precursor, the accent will be on maturation; and in my usage of the term prototype, the emphasis will be on development. The concepts of maturation and development, generally used in psychology, were introduced into psychoanalytic literature by Hartmann, Kris, and Loewenstein (1946).

Maturation refers to those processes of progressive change and of growth which are due to factors transmitted by genes and chromosomes. This growth and these changes take place both in the somatic and in the psychological

---

[2] It is debatable whether, besides prototypes, one should also speak of precursors of psychological phenomena, and differentiate the two. It might be argued that physiological precursors of later psychological phenomena develop in a straight genetic line and their unfolding is due to maturation. It remains somewhat questionable whether any such phenomena are demonstrable. Prototypes, on the other hand, serve as the physiological *models* for the later establishment of psychological functions and phenomena. In this process, development plays the major part.

sector of the personality. Besides those contributing specifically to maturation there are other innate factors operating from birth. The totality of innate factors is the infant's congenital equipment. The term *development* designates the modifications effected by the surround on the inborn congenital equipment. Accordingly, congenital equipment will be modified in the course of development by the organism's adaptation to environmental circumstances. On the other hand, congenital equipment is also modified by two kinds of stresses: (1) by those arising from maturational factors; (2) by those accompanying biological growth and function.

Before going into the substance of my argument, I feel it necessary to explain certain concepts used by me which to the psychoanalytic reader might appear self-evident. I am referring to the fact that in my explanations I am consistently speaking of phenomena connected primarily with orality and oral need gratification. I am using this approach for the purpose of simplifying my text. It should be evident from my previous publications (Spitz, 1955c, 1957) that I do not believe that the oral stage is exclusively concerned with the mouth and the perioral zone. The needs of the infant involve many other modalities besides the oral intake, some of them of equal importance. In those publications I have spoken of cutaneous, tactile, equilibrium, thermal stimuli, rhythms, and of deep sensitivity; there are many others, of which we are not yet aware.

I

Attempts to interpret the meaning of facial expression or behavior in the neonate as we do in the adult are bound to be misleading. Of course, when in the first five minutes after delivery silver nitrate is instilled under the closed eyelids of the quiescent infant and the infant responds with violent generalized prolonged excitation and facial contortion and screaming, we feel fairly safe in calling this an expression of unpleasure.

But when a smile appears on the face of the same infant, or what looks like a smile, we may not call this an expression of tension reduction or of pleasure. The circumstances in which infants at this age smile are far too variable for that. Far too often a facial movement which looks like a smile appears in circumstances accompanied by mounting tension, a condition experienced as unpleasure at any later age. Far too rarely, not to say exceptionally, does the neonate smile in circumstances which an adult would experience as pleasurable. It is no accident that our grandmothers used to say that when a newborn smiles, he has a bellyache.

The argument could be extended. One of the simplest demonstrations of the lack of correlation between overt behavior and the quality of experience in the neonate is the series of experiments performed by Jensen (1932). He demonstrated that a large variety of stimulations, including among others hair-pulling, pinching, pinpricks, and dropping from a height of one foot, elicited the sucking response.

This experiment shows that there is as yet no constant relation between a given stimulus and a response in the form of expression at birth and in the weeks immediately thereafter. It is an open question whether one can speak in the neonate of a reliable linkage between manifest behavior and the stimulus which appears to trigger it. When we find such linkages, they are very tenuous. And the behavior occurs in response to stimuli which are frequently vastly different from those which provoke similar expressive behavior at a later age. Similarly, the neonate will respond differently from older subjects to identical stimuli. We express this concisely by the statement that the neonate's behavior is neither stimulus specific nor response specific.

However, it is common knowledge that, in the course of the first year of life and later, certain forms of emotional expression become firmly linked to and associated with certain emotional experiences. The question is how this comes about. Three basic hypotheses can be formulated: (1) The developmental hypothesis, according to which the expression of emotion is *learned* in the course of infantile development; (2) the maturational hypothesis, according to which expression is *inherited* as an anlage and will be activated in the course of development; (3) some combination of these two propositions. The second and third hypotheses obviously involve phylogenetic factors. We may wonder how expressive behavior, be it of a mimetic nature or more generalized, has come to be linked with emotion-producing experiences in the course of *phylogenesis.*

However, a discussion of this problem would go far beyond the scope of this paper. I will therefore limit this investigation to the linkage between emotional expression and emotional experience in human ontogenesis. The excitation at birth (with the character of unpleasure) is clearly a discharge phenomenon. I will speak of this as a precursor of the emotions which will develop subsequently. We should certainly not regard this as an emotion, proposing, as I do, to reserve this term for a psychological experience with concomitants of a conscious nature. It follows that I consider the external manifestations of tension-increasing experiences in the neonate as indications of discharge processes. What is discharged is physiological tension without psychological content. Such manifestations occur reliably when stimuli succeed in breaking through what Freud called the protective shield against stimuli, the neonate's high perceptual threshold.

At birth the infant reacts to the surround only if a stimulus is sufficiently powerful to break through the stimulus barrier. That is the case when stimulation from the outside is overstrong; but also when normal discomfort originates from inside, because the newborn is not protected against stimuli originating inside as he is against those coming from the surround. Elsewhere (Spitz, 1957) I have discussed my concept of the nature of this threshold. In essence, I stated that at birth the psychic representations of the neural receptor stations are not yet energized.

So far I have said little about the behavior observable in the neonate when a stimulus is strong enough to overcome the barrier against it. I mentioned that we can observe excitation of a negative kind which is manifested through discharge phenomena. These are not consistent, not limited to given systems of the organism, but in the nature of overflow activity. They appear randomly, they are unorganized, diffuse, and should be considered total responses. Among these discharge phenomena are agitation, violent spastic movements, violent facial contortions, as well as vocalizations such as screaming, wailing, and whimpering.

In all this turmoil, we can nevertheless distinguish behavioral items which at a later age would be called expressive ones. Among the behavioral items enumerated above, vocalization has a special place in view of the role it will subsequently assume as the main instrument of human communication. At the neonatal stage the forms of vocalization I have listed above are in response to tension-increasing experiences. These are experiences which might be called painful or unpleasant, were it not that these terms carry a psychological connotation. However, we lack a sufficiently neutral term to designate tension-increasing experiences which do not involve the psyche. One of the peculiarities of the neonatal stage is that vocalization appears to be restricted to responses arising in the wake of stimulation we judge to be "unpleasure" provoking. Neonatal behavior patterns which I consider the somatic *precursors* of subsequently developing *expressions* of pleasure—the most conspicuous such behavior pattern is "turning toward"—do not appear to include vocalization. "Pleasure" vocalization in the neonate is probably nonexistent.

To my knowledge no investigation has been undertaken to establish at what stage of development vocalization other than that conveying unpleasure appears.[3] Nor are there any reliable observations on what this first vocalization of gratification consists of. We may suspect that it is developed from the more or less mechanical clucking sounds occurring during nursing activity, which lead to the "Mm . . ." sound, discussed both by infant observers and psychoanalysts (Spielrein, 1922; Greenson, 1954). It is debatable whether a vocalization of pleasure may be derived, for instance, from panting in connection with manifestly gratifying experiences. Whether this particular vo-

[3] See "Goma, das Basler Gorillakind." *Documenta Geigy Bull.,* 1–5, 1959–60.

calization might, for example, lead to the sounds of laughter ("he-he-he-he") will have to be verified through observation.[4]

II

I have not yet had an occasion to speak of the expression of emotion *proper,* for I was discussing the first six weeks of life. As stated above, emotions proper involve consciousness. During the first weeks of life conscious perception, in the sense in which psychoanalysis defines the term, is not present. At this time practically all activities of the neonate are uncoordinated and undirected, because a central volitional—that is, conscious—steering organization has not yet emerged. Physiological activities are the exception; they become increasingly coordinated and integrated into a functioning totality. But *intentional* skeletal musculature is not yet integrated under the direction of a *central steering and coordinating organization* and will only become so in the course of the subsequent months. It is this central steering organization to which we assign psychological functioning, both conscious and unconscious.

This organization, which we call the ego, will enable the infant to perceive his emotions and to relate their expression to sensations experienced and to stimuli received. It comes into being, at least in a rudimentary fashion, around the third month. Before this organization begins to function, I am unwilling to speak of emotion proper, only of its precursors. Even after the beginnings of the central steering organization are established, specific emotional expressions are still only loosely linked to specific types of experience. The infant's expression can still be interpreted (or understood) only in the context of an ongoing situation. In a certain measure, that remains true throughout a great part of the infant's first year.

It appears, then, that specific facial expressions as expression of emotions become meaningful as a result of a linkage. The linkage takes place between a specific facial expression and a specific experience, a coordination comparable to that which takes place in the conditioned reflex. The refinement and the progressively increasing specificity of the expression itself are acquired in the course of development. A great deal of research remains to be done in order to learn how this coordination is achieved. The fact that the negative expression is present from birth shows that it is inborn. It is presumably of

[4] To avoid misunderstanding I wish to go on record that all my statements on the ontogenesis of the expression of emotions refer to average, normal children. I am aware that deviations occur; for example, neonates who respond with unpleasure manifestations to stimuli which should be pleasurable. Such instances have been described by Escalona, by Solnit and Ritvo, and by others. They are the exceptions; my current task is to deal with the average. I will add that this average shows a rather wide range of individual variations which I will disregard here.

phylogenetic origin and has survival value. The demonstration of this proposition is one of the objects of the present paper.

The expression of pleasure is the next one to appear; in the infant its most conspicuous example is the smiling response. Beginning with the third month of life this is produced in response to a Gestalt signal, which comprises certain salient features of the human face. The constituent parts of this Gestalt are the eyes, the nose, and the forehead; moreover, the whole configuration must be in motion (Spitz, 1946d).

It should be clearly understood that I am referring exclusively to the smiling *response* and not to random activity of the facial muscles, which may look like a smile. The facial movement of smiling is probably present from birth—my earliest motion picture record for such a smile is of a three-day-old infant. This smile "movement" is a discharge phenomenon which occurs randomly; it cannot be reliably elicited by repeating the specific situation in which it had been observed, nor by situations which are the opposite of those eliciting the negative "displeasurable" expressions.

Among the few positive manifestations at birth, "turning toward" is the most relevant for this discussion. I consider "turning toward" as a positive expression because of its survival value, which is demonstrated by its phylogenetic history (Spitz, 1957). It is provoked primarily by eliciting the sucking reflex. In the third month of life this turning-toward response develops into reciprocity with the adult: the infant responds to the adult's face with a smile. I have considered this to be the expression of a positive *emotion* for the following reasons:

1. After the smiling response has been established, it ceases to be random and becomes stimulus specific. Beginning with the third month of life, it will be produced reliably in situations which have the specific character of initiating a need gratification. This linking of the smiling response to certain stimuli which adults would consider pleasurable or gratifying will continue throughout life in an unbroken line.

2. Conversely, the smiling response will not be manifested in situations which would provoke responses or emotions of unpleasure, such as pain, rage, anger, or boredom, in the adult.

3. The physiognomic characteristics of the smiling response are those of "turning toward."

4. Finally, when in the third month of life the infant achieves the smiling response, he has also achieved conscious perception and has become capable of rudimentary mental operations. This is evident not only from the smiling response but also from all his other volitionally directed, intentional activities.

III

The psychological concomitants of the smiling response at the level of the third month throw a new light on my findings about some responses at birth. They permit the conclusion that, from the viewpoint of structure, negative excitation at birth is fundamentally different from the turning-toward response. Negative excitation behavior is a nondirected, random, unspecific emergency behavior, in response to any stimulus *quantitatively* strong enough to break through the stimulus barrier. The turning-toward behavior, on the other hand, is specific, nonrandom, and occurs in response to a specific discrete stimulus. It is not a response to quantitative but to *qualitative* differences. At birth this is the only directed response to stimuli qualitatively differentiated from the surround. The turning-toward response has a positive value for survival. Consequently I feel justified in considering it one of the first positive behavior patterns in the infant, though not a psychological one.

Though the turning-toward response is present already at birth, it is questionable whether this applies also to the avoidance reaction. However, we know that the latter will soon emerge in the course of development, although its phenomenology has not been investigated in sufficient detail. We do not know when manifestations of unpleasure—e.g., screaming and random violent movements, which denote negative excitation—are transformed into movements of withdrawal and flight. In other words, we are unable to say at what point of infant development expressions of unpleasure are replaced by expressions of *fear*.

The inception and the sequence in the structuring of the expression of negative emotion parallel the development of the smile. In the neonate stage, negative experience results from a breakthrough of the stimulus barrier (either from inside or outside) and is responded to by increase of random activity, rise of tonus, and vocalization. In the subsequent weeks, though expression of negative emotions is still triggered by the quantitative factor of a breakthrough of the stimulus barrier, a qualitative factor is added. The stimuli for such a breakthrough become ever more specific. It becomes increasingly evident that this behavior of the infant will arise mostly in the hunger situation or in situations of intestinal discomfort. These are need situations, requiring discharge through gratification to insure survival. The development which now sets in adds *secondary needs* to the primary survival-insuring ones; I will call these secondary needs *"quasi needs."*

By the third month, the circumstances leading to and accompanying need gratification proper also begin to become specific. When they are withheld, the infant responds as if he were being deprived of physiological need gratification. In concrete terms, the infant now insists on being cuddled, on physical contact, on the presence of the adult.

By the fourth month of life, the infant reacts by screaming when the gratification of this quasi need is withheld, that is, when the adult leaves after playing with him; just as he reacts by smiling when the adult approaches him. It is at this point that the precursors of emotion are transformed into emotion proper. No other object (thing) will provoke these responses at the same age, though, of course, straightforward need deprivation or need gratification will.

It is regrettable that we do not yet possess findings on physiognomic differentiation between the infant's behavior when subjected to the frustration of a quasi need (such as the contact with the adult being interrupted), on the one hand, and the expression of fear resulting from the anticipation of pain on the other (Darwin, 1872).

IV

Before going on to the subsequent unfolding of the expression of emotion in the course of the second half of the first year of life. I want to mention some of the problems which arise from what I have presented so far. They can be summarized in three points:

1. How does the elaboration of the expression of emotion proceed from the physiological process to the psychological experience?

2. What elements in the expression of negative emotion and of the smiling response are innate?

3. What, if any, is the implication of these considerations for psychoanalysis and for psychoanalytic theory in particular?

I shall confine myself to the first question, the progressive shift of the expression of emotion from a somatic process to a psychological experience. Psychological stimuli (in the sense in which we apply the term to adults) do not provoke observable responses in the neonate; we must assume that he does not perceive them. He does not *perceive* physical stimuli either, but he *reacts* unspecifically to them when they are sufficiently massive. In this statement perception is defined as a function which involves an activity of the psychic apparatus. This activity comprises, among others, the dealing with and the processing of nervous stimuli with the help of psychic operations.

Our operational criteria for the infant having achieved perception are his capacity to *recognize* a percept previously experienced, or, at the earliest level, the demonstrability of a change wrought by the percept in the perceiving organism. This last statement includes the conditioned reflex.

But the conditioned reflex partakes of two worlds. As we shall see later, it stands on the borderline, reaching into the neurological on the one side, into the psychological on the other. This is why, on the one hand, chronologically, and in regard to consciousness, the conditioned reflex begins in the undifferentiated, nonconscious stage of life. On the other hand, however, it appears to form, many weeks later, the bridge leading over into the stage in which conscious and unconscious have separated from each other. It is my opinion that the conditioned reflex at the neonate level is largely responsible for maintaining those exchanges which eventually lead to the emergence of consciousness.

Conditioned reflexes can be set up in the neonate quite early, depending on the sensory modality which is used for the conditioned stimulus. In the first days of life it would obviously be impractical to try to condition through a visual stimulus; in the first days the neonate's eyes are mostly closed, and even when they are open, they do not react to visual stimulation, unless this be rather violent; in that case it produces the startle reflex. During the same period of life, however, conditioning with help of change of position, that is, deep sensitivity involving the coenesthetic system, is perfectly possible (Bühler, 1928).

Negative excitation which at the neonatal age requires discharge of a disorganized, random nature, will retain this negative connotation also at a much later stage, when psychological[5] functioning is already in existence—witness, for instance, the proverbial irritability and ill-humor which takes possession of us when we are kept waiting for food.

This is one application of Freud's proposition that, just as the birth experience is the physiological prototype for the psychological response of anxiety which appears much later, there exist other archaic experiences which become the prototypes for other emotions. It is my contention that the discharge of negative excitation is the prototype for the expression of unpleasure. I suggest that this proposition be applied in the first place to emotions consciously experienced as unpleasure; furthermore, that somatic and physiological responses to unpleasure stimuli should be considered to accompany in varying measure the whole subsequent gamut of psychological unpleasure both conscious and unconscious.

This proposition applies equally to the expression of pleasure; it follows that the feeling tone of the newborn's somatic response to pleasurable experience also will be recalled in the feeling tone of later psychological experience. I believe that there is a direct genetic connection between the feeling tone of the turning-toward response in the early feeding situation and the feeling tone attached to, first, following the face of an adult visually, and later responding to it with a smile.

---

[5] This statement should not be construed as implying that psychological functioning is predicated on consciousness. Consciousness is one of its attributes; consciousness and the central steering operations performed by the psyche offer us access to the nonconscious sectors and to their function.

It would be tempting to investigate the somatic origins of the feeling tone, expansive and at the same time all inclusive, which accompanies for instance such emotions as joy. But the expression of the opposite of unpleasure in the neonate is tenuous and not easy to observe. Darwin already remarked that it is much easier to observe expressions of suffering, pain, etc., than expressions of joy. I will therefore choose the easier road and take the negative responses as my point of departure.

In the course of infant care the neonate experiences a variety of stimuli as a disturbance of his quiescence; being washed, being exposed to cold, being disturbed in his sleep—these are the most common disturbing *external* stimuli. We are equally familiar with internal ones such as the baby's being hungry; and with his response to intestinal pain. None of these experiences has a psychological representation at this stage. It is to be assumed that they will acquire one in the following few weeks. How they do that, however, is unclear. It seems to me that at this point a series of experiments performed by Volkelt (1929), in a totally different psychological sector, that of perception, and the application of his findings to the feeding situation by Frankl and Rubinow (1934) are particularly enlightening. They investigated when and how the infant, in a series of successive steps, progressively recognizes the "thing" he most frequently sees, namely, his bottle with the food. These steps are the following:

1. The neonate responds reliably to the nipple when it *touches* his oral mucosa.

2. A week later he produces what these authors have called *Flaschener-kennungsreaktion,* which we can translate into English as "food-recognition reaction." By this is meant that when the *preliminaries* to placing the bottle in his mouth are performed (whatever these may be, e.g., putting a bib under his chin), he responds by this particular reaction. The food-recognition reaction consists in a conspicuous change of the infant's behavior, e.g., the crying infant becomes quiet; or the infant makes sucking movements; or he extends his lips, his tongue, etc. The precondition for the success of this experiment is that it must take place at the infant's feeding hour. The experiment shows that the response has been displaced from the unconditioned stimulus (food in the mouth), and that a conditioned stimulus (bib under chin) has been established. *Prolepsis* (the function of anticipation) has emerged in the form of a conditioned reflex—we may consider it the earliest *prototype* of psychological function.

3. The next step is a highly significant one. The *tactile* conditioned stimulus of "bib under chin" is replaced by a new, *visual* conditioned stimulus. The response is elicited already when a person approaches the infant's crib at the usual feeding hour. This means that the perception of a new conditioned

stimulus takes place both sooner and from a greater distance. The contact receptor has been replaced by a distance receptor. Anticipation, surely a psychological function, is more in evidence; in this experiment we have been able to record two steps in its development. However, the response still depends on the perception of a process going on inside the neonate, namely, hunger and thirst. Environmental perception as such is not yet established independently.

4. In the next step the outside world as the *perceived* stimulus, independent of the inner state of the infant, comes into its own; now the food-recognition reaction occurs in response to a thing, whatever its shape, which enters the infant's visual field. In this experiment the stimulus consists of two factors, namely, of the movement and of the object. In my belief, this is the point in development at which the earliest manifestation of *psychological processing proper* can be observed. It consists, in its simplest form, of a sequence of events in which *A* followed by *B* followed by *C* is remembered. Whereas in the preceding stage these different modalities were united in one summative sensation, now the modalities are distinguished from each other and their *sequence* is endowed with significance. This is the process of apperception; here it consists of two or more memory traces, in the present example, of the memory of an object and of its approach. They are used in a specifically psychological process, namely, in anticipation of that which will follow the perception of the approaching object.

The response to the percept of an *approaching object* could be called an "as-if" behavior of the infant. The infant responds in the terms of the need gratification which the percept food is *expected* to provide.

The inference that anticipation proves the functioning of a psychological process is not a stringent one. After all, anticipation of a sort is involved also in the conditioned reflex. But I believe that in the unfolding of the food-recognition reaction we witness a phenomenon of a different order. The rapid shifts in the physical nature and in the space-time structure of the response-evoking stimulus just described are not characteristic of the conditioned reflex. In the first three phases of the food-recognition reaction, the awareness of the stimulus was displaced successively to percepts both more distant in space and occurring earlier in time than the actual gratification of the need. These percepts are also very different in their physical appearance. The successive anticipatory percepts were first the bib under the chin and later a person approaching the crib.

In the subsequent stages, however, a new process sets in. Instead of re-sponding to a percept which is more distant in space and which also occurs earlier in time, the infant now disregards these previous percepts. It is as if a finer discrimination has begun, as if the three- to six-month-old infant has realized that "approaching person" could mean other things also, besides food. He now seems to wait for more "tangible" facts. Now he does not respond to the approaching person, only to the stimulus of a "thing" approaching his face, whatever the thing's general shape may be, within certain wide limits of size.

This is not the usual development in the establishment of conditioned responses; and the further steps in the unfolding of food recognition are increasingly directed toward the cognitive perception of essential attributes of the food itself; while the anticipatory recognition of the accompanying circumstances (e.g., the adult entering the infant's room, etc.) goes its own way. The subsequent steps in the achievement of food recognition are:

5. It is no longer sufficient that any object be approached to the child's face; the object has to be roughly cone-shaped and to end in a point.

6. A few weeks later the object's ending in a point is no longer sufficient; it must have a nipple at its point and must be filled with white liquid.

7. The final step, achieved somewhere around six months of life, is that the milk as such is recognized, whether in a bottle or any other container.

This sequence of steps in the development of the cognition of a visual percept also gives us the key to the ontogenesis of the expression of negative emotions—and, of course, positive ones as well. I postulated—and this certainly could be experimentally established—that in the beginning the expression of unpleasure takes place only in response to the unconditioned stimulus of experiencing pain or discomfort. In the course of the first few months of life this unconditioned response is modified. Unpleasure will be anticipated already in response to changes in the environment which in themselves, and at the moment when they occur, need not produce discomfort.

We do not possess as precise observational and experimental studies of the earliest development of negative emotions as those we have for the unfolding of the positive ones. There the meshing of the food-recognition reaction with the smiling response provides us with an unbroken genetic sequence beginning with birth. We can, however, advance a plausible hypothesis about the development of the expression of negative emotion. This hypothesis is based on direct observation as well as on the parallels between this development and that of the sequence observed in the expression of positive emotions. My hypothesis, which is presented below, is further supported by its consistency with well-established psychoanalytic propositions.

In the neonate the expression of emotion most in evidence is the one in response to unpleasure, caused by the unconditioned stimulus. This is in manifest parallel to the first stage of the food-recognition reaction, in which the response is to the nipple in the mouth. This would lead one to believe that later, more advanced expressions of unpleasure also develop in a straight genetic sequence from the original situation. But this does not seem to be the case.

In the weeks following birth the unconditioned stimulus of *somatic* pain, discomfort, etc., elicits manifestations of unpleasure, predominantly undirected and random. However, unequivocally clear manifestations of unpleasure in response to psychological stimuli do not develop in direct genetic derivation from these. To my mind, the first unequivocal psychological manifestation of unpleasure in the infant occurs when he begins to cry when left by the adult with whom he had been in contact. This behavior appears after the third month of life and is the counterpart of the smiling response of which I have spoken above.

This unpleasure manifestation can only be understood if we assume that the infant has integrated into the inventory of his need gratifications the *presence* of the adult as a quasi need. Accordingly the infant will react to the adult's moving away by expressing negative emotion in anticipation of being deprived of the gratification of this quasi need. There obviously is a parallel between this "negative" expression of emotion in response to a *receding* person, and the "positive" behavior manifested to the approaching person in the food-recognition response as well as in the smiling response.

One explanation of this paradoxical and circuitous line in the development of the expression of negative emotions may be found in the phenomenon of the stimulus barrier at birth.

The breakthrough of the stimulus barrier can be responded to only by an undirected total behavior, which is generalized, uncoordinated, and random. Such total behavior does not lend itself to structuring and further development within the individual ontogenesis. A gradual process of adaptation cannot be expected from a disorganized, decompensated emergency reaction, comparable to what Kurt Goldstein (1928) described as the "catastrophic reaction" in the brain-damaged adult.

However, in analogy to what I previously described for the "trauma of birth," elements of this reaction may be used for the expression of negative emotion, when at a later stage an experience of discomfort produces a shadowy, essentially physiological, recall of complete loss of control. The early physiological responses to unpleasure are random, uncoordinated, and often involve the autonomic nervous system. Some of them will enter into the later, organized expression of negative emotion. This holds true not only for infancy and childhood. Thus the adult may feel nausea under the impact of violent disgust. He commemorates, so to say, earliest infantile autonomic reactions.

Unpleasure experiences of two fundamentally different kinds will be expressed by superficially similar behavior patterns:

1. A form of unpleasure in response to the unconditioned stimulus of pain

and discomfort. The response to this is an uncontrolled behavior which will change very little in the course of development.

2. A form of unpleasure in response to psychological stimuli. This response is not present from birth. It has to be acquired by developing a *quasi need* on the one hand, and the *proleptic function*, that is, the function of anticipation, on the other. Both the need and the function are developed in the framework of object relations, primarily as the result of need gratification. Once the function to anticipate pleasure is acquired, it becomes possible for the child to perform also the psychological operation of anticipating unpleasure when *losing* the object. The infant displays this anticipation through the facial expression of negative emotion.

At this level at the age of three to six months of life the anticipation of unpleasure has acquired a *signal* function, the function described by Freud in *Inhibitions, Symptoms and Anxiety* (1926). The expression of this emotion increasingly acquires the function of communication. This communication comprises two bits of information, which are channeled in opposite directions:

1. The first is the mounting tension of the emotion. This is similar to the conditions leading to the breakthrough of the stimulus barrier. It is experienced as a danger signal, an information which is transmitted centripetally to the incipient ego of the three- to six-month-old infant.

2. The facial and behavioral expression of the same emotion. This is perceived by the surround as a communication. Though it is at first not intentional or directed, it nevertheless transmits information centrifugally.

At this stage the two components do not yet constitute an apparatus of the ego. They are not established as a discrete functional continuum, interconnecting with the different aspects of the personality. In the course of the following three months, these connections will be formed. They will become ever more suitable for triggering adaptive measures of the ego and for communicating with the surround. This process leads to the establishment of specific emotions firmly linked with their appropriate expression. The final outcome of this process is, in one instance, the "eight-months anxiety" (Spitz, 1946a, 1950a).

The eight-months anxiety marks the inception of an important stage in the child's development. It lends itself particularly well to the exposition of several psychological processes. In the present context I am discussing that aspect of the phenomenon which illustrates the next step in the ontogenetic development of the expression of emotion. Through the study of this step we gain insight into the further vicissitudes of what originally was an undirected state of excitation. For in the eight months anxiety we can observe how the subjective experience of emotion follows a different path from that of emotional expression. In what follows I will show how the *emotion* of anxiety (i.e., felt anxiety) assumes a centripetally directed function; at the same time the *expression* of the same emotion becomes effective in a centrifugal direction. The part directed to the inside acts as a danger signal, mobilizing the pleasure-unpleasure agency (Freud, 1926); thus the resources of the personality are marshaled in the service of defense against mental helplessness.

The other part is channeled into the efferent nervous system and sets in motion the gamut of the expressions of this particular emotion. These expressions serve as a communication to the outside: to the surround, to the libidinal object. They are perceived by the outside world as a sign of helplessness or as a signal, that is, as an appeal for help.

The successive stages of this development, beginning with the breakthrough of the stimulus barrier, are:

1. The unspecific, undirected, total emotional responses in the first three months of life.

2. The progressive integration of emotional responses with their facial and behavioral expression in the course of the next three months on the one hand; their serving as a communication to the outside on the other.

3. The establishment, in the third quarter of the first year, of a definitive link between felt emotion as a signal for the ego and the expression of emotion as a communication to the surround.

The process of organizing the original discharge into recognizably different expressions linked to specific emotions is initiated and carried on through the exchanges between child and mother in the course of object relations. The unfolding of the individual child's object relations parallels closely the ontogenesis of the expression of his emotions.

When infants are deprived of object relations, their emotional expression remains on the archaic level of the first months of life (Spitz, 1946a). The expression becomes rigid and vacuous. But when object relations are close and gratifying to mother and child, then the expression of emotions unfolds in a variety of patterns and eventually becomes a means of communication in the framework of object relations.

The proposition of the role of object relations in the ontogenesis of the expression of emotion is further borne out by two different observations: (1) the chronological sequence in the successive stages of the positive smiling response, which parallel those of the first specifically psychologically motivated expression of negative emotion; (2) the range of expressions accompanying the emergence of the eight months anxiety in the second half of the first year.

As to the first: the response of smiling, the expression of pleasure on perceiving the Gestalt signal of the human face appears approximately one month earlier than the response of unpleasure on being left by a partner. In other terms, a partner, at least in the form of a *preobject,* has to be established as a result of object relations before the consequences of the loss of this preobject can be anticipated. It is gratifying to find this argumentation confirmed by the facts of observation.

In regard to the second confirmatory evidence, we find that the phenomenon of the eight months anxiety varies in a wide range, and is dependent on the nature of the individual child's object relations. In my observations of psychopathological deviations in the first year of life, the appearance of the characteristic anxiety was significantly delayed and even completely absent when certain forms of inappropriate object relations were present during the preceding months. On the other hand, the eight months anxiety was replaced by uncontrollable manifestations of panic and fear in those cases in which object relations were extremely inadequate or the infant had been deprived of them altogether.[6]

Eight-months anxiety of the usual kind varies a good deal in its intensity. This phenomenon has not been sufficiently explored up to now.[7] The reason for this is that it requires thorough investigation of children in private family homes, in itself a major project. Added to this is the fact that children vary in their congenital frustration tolerance and that as yet we have no instrument suitable for evaluating this tolerance in the neonate.

We may say in conclusion that the ontogenesis of the expression of emotions is a function of the nature of the individual child's object relations as much as of the unfolding of an inherited anlage. To the psychoanalyst this finding is not unexpected. We were aware for a number of years and have been able to demonstrate (Spitz, 1946a) that the expression of pleasure is developed from an innate anlage in the course of the exchanges with the human object. We now find a similar sequence obtaining in regard to the expression of negative emotions. These also develop from an innate anlage, from disorganized, decompensated response to the breakthrough of the stimulus barrier, through object relations to the expression of negative emotions in response to the loss of the preobject and from there to the signal of anxiety.

I cannot discuss the further ramifications of the expression of emotions. Enumerating them as they appear in the course of the first year of life already

[6] Two different sets of circumstances can lead to this end result. One is a separation of the infant from his object at a critical age, resulting in a mourning process with regression to earlier, and often archaic modes of functioning and adaptation. I have discussed this picture elsewhere (Spitz, 1946a), and called it *anaclitic depression.* The second is the picture of infants raised from birth in institutions without opportunity to form any object relations whatsoever. Here the response remains unspecific, as in response to the unconditioned stimulus—a quantitative response, be it to the experience of pain or to the interruption of quiescence. I described this condition under the name of *hospitalism* (Spitz, 1945b).

[7] But see Benjamin's (1961) careful investigations and his distinction between "stranger anxiety" and "infantile separation anxiety."

shows that they also are differentiated in response to specific object relations. I need only mention jealousy, envy, possessiveness, demanding attitudes, anger, rage, love, amusement, laughter, boredom (yawning and fatigue), not to speak of the chronologically later, increasingly subtle expressions of doubt, hesitation, quizzical attitudes, trust and mistrust, and a whole gamut of others.

I am aware that in the ontogenesis of the expression of emotions it would be well to follow Darwin's example and to investigate the somatic components, the neuromuscular bases of these expressions, their connections with physiology, embryology, genetics, and phylogenesis. Such an investigation is not within my competence. It would certainly require the collaboration of several disciplines. In this study I have therefore kept within the limits of behavioral observation on the one hand, of psychoanalytic dynamics on the other.

SUMMARY

In the ontogenesis of the expression of emotions, both maturation and development, both the innate and the experiential, play their own particular roles. The innate factors in maturation are evident at birth in the two precursors of the expression of two diametrically opposed emotions, namely, negative excitation and "turning toward." These innate factors still play a major role in the ontogenesis of perception and in the inception of memory; however, both perception and memory traces are subject to the influence of development, as the latter becomes effective in the course of the formation and the conduct of object relations. At this point of my argument, I stressed a basic aspect of emotions and their expression, namely, their proleptic function. This function has survival value; hence, the potential for developing it is innate. Its unfolding, however, is predicated on a process of development taking place within the framework of object relations. This process leads to the endowment of emotions and their expression with two further important functions: (1) the signal function of emotions within the psychic apparatus; (2) the communication function of emotional expression directed to the surround. These functions, the proleptic function, the signal function, and the communication function, offer us an approach for further investigation of the subsequent stages in the ontogenesis of the expression of emotions.

Metapsychology and Direct Infant Observation

De Ajuriaguerra (1965) recently coined the epigram *"L'homme se fait en faisant"* ("Man is made by doing"). Maturation is certainly the basis of development; but without the exercise of function and the activation of behavior patterns (e.g., von Senden's 1932 report on operated blind-born individuals) maturation will be arrested. I described this phenomenon in children deprived of affective supplies (Spitz, 1945b, 1946b); Harlow's (1958, 1959) experiments on primates have recently furnished strong support for this assumption.

Once the stage of object constancy is acquired, a new dimension will be added to the relations of the baby with his mother. In the first half year of life, the preverbal dialogue between infant and mother takes place as a function of the child's needs, as expressed by Anna Freud's term of "need fulfillment." Once the memory image of the mother is established as a distinct integrated individual, of whom one can be certain, as an individual who provides the gratification of the libidinal drive at the same time as that of the aggressive drives, the mother-child dialogue acquires a wealth of novel possibilities. The baby will experiment with the consequences of alternately satisfying one or the other of his drives, and vary the proportions from experiment to experiment. His behavior can now be understood from the economic viewpoint.

Let us return to the developmental level before the fusion of the aggressive and libidinal drive has taken place and the significance of this archaic condition for developments in the perceptual area.

We have the good fortune to possess certain data gathered by von Senden (1932) on 66 subjects born with infantile cataracts who were operated upon when they were adolescents or adults. Von Senden's data suggest that at birth differentiation does not exist in the perceptual sphere, just as we have postulated the absence of differentiation in all other sectors of the personality. Von Senden's observations were recently duplicated on primates by Riesen (1965). Not only are visual stimuli not distinguished from each other, but

---

This is an abridged version of a paper reprinted from *Psychoanalysis—A General Psychology: Essays in Honor of Heinz Hartmann,* ed. Rudolph M. Loewenstein, Lottie M. Newman, Max Schur, and Albert J. Solnit. New York: International Universities Press, 1966, pp. 123–151.

[The first fifteen pages are not reprinted here since they review matters covered in other papers in this volume. The interested scholar, however, will want to consult the original for Spitz's integrated view of his work in relation to Hartmann's theory of adaptation. Ed.]

they are not even distinguished from stimuli originating in other perceptual modalities. Perhaps the most striking example in von Senden's book is an adult operated for infantile cataract who compared his first perception of color to the smell of varnish.

From this inchoate beginning visual and other percepts will have to develop as a function of the relations of the newborn with the outside world. I tried to show, and my findings were confirmed by the experiments of Harlow and others on primates, that the givens necessary for this development are mediated to the baby by the libidinal object. After birth, a relatively long period will elapse before the newborn becomes capable of recognizing a signal outside of himself, namely, the Gestalt signal inherent in the human face.

I have advanced the hypothesis that in the breast-fed infant (other rules prevail for bottle-fed infants), this signal owes the privilege of being the first one to be perceived to circumstances which correspond exactly to the postulate of Freud (1925a): "A precondition for the setting up of reality-testing is that objects shall have been lost which once brought real satisfaction" (p. 238). In the case of the first consistently established signal, the process is as follows: the nursing infant, as soon as he arrives at the stage where he keeps his eyes open during feeding, stares at the mother's face from the beginning to the end of his meal. Thus there are two percepts which become operative during nursing: one, the tactile perception of the food, of the nipple in the infant's mouth; and second, the visual percept of the mother's face. Of the two, only the visual percept remains invariable.

In contrast, the perception of the nipple is discontinuous. It is absent before the beginning of nursing and after its end. And when during nursing the nipple is removed from the mouth of the baby—a procedure which takes place frequently during every nursing—the percept of the mother's face remains unchanged. In other terms, the face of the mother is the stable element in an experience of need fulfillment interrupted by gaps of frustration, the loss of the part object, the nipple, which had responded to the need of the child.

The gratification of the libidinal drive during nursing insures the increasingly conscious perception of the Gestalt characteristics of the human face. Less obviously but no less powerfully, this conscious perception is enforced by the aggressive drive evoked through the loss of the nipple in the course of nursing. This is probably the first occasion in life when the two drives, only recently emerged from the stage of undifferentiation, will alternate in quick succession in a situation in which a large portion of the perceptual field (mainly the visual one) remains unchanged.

From this point onward the interaction of maturation and development brings about, by the second half of the first year, an extraordinary advance in the psychic apparatus, of which I have chosen to present the perceptual manifestations only.

In the perceptual field, between the third and the sixth months of life, the infant is exposed, again and again, to opposite emotions while contemplating his mother's face, which of course remains identical. In my opinion, this identity of the visual percept permits the infant to combine the "giving" mother's *face* with the "frustrating" mother's *face* into the unified percept of the mother's *person*. This development is a progressive one, and results from the maturation of the child's central nervous system and the unfolding of his psychic capacity.

This then is the road which the infant's development has to follow to arrive at the percept of the mother's *person* independent of the situation in which he perceives her; with that she has become different from any other being in the world, a unique and irreplaceable individual. In Hartmann's (1952) terms, this is the establishment of object constancy.

It is evident that this development starts with the inception of the reality principle. Furthermore, it is evident that the baby has to make considerable progress in applying this principle to achieve the above-mentioned results. The capacity to hold in suspense the gratification of the drive long enough to perceive and store the memory traces of the percept is indispensable. This means that he cannot give way simply and without concern either to his pleasure or to his unpleasure, but that he has to explore the percept, scan his memory traces, and recognize the person of the mother or reject the stranger.

With the achievement of object constancy we have arrived in the second half of the first year, at a level of structural development where we begin to discern important changes in the ego. During the first half year, what one could mainly observe of the ego was its equipment, which consists of what Hartmann calls "apparatuses" of the ego, that is, primary autonomy. In the course of development the ego apparatuses, which in the beginning were phylogenetically preformed innate ego nuclei, will acquire an archaic representation in the psyche. We are speaking here of extremely elementary functions, for instance, that of prehension, of grasping. I have described and filmed its development elsewhere, beginning with forced grasping at birth and its progress to intentional grasping directed by volition.

In the second six months, we can see subordinate systems being formed within the structural organization of the ego, prototypes as well as precursors of psychological functioning, such as the defense mechanisms of the ego (Spitz, 1958a, 1961). Prototypes appear to be innate somatic functions. Precursors, on the other hand, appear to be archaic psychological functions which in the beginning serve adaptation.

These archaic functions still take place in the conflict-free sphere of the ego, but toward the end of the first year a new form of adaptation will be set in motion. I am speaking of attempts to resolve intrapsychic conflict. It is at this point that the mechanisms of defense have their inception.

I intend to touch on only one of these mechanisms, the most obvious one and the one most widely used in the first year of life—the mechanism of identification. I wish to stress that until now, we defined identification as a process which takes place in the unconscious, hence is unconscious, and which consists in a certain redistribution of libidinal and aggressive cathexes. As a result of this redistribution a modification in the ego takes place.

Identification is the result of an unconscious process which takes place in the unconscious sector of the ego. It "represents a process of modifying the self-schema on the basis of a present or past perception of an object which is taken as model" (Sandler, 1960b, p. 150). I have found this definition helpful because of its emphasis on the self.

While Freud used this term in discussing "self consciousness," "self observation," "self criticism," the concept "self"—as a counterpart of "object"—was introduced by Hartmann in 1950. Since then many authors have contributed to it (Jacobson, 1954, 1964; Spitz, 1957; Spiegel, 1959; Lichtenstein, 1963). I single out Jacobson's (1964) beautiful formulation: the sense of self or identity develops as "a process that builds up the ability to preserve the whole psychic organization . . . as a highly individualized but coherent entity which has direction and continuity at any stage of human development" (p. 27).

My own view of the self is this: while the ego, one of the three psychic structures, is a theoretical construct, the self is a percept which stems from introspection, i.e., from our perception of ourselves.[1]

From my observations on infants and small children I have drawn the conclusion that the self is a product of awareness. Awareness in its turn is a function of the ego: like the ego, it develops. In the course of this process, the self develops as the cognitive precipitate of experience.

This cognitive precipitate, the self, begins to become manifest around the fifteenth month, about one year after the beginning of what I have called the awareness of the "non-I." The awareness of the "non-I" is achieved as a result of object relations in the feeding situation. The next stage will arrive when as a result of the infant's multifarious action exchanges with the "non-I" he becomes aware of his "I." These archaic relations and exchanges still remain within the somatic part of the personality. The exchanges themselves,

---

[1] In this context an interesting observation of Spiegel (1959) is worth mentioning. Staring fixedly at the regular interstices of a venetian blind, he noticed that when he moved his head from the vertical, the afterimage on the retina was modified by an angle corresponding to the inclination of his head. He explained this observation by distinguishing primary perception from the perception of the afterimage. *Primary perception* has as its frame of reference the external world and therefore remains constant. The afterimage belongs to the person, its frame is the body; that is, the images of the body which form the self. For this reason afterimages on the retina are variable.

the somatic relations with the "non-I," are invested with vast quantities of affect. For this reason these experiences are the first ones to mediate the perception of the surround.

In the course of the development which follows, the "I" will thus be perceived by the infant as a result of his perception of the "non-I." The inception of the self representation in its turn is the result of further affective exchanges experienced by the "I."

When after the eighth month the infant becomes the "executor" of his own wishes, he is also obliged to become his own "observer"; he becomes the observer of himself and as a result an observer of his self. Until then this was his mother's role, but now the child is obliged not only to observe his self, but also to judge it. This permits him to learn through experience in his attempts to understand, evaluate, and gauge the ever-changing tasks of daily living. This is a flexible, reality-adapted learning. It is quite different from the learning which preceded it, for up to that time changes in behavioral patterns were acquired thanks to the functioning of the law of effect and through the conditioned reflex. These two devices can elicit only reactive patterns, which are rigid in themselves; furthermore, being inflexible, they do not adapt themselves, or adapt only with difficulty, to changing reality during individual ontogenesis. The modification of such patterns can be acquired only in the course of phylogenesis, that is, over a long period, under the pressure of natural selection.

Conversely, those adaptive experiences which underlie learning take place in the course of reciprocal relations between the infant and environmental reality, be this alive or inanimate. Reciprocal relations and one-way relations involve either gratification or frustration or both, but the affective quality of gratification and frustration is of a much higher order in reciprocal relations than in one-way relations, and therefore more likely to lead to conflict.

Conflict in its turn expands, multiplies, and intensifies the relations themselves. This intensification then leads to the necessity of finding new methods of dealing with the situation. It seems to me that so many years after Freud had pointed out the seminal principle of conflict (and of defense against it), the creative role of conflict in development is still too little appreciated. We are ever inclined to stress its role in pathology and to neglect its positive side, namely, its vital role in the advancement of the individual and the species, its role in provoking the creation of adaptive devices. One of the great merits of Hartmann (1939) was his systematic research into this aspect of ego psychology.

In the case of the child, the most important among such conflicts occurs when the child clashes with the will of the mother. Furthermore, conflicts with environmental reality (be it animate or inanimate) force the child to become conscious of his limitations. The limits of the self will thus be progressively restricted and narrowed down, while at the same time the feeling of omnipotence will decrease.

It follows that the self is in part constructed from the residues of magic omnipotence. The traces of this origin of the self will never disappear completely in the course of life. One can notice them even in the adult. However, the adult's return to the omnipotence of the self is inhibited by reality testing. On the other hand, sleep permits the suspension of reality testing because in this state perception and hence judgment are eliminated. The arrest of motility in sleep makes reality testing unnecessary.

The suspension of the function which has the task of reality testing opens the road which leads to a return to the origins of the self, that is, to magic omnipotence. With that, hallucination of need gratification becomes possible, in the form of dream activity. Similar processes operate in psychosis.

Coming back to the distinction between the self and the psychic representation of the self, I wish to stress once more that the self is a concept which has its place in the theoretical framework of psychoanalytic psychology; the *representation* of the self has perceptual and cognitive attributes and thus is something of which we are conscious. I believe that in the future development of psychoanalytic theory we shall have to consider the relation of the self in respect to the three psychic structures on the one hand and the metapsychological viewpoint on the other. It will become necessary to determine the place of the self from the topographic, the economic, and the structural viewpoints.

It will be apparent that I have omitted the genetic viewpoint, because the distinction between the self and the representation of the self becomes delicate. In speaking of the origins of the self, I have already stressed that it is subject to development.

In my observations of infants, I distinguished the following stages: (1) The infant's capacity to distinguish something beyond that which he feels; he achieves this between the second and the third month. It is the stage in which he becomes aware of the "non-I." (2) The capacity to distinguish the "I" from the "non-I," which he achieves in the three months which follow the first stage. (3) The capacity to distinguish the libidinal object from any other person, a stage which he achieves in the course of the second half of the first year. In my concept the capacity to distinguish the object from the rest of the world marks the inception of the self in the psyche.

At this stage the infant becomes capable of experimenting with a host of new situations, behaviors, sensations. This change results from his increasing autonomy. At the same time, however, increasing independence also forces the infant to trace, or at least to retrace, the confines of his self representation.

These confines were established in the course of experiences with the realities of the outside world. Now the child can no longer permit himself to act as he did before; hallucinatory experiences cannot satisfy him.

Actually, these hallucinatory experiences are hardly distinguishable from dream experiences; this confusion will continue for a while, and the difference between the two will not become definite even at an age as relatively advanced as the oedipal stage. There is no doubt that children of five to six years still confuse dream experience with reality. The best proof of this is the frequency of pavor nocturnus and the tendency to sleepwalking, which is much greater in the preschool child and even in the early latency child than in older subjects.

I have described (Spitz, 1957) a number of phenomena which signal processes operating in the development of the self and its precursors. The first among these manifestations are certainly the so-called ''experimental movements.'' They can be observed during the fourth month of life (approximately): the infant raises his hands to the level of his eyes and slowly moves his fingers and hands, following these movements attentively with his eyes. However, one should really say that he *seems* to follow them; for when I attempted an experiment, the result was somewhat disconcerting. I interposed a piece of cardboard between the child's eyes and his hands while he was performing ''experimental movements''—thus making it impossible for him to see what he was doing with his fingers. In the majority of cases this did not stop the play of the fingers.

I conclude that this finger play contains an element which must be perceived by the infant in a coenesthetic manner. Recently I have learned from research conducted at the Hampstead Clinic that blind infants, though they are perfectly able to reach the stage of smiling, do not perform these so-called experimental movements.

It further follows that this behavior consists of two parts: (1) the coenesthetic sensations in fingers and hands; (2) a visual diacritic percept. One would be inclined to conclude that the visual percept of these movements represents a stimulus which triggers the repetition and that these are stimuli which the infant provides for himself, for his own enjoyment.

This finding has a parallel in the auditory sphere—the so-called babbling monologues, in the course of which the baby (beginning with the fifth month) imitates the sounds which he produces himself. Here again we encounter self stimulation—in a circuit requiring the hearing component to complete and elaborate the circuit. As mentioned previously, I would be inclined to accept such experiences and behaviors as precursors of the self.

Omitting the manifold developments which occur between the eighth and fifteenth month, we arrive at a much more advanced stage in the evolution of the self. This stage is marked by increased autonomy of the child, who now has acquired locomotion and the beginning of verbal communication.

Several behavior manifestations suggest that this is accompanied by a significant advance in the establishment of the self and of the self representation. I shall touch on only one of these, the negative head-shaking behavior, on which I have reported extensively elsewhere (Spitz, 1957). Around 15 months of life the child begins to use negative head-shaking for the purpose of expressing refusal and this signals an impressive progress in several dimensions. In the first place, this is probably the first abstraction of which the infant is capable and it takes place with the help of a series of drive displacements, drive modifications, and cathectic shifts. In the process a conspicuous role is played by the aggressive drive, the way in which it is manipulated, and the defense mechanism of identification with the aggressor.

In the second place, the infant has now acquired a semantic signal which will become the starting point for the development of the vast semantic system of language. The immediate consequences of this acquisition is that his dialogue, as I have called the infant's preverbal transactions with his surround (Spitz, 1963a, 1964, 1965a), will be enormously enriched.

This is an abridged version of a paper reprinted from *Psychoanalysis—A General Psychology: Essays in Honor of Heinz Hartmann,* ed. Rudolph Loewenstein, Lottie M. Newman, Max Schur, and Albert J. Solnit. New York: International Universities Press, 1966, pp. 123–151.

Third, he has acquired an instrument with which to differentiate himself from his surround; by this very act, he imposes on himself a "becoming conscious" of his personality or, to be more exact, of his self. Furthermore, he has acquired a new path for the discharge of surplus energy, which previously had to be discharged through motor pathways.

Fourth, the child has acquired a new, completely different and much more effective way of conducting his relations with his surround; now he can replace motor action with discussion.

At this point I would situate the beginnings of an *organized* self and self representation. This should be distinguished from the inception of the unorganized self (mentioned earlier) which emerges in the second half of the first year. And this shadowy self is in its turn very different from what I have tentatively spoken of as possible precursors of the self, e.g., the "experimental movements."

I realize that in speaking of inception, I expose myself to two diametrically opposite objections. The first of these is that I do not situate the inception of the self early enough in development, that it should be pushed back to the third month of life, and perhaps even earlier. That is the objection of those who take Jacobson's position; however, I believe that my previous discussion has sufficiently answered this objection.

The second objection could be raised by those who, following Erikson, place the establishment of the self (or identity) in adolescence or even later. I believe that in this case we are concerned mainly with semantics. It depends on what we call "the establishment" of the self, and what we mean by identity or self. No doubt, the self proceeds to incorporate and acquire additional and new dimensions throughout the individual's life history, hand in hand with the new acquisitions which his personality may achieve in the outside world, in relations with others (and also George Mead's [1934] "generalized other"), and in regard to the shifts and modifications taking place in his internal world.

It seems to me that as soon as the infant distinguishes objects from each other, and particularly as soon as he can choose and maintain in his memory his libidinal object, we should recognize the possibility and even the probability that the first rudiment of the self is also established. I am ready to concede that there are subsequent stations which will signal further progress in the organization of the self. In an earlier publication (Spitz, 1957), I mentioned, for instance, that around the eighteenth month one observes a phenomenon which reveals that a new step has been accomplished in the development of the self: the child begins to speak of himself in the first person or by using his own name. An interesting sidelight on this development can be found in Sanford Gifford's (1965) observation of a pair of monozygotic twins with different character formation.

Another particularly impressive example is that told by Clara and Wilhelm Stern (1907), whose classic book on the language of the child was published at the beginning of this century. Peter, their son, in the second half of his second year, saw snow falling for the first time in his life. He became exceedingly excited and shouted: "Kiok, Kiok!" His parents told him: "No, Peter, this is called snow!" But the child insisted and declared firmly: "Peter, Kiok!" With this declaration, he stated his autonomy; he referred it to his own person by designating this person with his given name. In other words, he was saying to his parents: "I, by the grace of God. Peter, I myself will call it Kiok, whatever you may say!"

Those who have the opportunity to examine a series of photos taken of the same person at intervals of approximately one year, beginning with his first year until he is grown up, may be interested in the following observations: it is very impressive to see the face and expression of the subject change from one year to the next and assume a directed, oriented, and from then on consistently maintained expression. During the first year the facial expression is vague, undetermined, and slightly disoriented; the eyes look somewhat lost, as if in a daze. Even in the course of the second year the eyes assume from time to time this lost expression, particularly in unfamiliar situations.

After a person's expression has assumed consistency, it may remain unchanged in the course of all the vicissitudes of the subject's life, right into adulthood and beyond. An exception should be made for certain transitional periods in the course of puberty and at the inception of adolescence, where sometimes the face may again lose its clearly directed and oriented expression. I wish to stress this phenomenon which seems to me to confirm Anna Freud's statement (1936) that during puberty pregenital problems are once again revived before the final formation of personality. I would be inclined to say that a revision of the perception of the self takes place here in puberty before the final decision.

The fact that the first change in the indeterminate, vague, lost expression takes place suddenly from one year to the next (and according to my experience, during the preoedipal, perhaps I should say pregenital phase) permits one to assume the occurrence of an event which has forced the child to seek a new adaptation; it seems that the child has lived through a basic experience, which he had never encountered before. I would not go so far as to call this experience traumatic, but it is certainly a decisive one.

In a number of my analytic cases I discovered that this experience was the birth of a younger sibling, a competitor. Evidently, this is an event which demands a complete reorientation of the child, a new individuation, as it is called by Mahler (1957). Such a development implies an effort to acquire autonomy and independence, to acquire confidence in one's self, and a certain amount of self control, a certain mastery and security; all these are processes which lead to the becoming conscious of one's own self.

A report on a five-year-old boy is illustrative; he was visiting his grandmother for a few days. On the first morning she came to take him to his bath and told him so; whereupon the boy replied in a peremptory tone: ''I am I, and I wash myself!'' One cannot, I believe, express at the age of five years one's awareness of the dignity of one's own self in a clearer manner. This is no longer merely a body self; this is the self of the total personality.

In conclusion, it should be realized that findings obtained through direct infant observation have numerous and far-reaching implications. These refer not only to the metapsychological viewpoint in its first formulation, but perhaps even more to the structural and genetic viewpoints, as well as to the problems presented by the introduction of the concept self. Clearly, only a very few aspects of these could be taken up here in detail. Furthermore, such factors as the adaptive viewpoint, substructures within the ego, the conflict-free sphere, were merely alluded to, while the important questions of primary versus secondary autonomy and primary ego energy and neutralization could not even be touched upon.

I mention them here as an ever-present concern in research on normal and pathological infant development. For the seeker, direct infant observation offers a huge mine of information, theoretical as well as clinical. The view-points I have discussed in my paper, and even more those which I mentioned above but was unable to deal with, provide the framework, the pointers, and the theoretical orientation in the new and fertile field of investigation of this *terra incognita,* the embryology of the psychic apparatus in man.

Further Prototypes of EgoFormation: A Working Paper from a Research Project on Early Development

with ROBERT N. EMDE, M.D., and DAVID R. METCALF, M.D.

For many years, separately and together, the authors have been conducting research with infants. These investigations have involved detailed observations of infant behavior, electroencephalographic studies, naturalistic studies of mother-infant interaction, and a number of theoretical explorations derived from these and other investigations.

Our recent research efforts have been inspired by Freud's trailbreaking work in *Three Essays on the Theory of Sexuality* (1905b). The principal theoretical statements which have guided us were formulated systematically in three publications of Spitz (1958a, 1959, 1961).

The following propositions form an overall framework for our research:

1. There is no aspect, activity, function, or structure of the psyche that is not subject to development.

2. Development is the resultant of the interplay of innate and experiential factors which themselves are often inextricably interwoven.

3. Innate factors include hereditary aspects and aspects pertaining to intrauterine and intrapartum events.

4. The role of the experiential factors in the inception, unfolding, and structuring of the psychic apparatus has two sources: exchanges with the surround and exchanges within the organism. The latter exchanges consist of interactions between incipient psychic operations and the innate physiological prototypes for some subsequently emerging psychic structures. The maturation of these prototypes takes place as an epigenetic unfolding; as a forward-moving, irreversible progressive growth and differentiation, programmed as it were by a maturational clock.

Reprinted from *The Psychoanalytic Study of the Child*, Vol. 25. New York: International Universities Press, 1970, pp. 417–441.

We have set ourselves the following tasks:

1. To collect experimental data which will test the correctness of the theoretical statements in question.

2. To construct appropriate models of the development and structure of the emerging psychic system on the basis of these statements. The value of these models should be tested further by systematic observation and experiment.

3. To demonstrate the explanatory power of these models within the framework of the system of psychoanalytic theory.

We would like to illustrate this approach by some initial findings from this rather ambitious program. These findings are psychobiological in nature and involve behavioral units which are common to every individual of the species. Examples from the current phase of our research include the following areas of development: (1) rapid eye movement states (REM states and REM sleep); (2) quiet, "deep" sleep; (3) effects of stress on neonatal sleep; (4) smiling; (5) normal fussiness.

METHOD AND SUBJECTS

The central strategy of our research project includes the weekly or biweekly study of individual infants from before birth through the end of the first year of life. In addition, cross-sectional studies, involving a larger number of infants, are used to explore hypotheses generated by our longitudinal studies. The design of our project includes alternating home visits and visits to our infant neurophysiological laboratory. During home visits, we make naturalistic observations of the infant, obtain a narrative account from the mother of changes since our last visit, and test the infant's responsivity to a variety of standardized stimuli.

The laboratory visits for electroencephalograms and observations are quite different. After the application of EEG and polygraphic leads, a laboratory recording session begins with a feeding of the infant and continues with a transition into sleep and through about 90 minutes of sleep recording. The recording includes direct observation of behavior, as well as continuous electroencephalogram, electro-oculogram, respiration, electromyogram, and evoked response recording.

To date, 22 infants have been studied longitudinally. Of these, 13 infants have been studied intensively during the first three postnatal months, and 9 infants have been studied through the first year. Over 500 have been studied cross-sectionally.

SLEEP INVESTIGATIONS

In common parlance, sleep and sleeping are considered equivalent: one is either asleep or awake. At best, the vernacular distinguishes light sleep from deep sleep with dreams ascribed to one or the other. Psychoanalysis has had, from the beginning, a different approach to the problems of sleep. At the outset, Freud (1900, 1901) was primarily interested in the exploration of dreams, which he recognized as the manifestations of the mental life during sleep. He demonstrated that determinism applies to dreams and all psychic activity in the same way as it applies to the physical world. But his differentiation went further than this. Being primarily interested in the problems of dreams and their elucidation, he noted from the very beginning the possible occurrence of dream states outside of the so-called sleep state, in the form of daydreams. He postulated that (1) sleep would be found to be different from the waking state in its physiological functioning and (2) that specific parts of the brain would be found to be involved in the dream process (1900). Furthermore, he dealt in the same period with a tangential but related phenomenon, that of memory. Freud anticipated modern brain physiology with his proposition of a double registration in the memory systems (1900, 1925b). It is interesting to note that, following Freud's investigations, Silberer (1911) discussed the importance of recognizing two qualitatively different kinds of sleep.

Physiological studies of sleep tended to follow two major investigative directions. One direction was that exemplified by the work of von Economo (summarized in 1929) on sleep centers and the neurophysiological work of Hess (1924, 1925), among others. The other direction was that explored for many years by Kleitman (1929). This culminated in the 1953 and 1955 reports by Aserinsky and Kleitman, which documented *in infants* the cyclic occurrence of episodes of body motility associated with rapid eye movements. This was soon followed by the reports of Dement (1955) and Dement and Kleitman (1957) indicating that a similar rapid eye movement–bodily activity cycle was seen in adults, and that rapid eye movement (REM) periods normally occurred about every 90 minutes throughout a night's sleep; furthermore, these REM sleep periods were found to be associated with a specific EEG and with dreaming. Much of the emergent physiological and psychophysiological research on sleep and dreaming, and its implications for psychoanalytic theory, has been reviewed and discussed by Fisher (1965).

As a result of these pioneering investigations, we now think of sleep as being composed of a number of different stages (I, II, III, IV, I-REM). Each of these stages is described by multiple criteria, which consist of the presence or absence of eye movements, EEG configuration, muscle tone, and some-times respiratory and heart rate patterns.[1]

From the psychoanalyst's point of view it is of primary interest that two of these criteria appear to correspond closely to propositions advanced 50 years earlier by Freud. The first of these is the finding of greatly reduced muscular activity (via active inhibition) during sleep as measured by the chin electromyogram. We remind our readers that Freud (1900) postulated that the inhibition of motility in sleep not only *facilitates* dreaming, but is also *necessary* for dreaming to take place. The second of these criteria is the regular occurrence of penile erections during REM sleep—a phenomenon which has been studied by Fisher, Gross, and Zuch (1965).

We have been intrigued to find that infant sleep and adult sleep show both significant similarities and important differences. This holds true for behavior as well as physiology. Our investigations of infant sleep were stimulated by these facts in conjunction with the central importance of sleep and dreams to psychoanalysis and the importance of Freud's genetic view.

REM "SLEEP" IN THE NEWBORN

An initial cross-sectional study resulted in a new conception of neonatal states (Emde and Metcalf, 1970). The combination of detailed behavioral observations and polygraphic recording provided us with information previously not available. In the adult we are accustomed to thinking of rapid eye movements as occurring in sleep. But the matter is not so simple in infancy. In newborns we observe rapid eye movements occurring in a number of different circumstances. Not only do they occur during the sleep cycle when the eyes are closed (*sleep REM*), but they also occur at times when the eyes are open and glassy *(drowsy REM),* during times when the infant is engaged in nutritional sucking *(sucking REM),* and during some times when the infant is fussing or crying *(fussing REM* and *crying REM).* We established that two trained behavioral observers reached better than 95 percent agreement in judgments of each of these behavioral states.

The states of drowsy REM, sucking REM, fussing REM, and crying REM have consistent electrophysiological correlates—correlates which are also present in the REM sleep of adults and older children. Even though the infant had his eyes open or was engaging in nutritional sucking, or was fussing or

---

[1] The concepts of light sleep and deep sleep are valuable but imprecise and do not refer to sufficiently invariant physiological correlates. Stage IV sleep, the deepest stage of quiet sleep in the human, is associated with very high and steady thresholds to arousal by sensory stimulation. Stage I-REM (REM sleep), associated with dreaming, is so unique as to be thought of as a separate state. It has, for this reason, been termed the "D State" by Ernest Hartmann (1967).

crying, he frequently had the same electrophysiology as the type of "sleep" during which the eyes were closed and rapid eye movements were conspicuous. We carried out an independent minute-by-minute study which compared a behavioral observer's interpretation of state with an EEG specialist's simultaneous EEG and polygraphic findings during the same period of observation. In the analysis of nearly 20 hours of data collection from ten normal newborns, the behavioral observer judged a total of 214 minutes to be either drowsy REM, sucking REM, fussing REM, or cyring REM states. In the independent judgments of the EEG and polygraph, the electroencephalographer judged over 98 percent of these (or 210 minutes) to be REM states indistinguishable from REM sleep.

We have used the term "undifferentiated" because drowsy REM, sucking REM, fussing REM, and crying REM disappear over the first three months of postuterine life (Metcalf and Emde, 1969). In addition, *neonatal REM* sleep shows a relatively high variability in physiological patterning which tends toward stability over the first three months. These changes are concomitant with another major change in the sleep cycle itself; by three months, sleep characteristically begins with a non-REM (NREM) instead of a REM period. This pattern of sleep onset will from here on remain the same. It is the adult pattern.

EEG DEVELOPMENT IN QUIET SLEEP

It is evident that our EEG studies relate at every step to our behavioral studies. The EEG is used here as one tool in a psychobiological, interdisciplinary research program based on the principles we have already stated. The study of the human electroencephalogram is recent, dating from the work of the psychiatrist Hans Berger in the 1920s and 1930s. Less well known is the fact that Berger quickly recognized that the human EEG undergoes progressive change throughout life. This is particularly evident from birth to three years. Because of this marked developmental change, the EEG provides excellent opportunity for the study of central nervous system maturation and development. Many workers, notably Ellingson (1967) in recent years, have contributed to knowledge in this domain; it has been our particular area of interest for some time.

In the neonatal period, although awake and sleep EEGs can often be distinguished from each other, this differentiation is sometimes difficult and unreliable, because REM sleep and undifferentiated "nonsleep" REM states share the same electrophysiology. The two main sleep stages, on the other hand, "active" REM sleep and "quiet" NREM sleep, show clearly different EEGs.

The EEG of REM sleep is one of extensive cortical activation and in many ways resembles the EEG associated with the alert, awake state. It shows a low amplitude pattern whose rhythms appear to be fast and irregular. During this state there is activation of many physiological systems as evidenced by extreme variability of pulse, respiration, and blood pressure, by a rise in brain oxygen utilization by REMs, by penile erections, and by increased body motility. Even the lack of muscle tonus during the REM state is not a passive phenomenon, but is a result of CNS activation; muscle tonus is reduced through the mechanism of active inhibition.[2] It is noteworthy that REM-state physiology, for all its inherent variability, changes very little throughout life once its characteristic integrated patterning, loosely present at first, becomes established at about three months.

Quiet sleep also shows many important changes during the first three months, and, in contrast to REM sleep, shows continued development throughout infancy and childhood. The quiet NREM sleep EEG shows wave-forms that are more regular, slower, and of higher amplitude than those of REM sleep. During quiet sleep there are no REMS, respirations are very regular, thresholds to arousal are high, and infants are generally motionless, except for occasional spontaneous body jerks or startlelike movements. It can, indeed, be surprisingly difficult to awaken an infant from this state. At about age three weeks, the quiet sleep EEG becomes more differentiated as a result of increased regularity of slow rhythms which replace the previously somewhat chaotic picture of this stage. Four to seven days later (at about five weeks), a momentous EEG change occurs, namely the onset of "sleep spindles." These EEG wave sequences are easily recognizable. We have shown that this seemingly maturational step can be accelerated by the impact of experience (Metcalf, 1969).

At about eight to twelve weeks, quiet sleep shows a further differentiation, the emergence of definable Stage II sleep. Stage II sleep is marked by the presence of well-formed sleep spindle bursts and a more characteristic, regular EEG appearance. The onset of sleep spindles probably indicates a complex maturational and developmental step. Existing and partially functioning excitatory and inhibitory brain systems become capable of integrated, self-regulating *interaction*. This step may have primary CNS integrative significance. Part of our research is concerned with searching for behavioral manifestations or correlates of this physiological development.

---

[2] During REM·sleep there is much motor activity, especially of face (smiles, frowns, etc.), hands, and feet as well as body activity (twisting, stretching, etc.). Muscle tonus reduction occurs concurrently and is most evident around the mouth and chin. REM-sleep body motility to this degree is not seen in the adult; the age when change from infant motility toward adult motility takes place is under study.

After the establishment of Stage II sleep at about three months, another kind of quiet sleep begins to emerge. We see here the beginning of adult types of deep, quiet sleep. This form of quiet sleep may be labeled "Stage III/IV." After this integrative patterning is complete, EEG development proceeds in a slower and apparently smooth fashion until about five or six months. When, as part of these developments, sleep Stages II, III, and IV become clearly distinguishable, three different kinds of deep sleep are formed out of what had been one undifferentiated kind of deep sleep. This is an often-overlooked and important developmental step, in the course of which a further major EEG pattern emerges, namely *spontaneous* K-complexes.

The K-complex is a specific brief series of waveforms, consisting of conspicuous deviations from the ongoing EEG tracing. K-complexes are similar to sensory evoked responses (Cobb, 1963), and can probably be elicited by sensory stimulation at earlier ages, but they do not occur *spontaneously* during sleep until after five months (Metcalf, Mondale, and Butler, 1971). When elicited at older ages, there is evidence that the patterned waveform of the K-complex varies according to the psychological meaning of the sensory stimulation (Oswald, 1962).

The K-complex may be considered to be an electrophysiological indicator of CNS information processing. This view is supported by many basic neurophysiological investigations such as those of Dawson (1958) and Barlow (1964). We are intrigued by the fact that spontaneous K-complexes are not seen before five to six months. This may be taken to indicate a new and important step in the capacity of the CNS to respond to itself; i.e., to respond in a patterned and perhaps selective way to processes arising in one part of the CNS and acting on other parts. Therefore, the emergence of spontaneous K-complexes may be connected with the increasing systematic manipulation of memory traces.

Somewhat apart from, but still connected with the preceding, is the question of drowsiness. Up to three months, the observational impression of drowsiness is not paralleled by characteristic changes in the EEG. The latter appear for the first time around three months. It would appear that drowsiness, an important psychological condition, has now acquired a specific EEG pattern. This linkage becomes clearer after six months and continues into the latency period.

Thus it appears that the age of three months is a period of critical developmental importance. EEG and physiological patterns become more clearly organized and systematically integrated with certain behaviors such as drowsiness, sleep behaviors, and sleep cycles. A further, rather abrupt change in the direction of increased differential organization is the development of spontaneous K-complexes during NREM quiet sleep at about five to six months.

Thus our attention is drawn to three nodal points in early EEG development. Our work, in broader perspective, utilizes the totality of EEG development in relation to a variety of behavioral developments, and focuses on these nodal points as "anchor points" of assumed special CNS maturational significance. The three points are aspects of quiet sleep development. They are the development of sleep spindles at four to six weeks, the development of Stage II sleep at about three months, and the development of spontaneous K-complexes at five to six months. A fourth nodal point (resting on the REM-state EEG) is the more complex integration of behavioral, physiological, and EEG manifestations, whereby at about three months undifferentiated REM states disappear and sleep-onset REM is replaced by mature sleep-onset NREM.

EFFECTS OF STRESS ON NEONATAL SLEEP

Normal hospital routine requires drawing blood from the newborn during the first three days of life. This is performed by pricking the infant's heel with a sharp stylette. We observed that this blood-drawing procedure is frequently followed by long, relatively motionless NREM sleep periods. Curiosity about this led us to explore the effects of such a stress-producing (painful) event at this age (Emde, McCartney, and Harmon, 1971). Hospital circumcision, done routinely without anesthesia, was chosen as an independent variable with sleep patterns following circumcision as dependent variables. Circumcision, done by plastibel technique, results in a gradually developing ischemic necrosis of the foreskin which could be expected to produce a continual bombardment of stimulation of pain pathways for many hours.

Results in two observational studies were dramatic. In the 12 hours following circumcision, most infants showed a primary increase in NREM or deep sleep. In a subsequent polygraphic study, normal male infants were observed for a 10-hour period on each of two successive nights. Continuous recordings consisted of electroencephalogram, eye movement recording, electromyogram, respiration recording, and behavioral observations. Twenty infants were studied on two successive nights beginning at 24 hours of age. One-half of the infants (control group) did not have circumcisions or heel pricks during the period of study; the other half (experimental group) were circumcised during the beginning of the second night's recording and observation. Eight out of ten circumcised infants showed a major increase in NREM or quiet sleep on the night following circumcision. Percentage increases of this deep NREM sleep varied from 41 to 121 percent. In contrast to this, in the undisturbed control group, the total amount of NREM sleep varied little from the first to the second night—the greatest single increase was less than 3 percent. These results are significant at well beyond the .01 level of confidence.

The cause of this phenomenon is not immediately understandable. A "common sense" guess about the effects of a continual disruptive stimulation at this age is that an infant would sleep less and cry more. Our results showed the opposite. Circumcised infants slept *more* and were awake less, and cried for the same amount of time as before circumcision. These results suggest an inborn adaptive mechanism which responds to stress by producing a quiescent state with high sensory thresholds. We are currently in the process of studying individual differences in regard to this phenomenon, as well as the endocrinological basis for it.

SMILING AND FUSSINESS

As derived from the *Genetic Field Theory of Ego Formation* (Spitz, 1959), our research project considers that there are certain periods during the first year when physiological and behavioral development progresses at an increased pace and in a definite normative sequence. It is inferred from that theory that these periods are accompanied by changing thresholds to stimulation and by *affective changes,* which are of crucial significance in the development of social relations. Because of this, we have paid particular attention to the behaviors of smiling and fussiness.

Our investigations have included detailed cross-sectional and longitudinal studies of smiling during the first three months (Emde and Koenig, 1969a, 1969b; Emde, 1970). In the normal newborn, smiling is linked to the states of sleep REM and drowsy REM and occurs as one of many well-circumscribed state-related "spontaneous behaviors." Since it is determined not by external stimulation but by intrinsic physiological rhythms, we refer to it as *endogenous smiling.* It is found with increased frequency in prematures (Emde, McCartney, and Harmon, 1971). We have reason to believe endogenous smiling is mediated through brainstem mechanisms since it was present in a microcephalic infant with virtually no functioning cerebral tissue (Harmon and Emde, 1971). In the normal newborn, endogenous smiling occurs at a mean rate of 11 smiles per 100 minutes of REM period. It is evenly distributed across successive REM periods of an interfeeding interval; thus, it cannot be considered an expression of a "tensionless" or hunger-free condition.

Newborn frowning, on the other hand, appears to be of two types. Like smiling, it occurs as a spontaneous state-related behavior. In addition, during later REM periods of an interfeeding interval and also during wakefulness, it occurs as an expression of distress. Endogenous smiling and endogenous frowning along with other spontaneous REM-associated behaviors wane sharply in the period between eight and twelve weeks.

Exogenous smiling, on the other hand, is not present at birth. It begins as an irregular response which is first elicited during wakefulness at about three weeks of age. It may occur to a wide variety of nonspecific stimuli in auditory, kinesthetic, tactile, and visual modalities, but it is unpredictable, rare, and fleeting. With ensuing weeks it occurs more often, but it does not become predictable until the eight-to-twelve-week period at which time it is best elicited by the visual stimulus configuration which Spitz and Wolf (Spitz, 1946d) termed the "essential sign Gestalt" (stimulus consisting of hairline, eyes, nose, and motion). This is commonly considered the time of onset of social smiling or of the "smiling response" (Ambrose, 1961; Polak et al., 1964a; Gewirtz, 1965). Within two weeks after its onset, however, the adequate stimulus for eliciting this response becomes more complex, as three dimensions are required (Polak et al., 1964b), and very soon after that the face of the mothering person becomes the most potent elicitor. In other words, soon after the eight-to-twelve-week period, exogenous smiling becomes more specifically social and endowed with meaning. As exogenous smiling is becoming more specific and enriched with psychological meaning, endogenous smiling, which is physiologically determined, is decreasing.

In parallel with this countermovement is still another countermovement. In one of our longitudinal research projects (Tennes et al., 1972) we have studied in detail the fussiness which normally occurs in most infants between three and twelve weeks of age. Extreme fussiness at this age has often been characterized clinically as "colic"; although its precise etiology is unknown, several groups have documented the fussiness of this age period (Spitz, 1951b; Stewart et al., 1953; Wessel et al., 1954; Brazelton, 1962; Paradise, 1966).

We found fussiness, unrelated to hunger, occurring in all of the infants studied during this age period. By twelve weeks the fussiness wanes and nothing else like it is observed through the first year of life. The time of waning of this fussiness is concomitant with the infant achieving capacities for being a more active regulator of contact with his environment, both in initiating stimulus contact and in terminating it. Again we are struck with the countermovement. As the capacity for mastery and active trial-and-error behavior is increasing, fussiness is decreasing.

Discussion and Psychoanalytic Conclusions

I

In the foregoing we have presented some data from our studies on neonatal development. These form one part of our research program and we selected them because of the developmental parallels and connections they present. These studies are:

1. Neonatal sleep and REM states of infancy.

2. The development of smiling.
3. The development of differentiation of the "mature" form of deep sleep.
4. The effects of stress on neonatal sleep.

Our findings support a number of Freud's theories and the principles he elaborated on the origin, organization, and functioning of the psychic system.

Our data impress us with the operation of two parallel lines acting and interacting in the progressive unfolding of the organism. These are the lines following maturation (the innate), and development (the experiential). They converge toward ever-increasing organization and regulation of the organism's functioning. The rates of change in the development of quiet sleep, the REM state, and smiling parallel each other in their progression. This progression is gradual from birth until the postnatal age of about six weeks, where we have found an important turning point in the nature of the interaction between maturation and development.

In the six weeks following this first turning point, the changes accelerate, with mounting evidence of incipient awareness and psychic functioning, to a second turning point in the third month. We have designated this turning point the emergence of the first organizer of the psyche. It is marked by clearly defined modifications in the behavioral pattern of the same three areas (quiet sleep, REM states, smiling). These modifications run parallel with a change in the EEG pattern, which has become organized and in which sleep spindles have appeared (see Table 1).

Until age six weeks the EEG pattern present when the above-mentioned behaviors were observed, was categorically different from the EEG patterns associated with a comparable behavior in the adult. After age six weeks, an increasing organization of the rather undifferentiated neonatal pattern begins to become rapidly evident. Sleep behavior becomes more specific; it approaches more and more the adult form. A good example of this is REM sleep, which represents 60 percent of total sleep in the neonate and only 20 percent in that of the adult. After the first turning point, the REM percentage decreases progressively. After the second turning point (age 2½ months) REM stages, which until then appeared indiscriminately during both sleep and apparently awake periods, disappear completely from the nonsleep periods.

The development of smiling is another example of this unfolding. We found that smiling shows that the endogenous physiological origin of this behavior decreases progressively during the first six weeks; in the second six weeks it is progressively displaced by a psychologically determined behavior. As endogenous smiling decreases, there is a proportionate increase in exogenous smiling. The stimulus for exogenous smiling originates in the surround, whereas the endogenous smile occurs as a function of innate internal rhythmic

TABLE 1.

	0–6 weeks	6–12 weeks	10–12 weeks
REM state	Occurs during behavioral sleep (eyes closed), drowsiness, nutritional sucking, fussing, and crying.	Occurs decreasingly during drowsiness, sucking, fussiness, and crying.	Occurs *only* during behavioral sleep and is more patterned from the physiological point of view.
Quiet sleep	*Neonatal Pattern:* Sleep begins with a REM state.	Continued neonatal pattern.	Neonatal pattern disappears; "adult" pattern of sleep onset is now present.
	EEG rhythmic activity becomes organized at 4–6 weeks. No EEG spindles before 4 weeks. Spindle bursts first seen at 5–7 weeks.	EEG rhythmic activity is poorly differentiated between "light" and "deep" sleep. Spindles become more defined.	Stage III/IV EEG sleep ("deep" quiet sleep) begins to differentiate from Stage II. Spindle maturation complete. Hypersynchronous drowsy pattern begins to emerge after 12 weeks.
Smiling	*Endogenous:* Occurs during sleep REM and drowsy REM at a rate of approximately 11 per 100 minutes.	Occurs at the same rate or at a slightly decreased rate.	Endogenous smiling wanes.
	Exogenous: Irregular response during wakefulness: elicited by a wide variety of stimulation in visual, auditory, tactile, and kinesthetic modalities.	Occurs with increased frequency, but is still irregular and in response to nonspecific sensory stimulation.	A regular response to the "essential sign Gestalt."
Fussiness	Endogenous nonhunger fussiness appears during the latter part of this period (3–6 weeks).	Intermittent bursts of prolonged nonhunger fussiness.	Prolonged nonhunger fussiness disappears.

processes. The exogenous smile begins as a response to a wide variety of stimuli and progressively is transformed into a specific response to the human face. After three months, the endogenous smile occurs mainly in REM sleep and is not a prominent behavior. In other terms, while the endogenous smiling had the characteristic of physiological rhythmicity, the exogenously determined behavior has the characteristic of awareness continuing into anticipation. Exogenous smiling represents a turning from inside perception (response to inner stimuli) to the perception of the surround. In terms of motivation, the progression goes from tension discharge to awareness with active exploration and anticipation. The latter is a specifically psychological process.

From the viewpoint of the psychic apparatus, we see at this age the emergence of a number of psychic structures (e.g., memory, anticipation, meaningful directed response). These psychic structures are modeled on neonatal physiological processes, which we have called "prototypes" (Spitz, 1958a). Each of these physiological processes has its innate phylogenetically predetermined maturational trajectory, and develops independently from every other one. Under the influence of the first organizer of the psyche, situated at age three months, they tend at certain maturational levels to form a range of predictable relationships with each other. They become coherent. But this maturation does not proceed alone, uninfluenced by other factors. At all developmental levels maturationally guided processes are turned into developmental processes as a result of the adaptations enforced by exchanges with the surround and the organism's response to them.

In this sense, postnatally, the concept "maturation" is a useful construct, even though *unrealizable: all is development.* For development is the resultant of the constant interactions between environment (or experience) and the innate: these interactions operate at all levels, whether molecular, cellular, or organismic.

Maturation, as a functional reality, is that aspect of development which provides potentialities on the one hand, and limitations on the other. Organizers, particularly in the context of this discussion, were first described (Spitz, 1959) as "emergent, dominant centers of integration . . . [forming a] field of forces from which a dominant center of integration, the first organizer of the psyche, will emerge" (pp. 33–34). Development is not blind. It is responsive to the surround in terms of the *law of effect*. In the ontogenesis of individual behavior the law of effect plays the same role as that played by natural selection (through survival) in phylogenesis.

Conversely, maturation is blind, for it is the product of phylogenesis over geological time spans. Development, through the impact of experience, is the means through which maturationally given potentialities are realized. It is one of the *inducers of organizers*. Organizers are formed out of species-specific, innate potentialities and directions, interacting with the species-unique demands of the surround.

Organizers introduce a new *modus operandi* into the psychic system. Indeed, we believe that *the psychic organizer is equivalent to the development of a new modus operandi through adaptive exchanges.* The organizer of the psyche is not a physical structure; it is not even a psychic structure. It is the emergence and establishment of a different way of processing the psychic givens. It introduces a better adapted way, which takes advantage of the opportunities offered by the surround. With this different way, the integration of these givens on a higher level of complexity becomes possible. From here on the new, more adapted *modus operandi* becomes predominant in the psychic processes. This will obtain until, at the next level, the growing complexity and number of elements achieved through the instrumentality of the organizer make a new step necessary. That step is the development of the next and more advanced *modus operandi* which will constitute the next organizer. As the term states, a more complex, more highly integrated reorganization of the psychic givens will now begin.

Postnatally the distinction between maturation and development becomes therefore increasingly constrained: by the same token a boundary line between psyche and soma becomes ultimately meaningless.

During the earliest postnatal days, approximately the first two to three weeks, physiological or somatic aspects of development are predominant as determinants of observable behavior. During this period, interactions between innate and surround become involved with an increasing variety of experience. The interactions increase in complexity and simultaneously become progressively more organized. These early patterned constellations of innate behavior and adaptive functioning, which culminate in volitional behavior and physiological adaptation, tempt one to speculate about their relationship to early ego or "pre-ego" development.

An outstanding example of the role of physiological prototypes for later psychic development and structure is breast-feeding behavior, and its "intaking" aspects in the neonate (Erikson, 1950; Spitz, 1957).

Examining this earliest physiological process and its interplay with differential experience sheds light on its emergence as the physiological prototype of an ego nucleus. Psychic structures will encroach on the discharge process which this nucleus provides. These psychic structures will in turn modify the functions of the ego nucleus to the point where their origin becomes unrecognizable, though they will continue to contain evidences of their somatic beginning.

In studying the prototype potentialities of neonatal sleep for subsequent development of the psychic system, of its structure, of its organization, of its activity, we have followed certain principles which have been outlined elsewhere (Spitz, 1957, 1958a, 1961, 1965b). These principles are:

1. Psychic activity, function, structure, etc., are not innate.

2. What *is* innate is: (a) the variable capacity for learning and adaptation; (b) the capacity for making use of neurophysiological and morphological givens for coping with the environment.

However, the physiological way the innate copes with its environment is not the way the psyche does it. The prototype is not a blueprint for a future psychic entity. It provides the available means for the later developing psychic structure and the limits within which they can operate. We realize that when we say "structure," we are taking liberties with this term. Though the subsequent development certainly is structured, it mostly is rather a *modus operandi* (e.g., defense mechanisms) and more rarely a coherent psychic structure (e.g., the superego). The *modus operandi* itself is not homologous with its physiological prototype. In view of the adaptive requirements of development, a direct continuation of the prototype is most unlikely. What will develop is an analogy that we must explore in the spirit of Robert Oppenheimer (1956): "One has to widen the framework a little and find the *disanalogy* which enables us to preserve what was right about the analogy." In this spirit, when examining neonatal sleep as a possible physiological prototype for later psychic functions, we shall stress more how it differs from sleep in the adult than dwell on the obvious similarities.

Furthermore, the neonate, during "nonsleep" periods, which could pass for "wakefulness" in the adult, shows undifferentiated REM states. The neonate begins behavioral sleep in a REM state; whereas the adult falls asleep in a NREM state. And while the adult shows a generalized diminution of motor activity during REM sleep, the neonate is behaviorally active despite paradoxical suppression of muscle tonus.

These differences suggest that REM sleep probably serves a different function in the neonate. In the adult, REM states are connected with dreaming. What, we may ask, would correspond to dreaming in the neonate? The very fact that the organism is compelled to adjust neonatal sleep to the adult pattern within the first three postnatal months suggests that the neonatal sleep pattern is probably not suitable for the function sleep will have to perform after the emergence of the first organizer. It is highly probable that an interference with this adjustment would encroach upon the development of a sharp demarcation of diurnal wakefulness and, concurrently, with the perception of reality.

The function of sleep and REM in the neonate is categorically different from their function in the adult. It is a good example of the uses of *disanalogy*, for it permits us to sense where analogies lie—not where we expect them.

For instance, the neonate's REM activity is triple that of the adult. Yet what can correspond in the neonate to dream activity, that rich mental life of the adult during REM sleep? And, even more significantly, in studies of premature infants, the percentage of REM activity increases in inverse proportion to the gestational age of the subject.

We need hardly argue that the psychic content, the material of dreams, is as yet nonexistent in the neonate, and *a fortiori* in the premature. We cannot therefore consider neonatal sleep and its REM activity in the same line as sleep REM in the adult. In the neonate's first three weeks of life, REM states are present, both during apparent wakefulness and sleep. We therefore come to the conclusion that they probably represent the operation of maturational processes in the CNS of the neonate, which are primarily related to physiological processes and hardly influenced as yet by experience. In our opinion, these maturational processes are part of an unfolding genetic progression, phylogenetically preformed for an average expectable environment. The processes involve the establishment, by practice and channelization, of the necessary connections within the CNS as well as in CNS behavioral integration.

What then does neonatal sleep represent? In our opinion, a physiological prototype for later function. It is sleep behavior in transition from an exclusively physiological phenomenon to adult sleep, a psychophysiological phenomenon. Neonatal sleep occurs during an existence practically devoid of interference from the surround, let alone exchanges with it. Conversely, adult sleep includes, among its functions, the enormously important psychic function of discharging the tension originating during the previous day's exchanges with a rich, varied, and ever-changing surround, probably with the help of the dream.

It is then not surprising that, by comparison with adult sleep, prototype REM sleep is poorly organized. But in the neonate it only takes three months of development to organize it. Three months is that developmental level at which a number of other psychic phenomena also converge, forming on the one hand a rudimentary ego organization, initiating on the other the preobjectal stage in the formation of object relations. And it is precisely at this level that the physiological patterning of the REM state becomes consistent. Now the REM state becomes firmly linked with behavioral sleep and can no longer be confused with wakefulness. Sleep spindles become definitely established in the sleep EEG.

If REM physiology in the adult belongs exclusively to behavioral sleep, then it has no place in the psychic life of directed, volitional action. After the three-month level, action, whether in the motor or mental sphere, will become increasingly incompatible with the REM state. Can this provide an explanation of the spectacular decrease of REM activity after the ego becomes established?

At the present state of our knowledge the linking of adult REM sleep with dreaming permits us only the assumption that during dreaming a CNS activity is going on. Some aspects of these linkages will become clearer when problems related to memory, object formation, and perhaps mental representation will have been adequately investigated.

One thing is certain: REM sleep is neither the cause nor a direct result of dreaming. That is evident from the difference of its role in the neonate and in the adult. REM sleep is the indication of specific ongoing processes in the CNS: in the neonate these processes are exclusively physiological. In the adult the vast realm of the psychological is added.

The ages at which REM and EEG pattern changes appear in the infant are quite suggestive through their convergence. The organization and structuration of sleep spindles in the EEG pattern and their maturation are coterminous with the appearance of the smiling response, the behavioral indicator of the first organizer. At the same period the REM states become limited to behavioral sleep. The adult "pattern" of NREM sleep onset also becomes established. Independently, as a result of certain theoretical considerations, we also situated the emergence of the preobject as well as of a rudimentary ego structure (Spitz, 1957) at this stage. Lastly, we may ask whether it is the progressive patterning of EEG and REM states which is one more indicator of the emergence and structuration of the first organizer of the psyche.

II

As happens so frequently, answering one question makes us aware of more unanswered ones. We concluded that prototype sleep in the neonate represents a transition from physiological sleep to sleeping as a psychophysiological function in the adult. But if REM sleep is an indication of a specific CNS activity in the neonate, then it may well correspond more to the adult's waking mental activity than to adult REM sleep.

What then would be the function of the neonate's NREM sleep in terms of prototypes? Should we assume that it corresponds to Engel's (1962) "conservation-withdrawal" to stress? Our finding that the neonate's response to circumcision consists in a spectacular increase in NREM sleep certainly supports this hypothesis. If so, of what is this the prototype?

Evidently there are quite a number of defense mechanisms of which one might think: denial, repression, withdrawal, regression, etc. One might even consider the neonatal NREM response as a possible prototype for defense *as such*.

However, in our opinion these initial observations are not sufficient for drawing such fundamental theoretical conclusions. Much more research will be needed to establish the further developmental steps which will follow this first one. We will have to observe the subsequent modifications of behavior in the course of the first year before drawing any conclusions.

The same can be said of the problem of the age of the onset of dreaming. Our work does not yet bear on this, inasmuch as we have not yet adequately investigated problems related to memory, object constancy, and mental representation. Furthermore, any useful speculations will require solution of the problems of dream reporting (or of reasonable inferences about dream experiences) during the first two years of life. We may remind the reader here that Freud's daughter dreamed the "strawberry dream" when she was 19 months old (Freud, 1900).

Recent dream and sleep research (some of which has been noted here) again raises the question from a different direction. Is there any evidence from the physiological study of sleep in general and REM sleep (associated with adult dreaming) in particular that sheds light on the age of onset of dreaming?

We do not know of any studies of infant REM sleep which explore this question. We have already mentioned our EEG work on the ontogenesis of quiet NREM sleep (Stages II, III, IV) culminating in the development of spontaneous *K-complexes* at about six months. We would suggest that the development of this CNS information-processing signal is a prerequisite for CNS readiness to support dreaming during sleep. It is known that there is occasional mental content also during NREM sleep. It may be that both kinds of sleep are necessary for dreaming. One possibility is that NREM sleep favors the more formal, secondary process aspects of day-residue processing, while REM sleep subserves the rich, associational, affect-guided psychic activity of dreams as generally understood.

These findings lead us to search carefully for the relation between developing integration of the physiological system and the development of psychic structures of ever-increasing complexity, i.e., ego development. We ask ourselves whether the appearance of *spontaneous* K-complexes can be brought into meaningful statistical relationship with behavior at somewhat more advanced stages of development, when object constancy is achieved (Hartmann, 1952; Spitz, 1965b), or insight behavior becomes manifest in problem-solving.

Many more problems confront us and the opportunities for research in the field of prototypes are numerous. We will not touch on them in our present report, reserving these problems for our future publications on the subject. But we will end with a brief discussion of the methodology of our research on prototypes. By this time, prototypes have a long history. After Freud, Hartmann (1939) was the first to take up the concept of prototypes as the explanatory principle for some ego defenses. As discussed elsewhere (Spitz,

1961), a number of authors approached the tempting problems of prototypes with very little actual definition of the term prototype. We therefore thought of establishing criteria for identifying a physiological entity as a prototype. Although it is easy to detect similarities in one respect or another between a psychic phenomenon and some physiological process, that does not make it a prototype.

We believe that in our present report we have demonstrated the usefulness of two such criteria, both genetic in character. One is the criterion of convergence of different developmental lines (Anna Freud, 1965). The process of psychological development of any physiological prototype or rather of its component elements, be they behavior, function, EEG, physiology, etc., will inevitably mesh with various other developmental processes, progressively converging to a point where they become coterminous and interact to form what we have called an organizer of the psyche. They are the constituents of the organizer and, at the same time, components of the subsequent changes in the development which arise from it. We believe that in a prototype such a convergence should be demonstrable as a developmental line—a line that leads from the prototype itself to the end result.

Our second criterion is equally genetic. For, to become a credible physiological prototype for a psychic entity emerging much later, the prototype must be the starting point of a developmental line. Accordingly, it can be observationally, mensurationally, and experimentally followed in its development. Decrease of physiological component elements can be quantitatively demonstrated. Their replacement through psychic devices, mechanisms, structures can be observed and the modification of the EEG verifiably be demonstrated.

This is what we have attempted to show in our present report. These are the principles we are applying to the other projects of our research program.

And this is indeed an application of Oppenheimer's recommendation to explore the disanalogies. For analogies can be found everywhere. But the genetically progressing series of disanalogies forms the meaningful coherent link for us, leading from physiological inception to psychological completion.

Accordingly, we would like to conclude by offering a whimsical recommendation for psychoanalytic developmental research: "Take care of the disanalogies; the analogies will take care of themselves!"

Bridges:
On Anticipation, Duration, and Meaning

MR. CHAIRMAN, LADIES AND GENTLEMEN, MY DEAR FRIENDS:

Twelve years ago you honored me by entrusting me with the Freud Anniversary Lecture at the New York Academy of Medicine. On that occasion I dared greatly and presented a systematic review of my scientific position in respect to psychoanalysis and psychoanalytic theory as a holistic developmental psychophysiological approach. It was published under the title: *A Genetic Field Theory of Ego Formation* (Spitz, 1959). Essentially it was based, on the one hand, on my understanding of Freud's and Hartmann's theoretical position, on the other, on my own research findings.

What I will present to you now are tentative ideas: speculations which have occupied my mind for a number of years: adventures and experiments of the mind which I am trying out, to see if they have merit—and what better audience could I find for such an attempt than this one?

Of necessity my approach will have to be a multidimensional one. At no later period of life do so many different levels of the personality meet for the first time as in infancy. I will take birth as my starting point—a starting point with nodal qualities. For at this point the newborn is at the parting of the waters, a being about whom we know a great deal retrospectively but very little about the enormous potentialities he is bringing with him.

I will make major use of three concepts introduced by Hartmann (1939): maturation, development, and the adaptive viewpoint.

Maturation is innate. It is a part of the newborn's congenital equipment and, as such, is of phylogenetic origin. It regulates the epigenesis of the infant's innate equipment in the course of its ontogenesis. What we often tend to forget is that the origin of the innate givens present at birth, as well as the evolution of these givens, were, at their phylogenetic inception, random processes. They originated at the beginning of life on this planet (at least 3½ billion years ago): they had certainly nothing to do in the immediate with the survival of the species, but only with that of the individual.

Reprinted from *Journal of the American Psychoanalytic Association*, 20:721–735, 1972.

This address was presented at the Plenary Meeting of the American Psychoanalytic Association, Washington, D.C. on May 1, 1971.

Nature, however, does not permit us to forget the stations of this stupendous adaptive struggle over unimaginable geological time spans. Complying with the biogenetic principle interpreted incisively by Haeckel (1867), *ontogenesis recapitulates phylogenesis*. In the course of this recapitulation, vestigial indications—e.g., the branchial cleft, the appendix, the pineal gland—mark the continuity of physical matter. At the same time, the phylogenetic history of such vestigial indications signals organizer-induced embryological changes from one evolutionary stage to the next.

You notice that I am stressing the continuity of substance and its transmission through heredity. It follows that the same constituent elements functioning in the vital processes of one embryonic stage will also form the constituents of the next stage. They will, however, be reorganized as an improved, better adapted organization on a higher level of complexity.

Embryological theory assumes that the successive steps in the development of the embryo are the result of induction evoked by successive organizers. The nature of these organizers, first assumed to be chemical, later physical, is as yet unknown.

In the monograph mentioned above (Spitz, 1959), I postulated that entities, analogous to those which regulate embryonal development, arise and operate at the successive stages of the development of the psychic system as well. Accordingly, I called these entities "organizers of the psyche." I will now add to this hypothesis the proposition that the organizer is neither a chemical nor physical substance; it is not even a structure. It adds nothing tangible to the continuity of embryonal substance in the course of the development of the embryo, and still less to that of the child's psyche.

I submit that in both cases the organizer is a modification of the regulatory procedure ruling the relations of the embryo's (and later the psyche's) constituents. Accordingly, in my concept the organizer is a model, a formula, which regulates the relations of these constituents with each other, as well as the constituents' relations with the surround. Every successive organizer in the further course of development introduces a new formula of regulation, successively more complex and better adapted. The new formula represents a more efficient *modus operandi*. This will be incorporated into the child's equipment, becoming available from here on for further regulatory purposes.

The substance, and quite often even the structure, of the constituent parts has not changed from one developmental level to the next. It is the method that changes, the manner in which the components of the vestigial remains in the embryo are related to each other and at the same time to the total individual, as well as their shifting valency at the given stage. Man did not have to invent legs—he, and his evolutionary predecessors, had them. What he invented is a *modus operandi* which transformed erect locomotion from a mode of orientation, of scanning, of defense in the nonhuman animal, into a way of life for man.

The unbounded inventiveness of the evolutionary process in regard to ever new, ever different, often wildly improbable formulas of somatic—and in due time also psychologic—adaptation—is witnessed by the whole of phylogenetic development, both vegetable and animal. I will just touch, for illustration's sake, on one of these inventions of our ancestors, the birds. Their predecessors had insured the continuation of the species through an astronomic number of offspring of which a few would survive. The bird eliminated uneconomical numbers and, instead, insured survival by replacing numbers with the armor of the egg shell—a passive protection.

At the next stage, in mammals, the protection was taken over by the parent, and the primeval process of cleavage (mitosis) was transformed into the formula of gestation *in utero*; in both cases, that of the egg and that of gestation, a transitional pause in the ontogenetic life of the individual was inserted, for the viviparous production of offspring had not proved adaptive enough. But neither had the armored protection of the eggshell—and for obvious reasons. That reason is to be found in nature's answer to the age-old jocular question, whether the egg was first or the chicken. To the Darwinian, the answer is obvious: the chicken was first. And the reason is simple: eggs do not adapt.

Ontogenesis proper begins with birth, when gestation ends. The maturation of the innate continues, programmed by epigenesis. Development, however, and developing behavior are triggered and their progression powered by the experiential, by the infant's reciprocal relations with the surround.

It is then hardly surprising to discover that the Darwinian principle of natural selection operates not only for the individual as organism, but applies as well to the postnatal development of that individual's behavior. True, in the case of behavior, the principle is not as harsh as in phylogenesis.

The principle of survival in the development of behavior operates according to the "law of effect" (introduced by Thorndike, 1913), which postulates that "successful or satisfying outcome of a response is remembered, whereas unsuccessful outcome tends to eliminate it." This formula was modified by K. Bühler (1918), who suggested that behavior is developed by retaining success-specific movements that achieve their goal, while relinquishing movements that do not. Thus, phylogenetic evolution through natural selection has a counterpart in the evolution of behavior according to the Thorndike-Bühler principle. Here also, adaptive movements survive, unadaptive ones are eliminated.

From the metapsychological viewpoint, behavior in the neonate is regulated by the Nirvana principle, which requires the discharge of tension and in its turn is regulated by affect. I will use the term affect in the same sense as Rapaport (1942), to include feeling and emotion as well as their prototypes, the affectively colored tension states.

During the perinatal and immediate postnatal weeks, affect is the device that regulates massive random tension discharge with relative adequacy. But after a few weeks, this primitive regulation becomes inadequate for coping with the increasing quantities of tension. The difficulty arises from the fact that not only is the progression of maturation nonlinear, but that it does not progress along chronologically parallel lines with development. The two are not symmetric nor are they consistently synchronous, but develop asynchronicities.

Indeed, by definition, maturation and development cannot progress synchronously. Maturation implements the rigid program laid down by phylogenesis over immeasurable time spans. Development, on the other hand, is the product of the constantly changing requirements of ontogenesis, of the unpredictably shifting adaptive demands imposed or withheld by the surround. Asynchronicities must therefore arise between the two in the course of their progression.

These asynchronicities will manifest themselves as a disparity between a rapidly increasing quantitative factor, namely the number, the valency, and the import of excitations received from the surround as the consequence of the decrease of the neonatal stimulus barrier. After the first few days of life, the crude regulation, according to the Nirvana principle (regulation through massive tension discharge), no longer provides adequate means of discharge. Tension mounts and accumulates, an engorgement with unpleasurable general excitation develops. I will call this state *critical quantity,* in analogy to the well-known critical mass. Activity, mostly random, increases. The situation can be resolved only through a more efficient way of regulation which would enable the system, the organism, to maintain homeostasis.

How will this more efficient way of regulation, the new, better, and different formula for dealing with critical quantity be achieved? An answer to this question is provided by a scientific discipline far removed from our own.

More than 100 years ago, Karl Marx, in an exchange of letters with a contemporary physicist on the subject of latent heat, stated the axiom that increase in quantity will reach a critical point, at which it switches into quality.[1]

---

[1] In the terms of present-day theoretical physics: scale change (increase in quantity) causes fundamental change (a shift into quality). This may change the original symmetry into a new symmetry, "broken symmetry," because the original symmetry is no longer evident. Broken symmetry can lead to functional structure, potentially an intermediate stage between crystallinity and information. Theoretical physicists consider the next stages being possibly a hierarchy, or a specialization of function, or both. Decreasing symmetry would then become increasing complexity, each successive level requiring a whole new conceptual structure (condensed from Anderson, 1972).

I may remind you at this point that this law became tragically familiar to all of us as the so-called "attainment of critical mass" on August 6, 1945—the day of Hiroshima.

The principle that critical *mass* (which, in psychoanalysis and psychology, we will speak of as critical *quantity*), imposes a switch from quantity to quality, has made its influence felt in an increasing measure in a number of other disciplines, as remote from one another as the social sciences from nuclear physics (witness the term "population explosion").

In my own epigenetic and developmental concept, achieving critical quantity enforces a highly increased, agitated trial-and-error activity which operates according to the Thorndike-Bühler law.

Redundant trial-and-error experimentation leads to the conservation of success-specific behavior, different in quality from the previous behavior that had failed. A new *modus operandi*—in my terms an organizer of the psyche—will emerge. The new formula modifies the relations between the psychic givens of the infant: it modified their relations to the whole person and, in turn, the relations of the infant to the surround. The new *modus operandi* is thus more adaptive than the previous one. In the course of the infant's development in the first year of life the sequence "increased (trial-and-error) activity—agitation—new *modus operandi*" is repeated at specific successive age levels. This behavioral sequence is the indicator of an ongoing psychic process, the outcome of which is the establishment of a new psychic entity, an entity that is a new and more adaptive regulatory formula, a new *modus operandi*. These new formulas I called *"organizers of the psyche,"* and I described the first three successive "organizers" in *The First Year of Life* (Spitz, 1965b).

The emergence of the first organizer of the psyche is preceded by an intermediate behavioral development in which innate neurophysiology and postpartum experiential factors share equally. I designate this intermediate entity as a *precursor* of the organizers of the psyche. It emerges at three to eight weeks of life, as a more or less functional *modus operandi,* as the behavioral pattern known as the conditioned reflex. At this age level the acquisition of the conditioned reflex becomes experimentally demonstrable during nursing at the breast: Witness the increasingly adaptive, goal specific, functionally precise structuration of the survival-ensuring rooting (orienting) reflex.

There is one aspect of the classical conditioned reflex which claims our particular interest: when the classically conditioned dog salivates upon hearing the bell, *as if* the food were already in his mouth, he anticipates the food (need) gratification. Anticipation is unquestionably a psychological process, involving, in the jargon of academic psychology, a *predictive hypothesis.*

Indeed, it is a psychological function without which we could not conduct even small parts of our daily life; we could not even cross the street. Thus the conditioned reflex forms the first bridge between somatic neural physiology and psychic activity, namely anticipation, the first observable behavior in life that is already governed by psychic processes and forces.

Compared to the stimulus reflex and the unorganized random discharge, which according to the Nirvana principle, operates at birth, the conditioned reflex represents a regulatory principle of a much higher order. Previously unmanageable quantities of tension are now being handled adequately by a qualitatively different procedure.

The advent of the conditioned reflex and its replacing the previously unorganized random discharge processes well exemplify the operation of a selective adaptation according to the Thorndike-Büehler principle.

From the psychoanalytic point of view, the conditioned reflex has, however, an even more important, perhaps I should say, a decisive significance. I have already stated that the conditioned reflex operates in both worlds, the soma and the psyche. From the interface with the soma it reaches into the psyche by introducing an outstandingly psychological function. That purely psychic function, however, mobilizes a typical somatic apparatus with which we are familiar from neurophysiology, namely, the alertness system. This in its turn activates the attention cathexis, which I, for one, would hesitate to assign exclusively either to psyche or to soma.

The conditioned reflex operates on a much higher level of complexity than its predecessor, the massive tension reduction through discharge operating at birth; for the conditioned reflex requires an intervention from the outside to trigger it. Triggered, it operates like a regulatory valve system, draining off stated amounts of tension at certain time intervals, activating a feedback that responds to a specific quantitative stimulus.

With the help of this valvelike regulation, reminiscent of the regulation of traffic by computer-controlled stop lights, the conditioned reflex can master the discrepancy between the input of stimuli and the means of discharge for a while. However, the asymmetry between input and discharge, development and maturation, keeps increasing steadily during the first year of life.

Accordingly, the engorgement of discharge-seeking tension is repeated at successive developmental levels. Asynchronicity and engorgement are characteristic preliminaries in the formation of each successive organizer. Furthermore, the period during which the organizer emerges and is established is also one of special vulnerability and of stage-specific disturbances. Sleep and feeding disturbances around the culmination of the conditioned reflex (the precursor of the organizers of the psyche) are familiar. Six weeks later the next disturbance to appear is the three months colic, which takes its name from the month in which the first organizer proper appears, with the smiling response as its indicator.

The second organizer after this appears in the second half of the first year, indicated by the stranger anxiety. Is that not also the age at which our parents used to complain about the teething problems of their children, and at which feeding problems also may occur?

Actually, the most conspicuous among the numerous changes indicating the inception of a new chapter in the first year of development is the appearance of the smiling response (the indicator of the first organizer proper), because it marks conclusively the infant's turning from endogenous experience to exchanges with the surround.

And this is the decisive turning point. Up to here the conditioned reflex related mainly to endogenous need, even though it did already involve distance perception. But in the smiling response, it is the human face which responds, and reciprocity, infinitely variable, begins and initiates quasi needs and the dialogue proper.[2]

But before the dialogue proper can evolve from the stage of undifferentiated primary narcissism, the "I" (primal self, Jacobson, 1964) must be separated from the "non-I."

Vision, or more specifically, distance perception is a central factor in this step, which constitutes the "I" and confronts it with the rest of the universe—with the "non-I."

This is the moment of Creation. The creation of the external world for the infant, the affective cathecting of the exogenous in the infant's psychic processes. The infant acknowledges this momentous step by the establishment of the smiling response.

The smiling response is indeed a very new, very different *modus operandi*. For this *modus operandi* enlists a powerful ally, a partner, who not only assists the child in the management of tension discharge with maximum efficiency, *but opens endless opportunities for expansion, going from communication to identification, to the buildup of the self, to personality, and ultimately to that of joining society.*

Having thus made a first and tentative attempt to conceptualize how we might conceive what an organizer is—namely, the achievement of a new method, a new formula for coping with somatic demands in the beginning, and later with psychological problems—I return to the precursor of these organizers, marked by the appearance of the conditioned reflex.

---

[2] I have introduced the concept of "action dialogue" (dialogue for short) to designate the ongoing action exchanges within the dyad. I described this first as "a reciprocity" (Spitz, 1962) and elaborated the concept in my successive papers in which I gave it the name of "dialogue" (Spitz, 1963a, 1964, 1965b).

As maturation progresses in the course of the postnatal days, the effectiveness of the stimulus barrier decreases. There comes a point at which random discharge according to the Nirvana principle becomes insufficient for coping with the increasing quantities of excitation. Unmanageable, critical quantities of tension accumulate. In compliance with the constancy-ensuring Nirvana principle, this tension has to be discharged.

Let me remind you of Freud's (1926) discussion of the birth situation as a danger situation, as a threat to survival, which produces an affect of severe unpleasure that he considered the prototype of all later anxiety.

It is a momentous event, this first meeting of affect and percept in the experience of the birth cry, the desperate gasp for survival. And yet there remains no memory of it—for the affect is still only unpleasure tension, while the percept is endogenous and nonexistent in the terms of conscious experience.

What does this experience consist of that can serve as prototype? Freud commented on its somatic aspects. I wish to add that the birth cry marks not only the first meeting of percept and affect in the individual's life, but also the first experience of *time* in the form of the duration of unpleasure. This duration comprises a sequence of increasingly violent, ultimately survival-endangering unpleasure experiences, which, however, culminates paradoxically in liberation from this very suffering. This is a liberation from an actual threat to survival. The process taking place is an irreversible sequence, unidirectional; it is an irreversible progression having all the attributes which characterize the time dimension.

May we then argue that the meeting of the percept and affect with a "happy ending" will introduce an affective bias for survival-connected percepts? That this bias will extend to all unpleasure-connected experience? May we argue that the factor of duration which moves in the opposite direction to the Nirvana principle's demand for immediate discharge, represents at the same time a gradient in the direction of *reducing* duration; a gradient that will lead to anticipation; a gradient that thus promotes an affective preference for percepts with survival value in the surround? You realize that I am not speaking of individual performance, but rather of the phylogenetic evolution of a programmed code, ensuring survival of the species, an evolution propelled by the avoidance of unpleasure.

With this in mind, I will now advance two propositions on the nature of memory: (1) I believe that no memory trace can be stored in the psychic system without involving affect at some point; (2) that perception in the sense of the possibility of the perceived becoming conscious cannot take place without the intervention of affect.

In my concept, affect has a selective function in the process of perception.

In the weeks following birth, affect forces the neonate *to select* from the "continuous barrage of environmental stimuli" (Kety, 1972) composing our universe only those which are survival specific. They are the ones which offer the possibility of orienting ourselves in the time-space continuum with the help of our five senses.

Therefore, when the infant acquires a coherent conditioned reflex by the end of the first two weeks of life, he has begun his first step in orienting himself in the space-time continuum of his surround. He performs this step in the course of achieving need gratifications; the need that he is gratifying as a neonate is liberation from unpleasure.

I consider, furthermore, the conditioned reflex the first implementation (the first on the psychic level) of the tendency to coherence, that tendency which is present in all congeneric living matter. The conditions for such coherence are coextensiveness and simultaneity of percept and affect during one and the same process. Under the pressure of the need to survive, this affective coextensiveness introduces the time-binding factor of duration.

At birth the input from any one of our sense organs is discrete, unconnected, and without affective relation to any other sense in the infant's system. The visual input of a ringing bell swinging before the eyes of the neonate is received, but remains separate from the coextensive auditory input from the same source.

Selma Fraiberg's observations and experiments (Fraiberg and Freedman, 1964; Fraiberg, 1968) demonstrated in blind-born infants that this separateness is a condition which extends far into the first years of life.

Accordingly, for the infant, the visual bell by itself will not be identical with the auditory bell by itself, or with the touchable or the taste bell, or the temperature bell, etc. Only when affect creates a durable bond between them can they become a coherent, unified, plurisensory Gestalt endowed with a completion gradient.

There is nothing durable in the sensory input as such: the affectless sensory input is characterized by its impermanence. The perception through our sense organs causes modifications only in the sense organ itself, I remind you here of Freud's "Note upon the 'Mystic Writing Pad' " (1925b), which he concludes with the remark that the discontinuous functioning of the systems *Pcs.* and *Cs.*[3] lies at the origin of our concept of time. Sensory input alone does not appear to modify the CNS, and leaves no evidence, cellular or otherwise, of its passage.

In the case of the conditioned reflex, a specific percept, say the bell, has been endowed with meaning. That is not surprising in the classical Pavlov

---

[3] [Preconscious and conscious. Ed.]

experiment with the *adult* dog, which has learned to endow sounds with meaning. But in the case of the newborn in his first two weeks, nothing is meaningful outside of the endogenous, need-connected bell. Therefore, if we condition a three-week-old to a bell, this need will be the first environmental percept to be endowed with meaning. The meaning is food, or rather "drink-in-the-mouth," of the neonate. This meaning is arbitrarily imposed by us, for in the absence of this experimenter-created coextensiveness there is no connection between the bell and the food.

This coextensiveness of the bell being simultaneous with the food combines with the *affective* unpleasure of the hunger situation to create a bond between the two; from here on, the bell will have the meaning of food as the consequence of this first psychological sequence. Furthermore, this meaning has a certain permanence, it becomes a memory trace at an age level when other memory traces are nonexistent or acquired by other means.

True, the permanence is only relative. In the classical Pavlov experiment, permanence is a function of the number of repetitions of the experiment. If not reinforced through later repetitions (and repetition again introduces the time element), the permanence will be lost. Classical conditioning remained impermanent because it was relatively low in affect and certainly did not include an "immediate danger situation plus affect" like the birth experience.

However, in affectively very highly cathected danger situations, as, for instance, in traumatic neurosis, absolute permanence is imparted to the percept even if it is experienced coextensively only once, as in the so-called "one-trial" learning. In analogy to the prototypic experience of birth, it appears, then, that the quantitative aspect of violent affect accompanying coextensive percepts is capable of ensuring the permanence of the traces in the memory, though mostly in a somatic and not in a cognitive form. Evidently intensity can replace duration and vice versa.

An explicatory hypothesis on the reason why affect has this power can be developed from Freud's remark on the relation of the preconscious to the intermittent nature of perception in relation to time, as I have tried to elaborate in the ideas I have presented above. I will have to limit myself here, however, to a few remarks about coextensiveness, before concluding my presentation.

Coextensiveness is often used in a spatial sense only. But as we have shown above, the engram in the CNS is not only a spatial process in the proper sense of the term, its scribing is equally a question of duration, of coexistence in time. For while percepts of the most different nature can coexist in the same time, no two spatial percepts can occupy the same space.

It is here again that we run into the antinomy of the space-time continuum. For space is three dimensional, and so is our central nervous system. Biologic time, however, has one dimension only, and it is not reversible. Biologic time corresponds to a process; and while spatial displacements are reversible, biological processes are not reversible. Duration is necessary for the unrolling of an affective process. Time goes on inexorably and so do the living processes in the central nervous system—irreversibly!

Piaget's reversibility (1936b) is not possible in the concrete. It is an ideational operation of displacements in space or, alternatively, an abstraction comparable to mathematical operations. Piaget's reversibility is an epistemological operation, not a process involving living matter, which can only be displaced in space, not in time. For, as Heraclitus said, "You cannot cross the same river twice."

For the newborn to cross the river at all, affect must quicken the percept. The percept can only acquire existence after affect had endowed it with duration, with biological time. Only then can cohesion develop as a bond between percept and percept, as well as between percept and affect.

We lack the concepts, we still lack the very words with which to describe the no man's land of human beginnings. We do not yet know how to speak of the newborn's psyche, of the first stirring of the newborn's mind in the twilight zone before dawn.

Forgive me if in my attempt at orientation I stumble over my own mixed metaphors when I speak of the bond between affect and percept as a bridge, made of duration, anticipation, and meaning; a bridge to span the void across the chasm in front of the soma, a bridge reaching toward the shore of an as yet nonexistent psychic system—toward a shore which anticipation and meaning are in the act of creating and fashioning; and on which duration uses predictive hypotheses to mix the cement for the engrams of the first landing stage.

PART 4

AGGRESSION IN EARLY
DEVELOPMENT

Editor's Introduction

The three papers in this section deal with the early development of aggression and its regulation. In "Aggression: Its Role in the Establishment of Object Relations," Spitz describes his observations of aggression in normal infants and in infants who have suffered prolonged separation from their mothers. Self-destructive behaviors occur during separation, and other-directed aggressive behaviors occur during reunion. Spitz interprets these observations in terms of psychoanalytic drive theory and in terms of his own emerging theory of object relations. The formulations are harbingers of today's interest in the meaning of anger expressed during reunion after brief maternal separations in those infants who are assessed in the "strange situation" (see Ainsworth, Blehar, Waters, and Wall, 1978). They are also relevant today to assessment of infants suspected of being neglected and abused (see Gaensbauer and Sands, 1979) and to the study of the development of anger itself, currently a topic of renewed interest (Stenberg, Campos, and Emde, 1982).

"On the Genesis of Superego Components" is the central paper of this section. In it, Spitz crystallizes the arguments of *No and Yes* (1957), which he had just published; focuses on the period between 15 and 18 months as a time of momentous developmental transformation; and attempts the construction of theory in a psychoanalytic area of considerable uncertainty—the origins of the superego. In tracing the development of aggressive drive during the first two years, he takes note of a process of internalization—a progression toward increasing self-regulation in certain areas of behavior in which regulation had previously come from the outside. Spitz conceptualizes three "primordia" or early components of the superego that arise during this time.

The most dramatic aspect of this development is the process which culminates in the emergence of the "semantic no." The "semantic no" is a milestone in the beginnings of communication. It represents a shift from the passivity involved in obeying a prohibition to the activity involved in constructing a negative. The central emphasis Spitz gave to this development is best indicated by his own words:

> Up to this point the possibilities for discharge of aggression were limited to fight or flight—to repression at best. From now on discussion has entered the scene. Communication opens up an avenue of discharge so new that it represents the major turning point in phylogenesis: it is the humanization of man.

Spitz uses Anna Freud's concept of "identification with the aggressor" to explain this development, but it is a partial explanation at best. Spitz also takes note of the role of maturation in this process, and writes of the "mushrooming" of imitation and identification. He cites Myrtle McGraw's (1935) model of development wherein the proliferation of a behavior is inevitably succeeded by an exaggeration of that behavior, which then becomes checked or inhibited by the emergence of newer behaviors. If this model is applied to psychological functions, the emergence of inhibition would be expected after the period during which imitation and identification proliferated. Curiously, this line of thinking—about developmental emergence, inhibition, and "discontinuity"—has a rich tradition that is often forgotten; it is very much alive among today's "systems theorists" (see Sameroff and Harris, 1979).

From a psychoanalytic standpoint, it is important to realize that Spitz's discussion of superego origins does not include the formation of the superego per se. His discussion is based on observations of children under three years of age who have not yet formed this structure and who would be considered preoedipal. (For reviews of the psychoanalytic theory of superego formation written since Spitz's discussion, see Sandler, 1960a; Furer, 1972; Arlow, 1980). That many issues Spitz raises are still unsettled is indicated by a recent international colloquium held at the Hampstead Clinic in London in November 1980, devoted to "The Superego: Its Early Roots and the Road from Outer to Inner Conflict as Seen in Psychoanalysis."

"Aggression and Adaptation" includes a discussion of Lorenz's ethological concept of ritualization and its possible parallels in human development. Spitz is mindful that more can be learned from disanalogies than analogies as one compares ontogenesis with phylogenesis. Still, thinking about ritualization in other species leads to some generative speculations about the interrelationships among several developmental processes, including aggressive and affective processes, early forms of learning, and communicative processes. (For a recent review of infant learning research, see Sameroff and Cavanaugh, 1979; for a recent integration of learning, affective processes, and psychoanalytic notions of adaptation, see Greenspan, 1975).

Aggression: Its Role in the Establishment of Object Relations

The numerous articles published in recent years on the role of aggression in psychological development have been mainly concerned with elaborating that reformulation of the theory of instincts which Freud presented in *The Ego and the Id* (1923). Two of these articles—"Comments on the Psychoanalytic Theory of Instinctual Drives" by Hartmann (1948), and "Notes on the Theory of Aggression" by Hartmann, Kris, and Loewenstein (1949)—have been selected by us as the most exhaustive and the most advanced presentations of the theory. The authors examined the adaptive and the organizing aspects of the aggressive drive. They discussed the psychological aspects of the manifestations of both the aggressive and the libidinal drive and their vicissitudes. They have expanded Freud's concepts by suggesting the existence of a neutralization of aggressive energy.

This approach resulted in several conclusions, one of which is that while the internalization of libidinal energies leads to neurosis, the internalization, without neutralization, of aggressive energy in the ego must lead to some kind of self-destruction (Hartmann, Kris, and Loewenstein, 1949, p. 24). The authors suggest further that "internalized aggression plays a relevant role in the etiology of illness" (p. 22).

As for the constructive aspects of the drive, the authors find that "the musculature and motility, apparatuses for the discharge of aggression, contribute decisively to the differentiation between self and environment and through action, to the differentiation of the environment itself" (Hartmann, Kris, and Loewenstein, 1949, p. 23). Objective danger situations require motor discharges (fight and/or flight); the enforcement of passivity is made responsible for the probability of pathological disturbance.

The opportunity in the adult for the direct observation in relatively pure form of the total inhibition of the discharge of aggression is rare in psychiatric experience; its best example is probably offered by the so-called combat neurosis (Spitz, 1946c). Such observations can be made with much greater facility and exactitude during the early development of the personality, i.e., during infancy.

Reprinted from *Drives, Affects, Behavior*, ed. Rudolph M. Loewenstein. New York: International Universities Press, 1953, pp. 126–138.

Given the parallel between similar findings of our own, as presented in our past publications, and the propositions advanced by Hartmann, Kris and Loewenstein, it appears desirable to complement the data derived from psychoanalytic reconstruction, on which theoretical deductions like those of the authors must of necessity be based, with the data of experiments and direct observation.

We believe that an attempt to apply the significant propositions of Hartmann, Kris, and Loewenstein to our findings in infancy should yield useful viewpoints for the clarification of the genetic picture of the aggressive drive and important suggestions in regard to prophylaxis and treatment of early psychiatric and psychosomatic manifestations.

We will begin with a fundamental question: Psychoanalytic theory assumes that the aggressive and the libidinal drives are primal ones. We will ask whether they are already present at birth and, if so, whether they are distinct from each other and capable of being differentiated.

Our observations and those of others indicate that at the outset the infant is in the narcissistic stage (as formulated by Freud, 1915a), during which the total energies at its disposal are at the service of the vital processes. Actions and reactions do not take place in response to outer stimulation, but by and large to the afferent impulses generating in the interoceptor system. The young organism is protected against outer stimuli by its high perceptive threshold, by the stimulus barrier, which Freud considers the prototype of repression. Perception is directed toward the organism's own processes; it responds nearly exclusively to proprioceptive stimuli.

In the following few weeks, the development of the exteroceptive organization is paralleled by the progressive appearance of conditioned responses. This supplements the interoceptive behavior which persists. It is only after about two months that a behavior going beyond this elementary pattern becomes visible. An example will illustrate these points. During the first few weeks of life the infant in the hunger situation will not react to the offer of food, *for it does not perceive it.* At this stage, perception of the food object is predicated on the presence of a proprioceptor stimulus, namely, the hunger sensation; without the proprioceptor stimulus the exteroceptor perception is not possible. It is only progressively that the infant in the course of the first three months will develop to the point where it will recognize the signal of proffered food *outside* the hunger situation (Frankl and Rubinow, 1934). It should be added that even in these circumstances the infant does not perceive in food an object, but a signal, that is a part-object (Klein, 1935, p. 283).

At this point (i.e., after about two months of life) we can begin to distinguish manifestations of pleasure in the child from manifestations of unpleasure, and frequently of rage. Phenomenologically we can speak of observable manifestations of the libidinal drive on the one hand, and of the aggressive drive on the other. Of course, before that, libidinization of certain areas, of certain situations, of certain behavior patterns has been proceeding in the oral, acoustic, and optic sectors (also in regard to thermal stimulation and the enjoyment of freedom of movement).

When we speak of a differentiation of the two drives, we are referring to their functional aspects.[1] My concept of the differentiation of drives is that of a developmental process, in the course of which the two primal drives, libido and aggression, are functionally differentiated out of the great energy reservoir of the narcissistic stage. The differentiated drives are directed in the beginning toward what I have called the preobject (Spitz, 1950a)—an object which is a precursor, not very firmly established and not too clearly differentiated, of the libidinal object itself. The integration and structuration of the ego, on the one hand, the emotional expression of the drives in response to environmental influence on the other, interrelate in the course of development. This is a circular interrelation (similar to, though not identical with, a feedback process), in which the infant's actions and the emotional expressions of his drives provoke responses from the environment. These responses then will shape the infant's further development and responses.

Definite manifestations of the aggressive drive can be observed at the time when the infant becomes capable of goal-directed actions, however primitive the action may be. Around three months, angry weeping and screaming can be observed when the infant is deprived of its human partner.[2] Withdrawal of food provokes screaming, which is no longer the expression of helpless discomfort but of specific resentment. The aggressive drive finds its generalized discharge in the relatively meager skeletal musculature of the infant. Specific aggressive acts, however, are still absent.

It is in the period of the transition from what I have called "preobject relation" (Spitz, 1950a) to real object relations that aggression and aggressive manifestations become specific. Like Hartmann, Kris, and Loewenstein (1949) we believe that the collaboration of the aggressive drive with the libidinal drive is a prerequisite for the formation of object relations. These authors have formulated in a more general manner that libido and aggression are not distinguishable from each other in the stage preceding object relations. On the other hand, they state that, at an unspecified age, aggression is directed at an object labeled "bad" (the non-I), while at the same time libido is directed to an object labeled "good" (the I). They obviously imply that at

[1] Differentiation of a drive should not be confused with "defusion." The latter is a pathological process, the former a developmental process.

[2] Any such dating of observed phenomena refers to statistical averages; actual appearance of the phenomena can be delayed within a rather wide range of a month or more.

this age perception has already been achieved and the percept differentiated into good and bad. Between these two stages is situated what we have called the *inception* of object relations, when the object is in the twilight area between conditioned reflex and preobject. At this stage the nascent object is the target of the simultaneous manifestation of both drives, the aggressive and the libidinal drive. It is the delimitation of the I from the non-I which marks the emergence of an object (preobject), it is with the help of this delimitation that the aggressive drive is differentiated from the libidinal drive.

In the second half of the first year we see progressively destructive activities appear. Hitting, biting, scratching, pulling, kicking, are used in the manipulation of "things," be they inanimate or human. This manipulation serves many purposes, primarily that of perceptive orientation and of manipulative mastery; at the same time, it establishes relations, earliest object relations, between the infant and the "thing" (and this includes the libidinal object!) in question. These relations will be established as a result of the "thing-reaction" (of the infant), as a result of the attacks directed at the object. In this way, then, beginning with a distinction of self and nonself,[3] a further distinction between the animate and the inanimate, and finally a distinction between friend and stranger, between libidinal object and the object as conceived by academic psychology will develop.[4]

Therefore we are of the opinion that a sublimation of the aggressive drive necessarily must be preceded by the *functioning* of this drive; in relation to preobjects, "things" and persons, this implies object relations of a preambivalent nature (Abraham, 1924), in the course of which the functions of the drives will be mastered and related by the infant to the object it is exploring.

We consider, furthermore, that long before sublimation can begin, the understanding of prohibitions and commands must be established.

Up to here we have followed the development of the aggressive drive in the first year of life, but have only touched upon its modifications, of which Hartmann, Kris, and Loewenstein mention four: displacement, restriction of aim, sublimation, and influences of libido (of which fusion is one).

The articles of Hartmann, Kris, and Loewenstein, basing themselves on a hypothesis introduced by Freud, state that the formation of permanent object relations is "dependent on the capacity of the individual to bear frustration"

---

[3] "Self" and "I" will be used interchangeably in this paper, because defining the two would require a digression and is unnecessary in this context.

[4] I have found it useful, in studying the genesis of the formation of first object relations, to make a clear distinction between "things" and the libidinal object (Spitz, 1949,). Things—that is, objects as conceived by academic psychology—can be described in terms of spatiotemporal coordinates; they remain identical with themselves. The libidinal object, as defined by Freud, is described by its history. It does not remain identical with itself, it is not described by spatiotemporal coordinates, but by the drive structure directed toward it.

(1949, p. 21), a view with which I fully concur and which I have frequently expressed. This capacity to bear frustration, or, as Freud expressed it, to "effect the postponement of satisfaction" (1920, p. 10) is more generally referred to as the reality principle. I postulate on the grounds of my interpretation of experimental findings that the infant must achieve the reality principle before any objective perception can take place. This, by the way, is also in accordance with Freud's (1900) formulations on the detour function of the two systems.[5] For example, only when the infant becomes able to postpone the gratification of the hunger drive, communicated to it by the proprioceptor stimulus, will it become free to direct its psychic energies to its environment and perceive the environmental world, that is, the food object. This capacity to tolerate frustration is slowly acquired and develops step by step to an ever-increasing liberation of perceptive activity in the course of the first six months of life. Exact experiments (Ripin and Hetzer, 1930; Kalia, 1932; Frankl and Rubinow, 1934; Spitz, 1946d) have shown the successive steps in this environmental discrimination. Thus the postponement of gratification of the drive leads to: (1) a cathexis of the percept; (2) a confrontation of the percept with a memory trace; (3) "thought," that is, "essentially an experimental way of acting, accompanied by displacement of smaller quantities of cathexis together with less expenditure (discharge) of them" (Freud, 1911).[6]

Perception and thought initiate the discharge of the drive into aim-directed activity. Sensory organization, musculature, and motility here function as apparatuses for the discharge of aggression. Aim-directed aggression is now placed in the service of acquiring mastery over objects of the environment as well as for the acquisition of skills, among which grasping is one of the first and locomotion the second.[7] The function of grasping in the discharge of aggression becomes clearly evident in the second half of the first year.

By the time the baby is eight months old, it has acquired an orientation and coordination of the different parts of its body, thanks to the body image formed with the help of the distribution of the aggressive drive into the most varied systems. Around that time the aggressive drive can be directed toward the objects with the help of the effectors. The beginning of locomotion in the infant marks the conquest of space by the child.

----

[5] I do not share Hartmann's view that both "the turn towards the external world and the compulsion to recognize it are still under the auspices of the pleasure principle" (1939, p. 90). This view of Hartmann's is based on Freud's assumption that the narcissistic stage is abandoned and object-libidinal cathexis formed for libido-economic reasons.

[6] [Spitz is quoting from "Formulations Regarding the Two Principles of Mental Functioning," *Collected Papers*, Vol. 4, London: Hogarth Press, 1925. The *Standard Edition* translation appears in Vol. 12, p. 221. Ed.]

[7] In a 1949 motion picture, *Grasping* (Spitz, 1951c), and in an article "Purposive Grasping" I have dealt with the steps involved in the development of grasping.

Developmentally this is preceded by the perceptual acquisition of an orientation in space. Motility, of the upper limbs at least and frequently also of the trunk, has been coordinated and has come under central control. Psychologically, what I have called "crib space" is expanded into the space surrounding the crib. It should be noted that this takes place at an age when locomotion in the sense of walking has yet to be achieved, and even directed crawling is often as yet not too successful. Before this orientation in space the infant, though perfectly able to grasp an object inside the crib, is unable to grasp an object held outside of it. For the space of the infant at this stage is circumscribed by the limits of the crib. And it is the breaking down of this barrier with the help of the aggressive drive which represents the inception of the conquest of space by the infant in its eighth month.

This age also marks the time when the infant differentiates "things" from human beings, friends from strangers; it marks the inception of full-fledged objectal relations.

It is at the inception of object relations that we will examine more in detail the manifestation of aggression; for we believe that it is here that we are able to see on the one hand phenomena of neutralization of aggression, on the other hand a turning of the aggression toward the self.

Such observations have been made by us in our studies of a nosological picture which we have called "anaclitic depression" (Spitz, 1946a).

In this disease the etiological factors are simple and well known. Children who, during the first six months of their lives have been in good relation with their mother, respond to the loss of their love object by a progressive mourning reaction if no adequate substitute is provided. They begin by showing greater restlessness, weepiness, clinging to chance visitors. In the further progression of the disease, apathy sets in. The manifestation of aggression common in the normal child after the eighth month, such as hitting, biting, chewing, etc., is conspicuously absent in the depressed children. How can this be fitted into the conceptual framework of the theory of drives?

We believe that similarly to every other sector of the infant's development, the development of the drives, both libidinal and aggressive, is closely linked to the infant's relation to the (libidinal) object. As far as the libidinal drive is concerned, we have shown this in our article on autoerotism (Spitz, 1949). It is equally so with regard to the development of the aggressive drive.

It is the relationship with the love object wich gives the infant the opportunity to release its aggressive drives in all the activities provoked in it by the actions of the object. That, after all, is well-known to nursing mothers who suffer from the tendencies of their infants to bite the nipple. It should be understood that we include in the manifestations of the aggressive drive also those activities which are not experienced as hostility, for instance grasping, etc. When the object-formation period is reached in the second half of the first year, all these manifestations become more and more evident. At this early stage of infantile ambivalence, no real difference is made by the infant between the satisfaction of one drive or the other; they are manifested simultaneously, concomitantly, and alternatively in response to one and the same object, the libidinal object. If the infant is deprived of the libidinal object, both drives are deprived of their target. This is what happened to the infants affected with anaclitic depression.

Now the drives hang in mid-air, so to speak. If we follow the fate of the aggressive drive, we find these infants slowly becoming self-destructive. It is in such cases that we have found the frequent manifestations of head-banging, well known also in animals.

Hartmann, Kris, and Loewenstein express doubt whether unpleasure resulting from self-infliction of damage is already recognized as signals warning of danger, in view of the incomplete awareness of the bodily self and the incapacity to distinguish between self and external world.

We have a motion picture of an infant who, at eight months, after prolonged separation from its mother, would violently hit the left side of its face with its fist by the hour in a rhythm comparable to that of head banging. This child directed its blows always at the same spot on the left side of its face under certain specific circumstances which aroused its resentment. The blows were well coordinated, and it is difficult to assume that this child was not distinguishing the self from the outer world, that it did not realize that the pain inflicted on its face originated in its own action.

Perhaps we may compromise in assuming a transitional stage in which the infant has already delimited the self from the outer world under routine conditions. However, when circumstances of suffering arise, in which it cannot vent its aggression on the outer world, then the boundaries again become fluid and the aggressive action is directed against the only object available, i.e., its own body.

Similar assumptions have been made in the past by Pierce Clark (1932). From all my observations on infants I am very much inclined to assume that the deprived infants' aggression, which cannot be directed against an outer world object, is returned against the self.

A counterpart of this phenomenon arises when the libidinal object, that is, the mother, has returned to the child after a limited period of depression. Then we have observed that all functions expand in an exuberant fashion. That applies both to the libidinal drives and to the aggression. Particularly the manifestations of the latter are conspicuous: after coming out of the anaclitic depression the restored infant no longer hits or scratches itself. It now begins to bite, to scratch, to kick *others*.

In other terms, as long as these infants were deprived of their libidinal object, they became increasingly unable to direct outward, not only the libido, but *also* the aggression. Although one cannot observe phenomenologically what happens to the two drives during the period of deprivation, one gets the impression that the aggressive drive is the carrier, as it were, not only for itself, but also for the libidinal drive. If we assume that in the normal child of that age (second half of first year) the two drives are fused, we might postulate that in the deprived infant a defusion of drives occurs.

How does this come about? When the separated infant cannot find a target for the discharge of its drive, the infant first becomes weepy, demanding and clinging to everybody who approaches it: it looks as though attempts are made by these infants to regain the lost object with the help of their aggressive drive. Later on visible manifestations of the aggressive drive decrease; and after two months of uninterrupted separation the first definite somatic symptoms are manifested by the infant. These consist of sleeplessness, loss of appetite, loss of weight.

An attempt to explain the loss of appetite and the loss of weight has to take as its starting point the libidinal stage at which the infant is at this period. It is the oral stage; one of the attributes of the lost love object is the gratification of the oral zone. The mother is the very source of food, and, psychologically speaking, food itself. When the infant is deprived of this love object, the libidinal and the aggressive drives are denied the opportunity for discharge. They are dammed up and turned against the self. After a brief period of transition we can observe that the infant withdraws and rejects everybody who lacks the attributes of the love object. Similarly food alone lacks these attributes and will be rejected. Loss of appetite would then represent a behavior of withdrawal and rejection; loss of weight its consequences. As in the withdrawal behavior toward persons other than the love object, the libidinal and aggressive drives normally acting in the intake of food are withdrawn and dammed up. The dysfunction of food intake and utilization is the result.

An explanation of the second disturbance, the insomnia in the infant—the dysfunction of the sleep center—will have to be made with the help of extremely tentative hypotheses.

Let us begin by positing that it is perhaps not so much the act of *sleeping* which is disturbed, but the process of *falling asleep* which is obstructed and halted. The infant falls asleep when its needs are gratified; at the breast, when its hunger is satiated. This is a picture of complete narcissistic equilibrium, of the still undifferentiated unity of object and subject.

It would seem to us that the infant's sleep disturbance, when separated from its object, is a physiological manifestation of the disruption of this narcissistic equilibrium. The healthy infant which is able to gratify its libidinal and aggressive drives during its waking period and discharge them in actions will, after this discharge, be able to return to the narcissistic equilibrium of sleep. The infant which has been deprived of its object will first attempt to use its drives to recreate in a hallucinatory manner the object with a progressively increasing measure of frustration, like in all hallucinatory processes. This continuous frustration will finally end in the predominance of the disappointment and in an avoidance of sleep and the concomitant attempts at hallucinatory gratification through dreams.

These explanations, however, do not demarcate the manifestations of the aggressive drive from those of the libidinal drive. The two were fused and, therefore, difficult to distinguish. Some light is thrown on this question by our observations on infants suffering from hospitalism: they present a tangible demonstration of the defusion of the two drives. It can be observed in the unchecked progression of deterioration in these children who were subjected to long-term deprivation of emotional supplies. The result is a progressive destruction of the infant itself, eventually leading to death.

The obverse of this defusion can be observed in anaclitic depression, when the pathological process which follows deprivation is halted by the return of the love object. Then we can witness the manifestations of a partial refusion of the drives in the rapidly returning activity of these children, in their becoming gay, playful, and aggressive.

In the first case, when the deprivation syndrome goes on unchecked and the children are separated not for months but for years, those children who survive offer pictures reminiscent of brain-damaged individuals, of severely retarded or downright imbecile children. In the due course of events these will probably become either the inmates of institutions or, under "favorable" conditions, they will offer, according to the specific individual circumstances, the manifold problems of the "asocial" (Aichhorn, 1935), of the "atypic development" (Rank, Putnam, and Rochlin, 1948), of the "schizophrenic" (Bender, 1947), of the "hyperthymic" (Bowlby, 1944), of the "turbulent" (Wallon, 1925) child—in one word, of the severely disturbed problem child. Theoretically we may posit that in these children the aggression has been turned against the self, resulting in the shockingly high percentage of deaths; and becoming manifest, that is, turned toward the outside world again, in the surviving children. In these, however, the aggression is mostly not directed at a specific object, libidinal or otherwise. It is directed at everything and everybody and takes the form of a generalized and mostly senseless, that is, "objectless," destructiveness.

In the second case, when the process of deprivation is interrupted within a reasonable length of time—that is according to our experience after not more than three to five months—by the return of the love object, the result is different. When the mother is returned to these infants within this period, they become not only gay and lively, happy with their mothers, with grown-ups, with other children, and active in their games in general. They also become more aggressive against others, for a while at least, than any normal infant of the same age. They may become actively destructive of objects, clothes, bed clothes, toys, etc. But this destructiveness does not compare with the contactless destructiveness of the child who survives prolonged deprivation of emotional supplies.

It is also among these infants whose mothers have been returned to them after several months of absence that we found the biting children and those who tear out other children's hair—not their own.

We have a film (No. 264)[7] which shows one such infant systematically tearing a piece of skin off another child's instep, leaving a bleeding lesion.

But what has happened to the two drives during the period of deprivation? Why have they become defused, why does it appear as if the aggressive drive had been subjected to a different fate from that of the libidinal drive?

Our present state of knowledge does not permit us to formulate a conclusive answer at this stage. Our own speculations have led us in the direction of suggestions expressed by Freud in various forms throughout his publications, beginning with the *Three Essays on the Theory of Sexuality* (1905b), regarding the affinity of the libidinal drive to the organ systems. Elsewhere, particularly in "The Economic Problem of Masochism" (1924), he has remarked on the musculature as the organ of discharge for the aggressive drive. Organ systems are considerably slower in the function of discharge than the skeletal musculature. It is to be assumed that they have the capacity of holding energy in a bound state. This is not the case for the skeletal musculature which discharges energy rapidly, completely, and in bursts of brief duration.

We might, then, speculate about the existence of an organic, a physiological basis, which in the case of pathological processes of discharge-inhibition would produce the defusion of the two drives. Once the libidinal drive becomes separated from the aggressive drive, the difference between the rhythm of discharge in the organs from that prevailing in the skeletal musculature could lead to a different fate for each of the drives. Perhaps some of the propositions of Cannon (1934) might find application in this context.

Any such statements can only indicate one of the possible directions of our thinking. Much careful research will be needed before we will be able to advance any less tentative statements.

Regarding the suggestions for prevention and treatment of early psychiatric and psychosomatic manifestations of which we have spoken in the beginning

---

[7] [This film is available in the René Spitz Film Archives. See Part 7. Ed.]

of our paper, we believe that they follow logically from the preceding considerations. As stated previously (Spitz, 1950d), prevention can be achieved by avoiding at all costs any disturbance of the formation of object relations during the critical period (beginning with the sixth month of life). If the original libidinal object, the mother, has to be separated from the child, an adequate and acceptable substitute has to be provided.

As for the therapy of already damaged infants at this age level, the discharge of aggression combined with the discharge of the libidinal drive should be facilitated in every possible way.

This is not the place to go into the details of these procedures. We will come back to this point in a more extensive publication which we are preparing on the subject of the aggressive drive.

On the Genesis of Superego Components

The structural concept of the psychic organization in its final form was laid down by Freud in his book *The Ego and the Id* (1923). Its formulation had been developing since 1914 when he first introduced the concept of the ego ideal and described its self-observing function in the article "On Narcissism: An Introduction." He continued his exploration of a self-criticizing part of the ego, which is split off, in the paper "Mourning and Melancholia" (1917b). In *Group Psychology and the Analysis of the Ego* (1921), the superego was for the first time formulated as a "differentiating grade in the ego." In these publications the formulation of the concepts is derived, by and large, from the clinical observation of pathological phenomena and not through a genetic investigation. The exception to this is to be found in the ultimate formulation in *The Ego and the Id* (1923), which takes up the original propositions of the origin of the ego ideal as stated in the paper on narcissism.

The close linkage between the emergence of this differentiating grade in the ego and the fate of object relations has directed our attention to the early stages of personality organization which constitute what one might call the *primordia* from which the superego ultimately will be formed.

In the following, I propose to investigate the emergence of certain behavioral phenomena in the course of the first and second year of life. Their appearance seems to indicate the formation of corresponding specific psychic structures. In the beginning, these structures are observable as physical and psychological behavior patterns. Several years later they are destined to participate in the formation of the superego and to become component parts of its organization.

We will attempt to explore the role of object relations in the establishment of these behavioral and psychological entities on the one hand, the function of the entities in the formation of psychic structures on the other. These psychic structures in their turn will determine decisively the formation of object relations of increasing complexity in what impresses the observer as a circular process, a feedback as it were. The continually progressing circular process culminates eventually in the formation of the superego, which establishes man as a member of the particular form of human society in which he

Reprinted from *The Psychoanalytic Study of the Child*, Vol. 13. New York: International Universities Press, 1958, pp. 375–404.

is raised. At the same time it establishes a clear differentiation between human and animal societies, or perhaps one might even go further and say that the difference is between societies with a historical tradition and ahistoric societies.

In the interest of clarity we will begin by defining the terms which we use. Without reviewing the literature extensively (Fenichel has done this in his usual thorough manner in the article "Identification," 1926), we will differentiate two approaches to the problem of superego formation.

The first of these assumes that the superego is present in an archaic and rudimentary form from the beginning and that its functioning is evident already in the first months or at least in the first year of life. Various authors differ rather widely in the evaluation of the role and importance they are willing to assign to this archaic superego. They also differ as to those manifestations of early childhood which they consider as being indicative of the archaic superego's functioning, as well as in their opinion regarding the age at which the infant acquires it.

The second approach has been most clearly formulated by Glover and summed up in his paper "The Concept of Dissociation" (1943). In brief, he believes that primitive ego structure is multinuclear and that the ego will be formed through the unification of these nuclei. This process is brought about through a synthetic function of the psyche which operates with progressively increasing strength. He also assumes that a rudimentary division gradually occurs in the individual ego nuclei, which will merge only when the ego itself is synthesized. He sharply distinguishes these rudimentary formations in the psyche from the highly organized mental institution of the superego. The latter can only appear as a differentiation in the total ego when infantile instinct has reached its final development. On the other hand, he ascribes a partial autonomy to these ego nuclei and, I presume, to the rudimentary division within them.

I have come to very similar conclusions in my own approach based on direct infant observation. I have examined in various studies the formation of such nuclei which are destined to become, through the operation of the synthetic function, the constituent parts of the ego. In the present paper, we will turn our attention to those developments and differentiations which are destined to become constituent parts of the superego. We will speak of them as primordia or building blocks of the superego. The latter will be integrated as an organized structure at the time of the passing of the Oedipus complex.

EARLY IDENTIFICATION AND ACQUISITION OF LANGUAGE

In the course of a recent publication (Spitz, 1957) I investigated early identificatory processes, which lead to the acquisition of language, that is of semantic communication. I investigated particularly the dynamic and economic processes underlying the inception of those semantic gestures which are the precursors of words proper. Language originates from words which express needs. I have called these words variously global words, sentence words, or need words. The first word of the child, like "Mama," expresses, according to the situation, "I hurt"; or in another situation, "I am glad to see you," or "I am pleased," or "I am hungry," "I am uncomfortable," etc.

These need words appear sometime between the eighth and twelfth month. Until the eighteenth month of life, they multiply slowly to the point where the baby has at its disposal about 15 to 20 of them and even begins to combine 2 of them with each other. Around the eighteenth month a momentous change takes place. The need words are replaced by word symbols. These are specific, individual words which are used for specific, individual objects in a one-to-one correlation.

Somewhere in the course of the six to ten months which elapse between the emergence of the need words and the inception of the word symbols, approximately around the fifteenth month of life, a gesture can be observed which, in our Western culture, is used for semantic purposes and which expresses a specific semantic message. This gesture is the head-shaking "No," the gesture of negation. A few months later it will be combined with the word "No."

I have elaborated in the above-mentioned monograph many aspects of the significance of this gesture and can therefor forego repeating these arguments here. Suffice it to mention that in his article on "Negation" Freud (1925a) stated that negation is a judgment; and that from the beginning he spoke of the differentiating grade in the ego as that structure upon which devolves self-criticism. It follows that the function of self-criticism will avail itself for its purposes of the function of judgment; this can be expressed through negation, the semantic expression of which is head-shaking and/or the word "No."

We need not go extensively into the history of the concept of the superego in Freud's thinking nor into the propositions on its formation. It will be sufficient to state that the superego is formed with the help of identifications with the parental objects. On the road leading to these identifications, the child incorporates the "do's" and the "don't's" of the parents into his ego. In the course of this process and particularly during the so-called period of stubbornness, the parent may be confronted with generalized negativistic attitudes of the child. A struggle takes place between the "do's" and the "don't's" of the parents' wishes and the child's wishes. In everyday terms, the struggle takes place between the parental prohibitions and commands and the child's resistance.

PROHIBITION AND COMMANDS

The inception of the period of stubbornness is heralded by the child's first understanding of the meaning of prohibitions and commands. This understanding begins between the ninth and the twelfth month of life. If at this stage one interrupts an activity of a child by saying "No, no" to him and shaking one's head at the same time in a gesture of denegation, the child will mostly stop what he is doing. This is a statement which obviously applies only to our Western culture. In other cultures this may take different forms, though we suspect that the essence will remain the same.

The understanding (and obeying) of commands and prohibitions should be clearly distinguished from compliance with the dictates of the superego. Obeying commands and prohibitions is a submission to another individual as a consequence of something perceived outside. Compliance with the dictates of the superego is something quite different. These dictates originate inside, not outside. The individual complies with them not in response to an external physical percept, but in response to an inner percept of an emotional nature, be this in the nature of guilt, of anxiety, etc.

The understanding of prohibitions and commands is probably achieved in the first place with the help and the instrumentality of the conditioned reflex. Undesirable actions of the infant are inhibited by physical means. This intervention is accompanied by appropriate words of the parent, in the appropriate tone, with the appropriate facial expression and gestures. In the course of events any or all of these accompanying epiphenomena of the prohibition will come to stand for the intervention itself and will be reacted to as such. That is, they will be understood as prohibitions and obeyed. Needless to say, we are not overlooking the fact that this development parallels the unfolding of object relations, that is of intrapsychic processes, and is inextricably intertwined with them.

In the process of this interchange, the child has received a communication, a signal has been given by the prohibitor; and the child has understood this signal. However, at this stage the child is unable to communicate his refusal in the same way to the grown-up; the child cannot express refusal at the age of 9 to 12 months by shaking his head, and still less by saying "No, no." It will take him another 6 months to acquire this gesture or this word and to endow them with meaning. Imitation and identification will play a dominant role in this process.

Identification and imitation form one of the major contributions of the child in the formation of object relations. Indeed, Freud's assumption was that the object choice is achieved with the help of identification and that identification is the earliest of the mechanisms of the psyche. In direct observation we find imitation as early as the fourth month of life. A fraction of all infants observed, which we may put tentatively at about 10 percent, show a tendency to imitate conspicuous facial movements. As could be expected, even in these cases the imitation is in the nature of crude totality configuration, just as perception still takes place in terms of totalities. True imitation of parental gestures appears toward the end of the second half of the first year. These are echo-like reproductions of the grown-up's gesture. They occur in the course of the unfolding object relations, mostly as games between the adult and the infant. They are immediate responses and mirror a gesture initiated by the adult.

Several months later, at the beginning of the second year of life, the child takes the initiative. In his games, he uses behavior observed in the libidinal object even in the absence of the grown-up. His spontaneous actions are replete with gestures borrowed from the adult, and he can be observed to experiment extensively with such behavior patterns.

It is evident that identification proper is at work in this performance. The infant has incorporated the percept of actions observed in the libidinal object by laying down the memory traces of his observations in the "Mem-systems" of his ego. A modification of the structure of the ego is the result.

The mirroring of the grown-up's gesture, the primitive identification with the gesture develops at the same period as the understanding of prohibitions and commands is acquired, between the ninth and the twelfth month of life.

In the nature of things at this age, prohibitions are vastly more numerous than commands. They are expressed by the grown-up mostly verbally and given emphasis by appropriate gestures, like head-shaking and finger-wagging.

At the same age level locomotion, first on all fours and then erect, is acquired. As a result, the child's independence is rapidly increased. Concomitantly, prohibitions in the form of the "No, no" of the grown-up become more and more frequent in more numerous and more varied situations.

These prohibitions are understood only dimly at first by the child as obstacles in the fulfillment of his wishes. They are constantly repeated, they are experienced and reexperienced in the exchanges between the growing child and the grown-up love object. From purely material obstacles they will be transformed in the course of these exchanges to part and parcel of object relations. Their memory traces are accumulated in ever-increasing numbers in the course of the subsequent months.

Each of the prohibitions expressed will consist of two parts: (1) the act of the child which is prohibited; and (2) the adult's prohibiting behavior, both verbal and nonverbal.

1. The child's act is infinitely variable. The actual physical circumstances in which the child's act takes place, the intentions which the child has toward the single constituents of the situation will vary from occasion to occasion.

2. The grown-up's prohibition has an invariant quality, be the occasions ever so dissimilar. It is the quality of frustration, of being an obstacle, which remains invariant. And its invariance is expressed in the word, in the gesture performed by the grown-up, both of which communicate his intention.

THE ACQUISITION OF "NO"

The invariance of the "No" gesture, of the word "No," of the intention within the multiform experience would appear sufficient to insure a lasting memory trace through the cumulative effect of repetition.

As I have pointed out elsewhere (Spitz, 1957) this oversimplified and mechanistic approach will be greatly enriched if we apply to it experimental psychological findings and psychoanalytic considerations.

In 1927, Zeigarnik, a Gestalt psychologist, proved experimentally that uncompleted actions are better recalled than completed ones. Applying this finding to the child's remembering the adult's prohibition, it becomes evident that each prohibition, verbal or by gesture, or a combination of both, inhibits an action initiated by the child. Accordingly, each prohibition leaves in its wake an uncompleted "task." The common element, the invariant, of these uncompleted tasks is the "No," the prohibiting gesture and word. This Gestalt psychological observation adds a motivational explanation to the mechanical cumulation of an invariant element, that of the uncompleted task.

Psychoanalytically we are still inclined to consider this as too narrow a basis for the explanation of the spectacular feat which the child performs when he takes over the "No" gesture from the adult and turns it against him. It is obvious that the psychological processes involved in this complete reversal of the situation must be more complicated ones. Were it not so, we would for instance find animals using such gestures in refusal of their masters' wishes, yet we know of no animal which has ever done this.

From the psychoanalytic viewpoint each prohibition involves a frustration of the child's id drives. Whether we make it impossible to get a thing which he desires, or whether we disagree with the particular form he happens to give to his object relations, we are imposing a drive frustration. The memory traces connected with such prohibitions, the gestures and the words in which they are expressed, will therefore be endowed with the specific affective cathexis of frustration. This specific affective change will therefore be the first insurance of the permanence of the memory trace of the prohibiting "No."

This is an explanation which does not go much beyond the Gestalt example of the uncompleted task, though it does introduce the qualitative element of the affect and the quantitative element of its charge.

Furthermore, in terms of development, the child at this stage has just completed the transition from infantile passivity to the toddler's full-blown activity and is fascinated by the newly acquired possibilities. Prohibitions interrupt this activity and invite a return to the passivity of the previous stage. They also enforce a regression in the direction of the passive or passive narcissistic organization of the ego, whereas the child at this stage is enjoying volitionally directed object relations which he initiates himself. Obstacles put in his way, which force him back into passivity both in action and object relation will not be readily tolerated; he will attempt to overcome the obstacles in the path of his progress. This, incidentally, is a general law of animal behavior formulated by Eibl-Eibesfeldt (1957).

The child directs an aggressive cathexis against the "presentation" of the obstacle in his path. The affective charge associatively connected with the frustration experience will reinforce this aggressive cathexis. This charge invests the memory traces of the prohibition. Now the "no gesture" becomes suitable to be turned against the prohibiting grown-up.

IDENTIFICATION WITH THE AGGRESSOR, A PRIMORDIUM OF THE SUPEREGO

At this point the child is caught in a conflict between the hostile, aggressive reaction to the prohibition on one hand, and his libidinal attachment to the love object on the other. This is an intrapsychic conflict between the two drives with which the ego has to deal. A defense mechanism of the ego is called into action, specifically the one described by Anna Freud in 1936 as "identification with the aggressor." The manifest conflict involved takes place essentially between the *external object* and the *ego*. Identification with the aggressor, however, leads to internalization of the conflict.

The examples given by Anna Freud are at an age level at which we may assume that the superego, or at least its immediate precursors, have begun to operate. In our 15-month-old, who acquires the "No gesture" from the adult, this is not the case. He also finds himself in a conflict between the ego and the external object. However, no superego nor its precursors are present at this stage. The libidinal object at one and the same time is also the prohibiting authority. Only several years later will the introjected imago of the libidinal object be destined to be transformed into the superego. Actually we are not dealing with a process involving the superego—we are dealing with the dynamic process of early secondary identification.

I have advanced the proposition that the dynamics operating in this process are as follows: The libidinal object's "No" inflicts a frustration on the child and causes unpleasure. In due course, the "No" is laid down in the ego's "Mem-systems" as a memory trace. The affective charge of unpleasure, separated from this presentation, provokes an aggressive cathexis in the id. This is attached by way of association to the memory trace in the ego.

Freud stated that when the child identifies with the libidinal object, "he passes from the passivity of the experience to the activity of the game." Anna Freud elaborated this finding in her statement: "Identification with the aggressor is succeeded by the active assault on the outside world."

The identificatory link with the libidinal object is the "No," both in gesture and word. The aggressive cathexis with which this "No" has been endowed in the process of the numerous unpleasure experiences connected with these memory traces has made it a suitable vehicle to express aggression. It is thus that the "No" becomes such an important device for expressing aggression in the defense mechanisms of identification with the aggressor. The aggressor in the case of the 15-month-old is the frustrating love object against whom his own "No" is returned.

In discussing identification with the aggressor, Anna Freud showed that it is a preliminary phase in the development of the superego. That becomes quite evident in the course of the second year of the child, who has acquired the semantic "No," for at this stage the child turns this device also against himself in the so-called role-playing games.

All observers are familiar with the role-playing games of toddlers. Beginning early in the second year of life, the child assumes the role of the grown-up in his games. He may, for instance, dial a toy telephone and conduct an imaginary conversation. He may imitate a nurse and hand out diapers and feed his doll, etc. In these games, as every observer knows, imagination plays the major role. A stick can play the role of the doll, a teddy bear can become alternately the child himself or the parent, a box can play the role of the telephone.

But already in the first half of the second year, you can observe the child saying "No, no!" to himself in such role-playing games, or shaking his head in denegation at some of his own activities. It is obvious here that he has assumed the mother's role. It is an example of what Anna Freud (1952b) described in another context with the words, "The child . . . adopts the mother's role, . . . thus playing 'mother and child' with his own body" (p. 79).

I consider this form of identification with the aggressor, in which the child plays the mother's role and applies the prohibition to himself, as one of the primordia which will go into the later formation of the superego.

THE ROLE OF VERBAL IMPRESSIONS IN SUPEREGO FORMATION

It might be objected at this point that Freud (1923) postulated that, no less than the ego, the superego is derived from verbal impressions. Its cathectic energy, on the other hand, is provided from sources in the id. The derivation of the superego from verbal impressions would be in perfect agreement with our findings if, at its inception, the child's identification with the aggressor (one of the primordia of the later superego) would take place in response to the parent's *verbal* "No." This, however, is not the case, as evidenced by the fact that the child manifests its identification with the aggressor by taking over first the semantic *gesture* of the head-shaking "No, no" from the parent. At this age level, the diacritic discrimination in the auditory sphere and the processing of auditory perceptions is not yet as differentiated as in the visual or in the tactile sphere. Accordingly, by and large, the use of the verbal "No, no" appears somewhat later in the child's life than the head-shaking sign of negation. From the viewpoint of the infant's perceptive discrimination, at the age at which the head-shaking "No, no" is understood as a prohibition, verbal impressions are only epiphenomena of the parental prohibitive interference with the child's activity. It will be several months later, in the second year of life, when locomotion imposes distance between parent and child, that verbal impressions assume a major role as prohibitions and commands. Even at this age one may suspect that verbal prohibitions will be understood earlier than commands, just as the use of the head-shaking "No" is acquired earlier than that of the head-nodding "Yes."

Physical Restraint and Facilitation, an Archaic Primordium of the Superego

This suggests that among the primordia which will form the superego there are some to which we have paid little attention up to the present. They belong to the perceptual sector of tactile and visual impressions, such as restraining the child physically on the one hand, the facial expression, as well as the tone of voice which accompanies such prohibiting interference, on the other. Similarly, imposing physical actions on the infant, whether he likes it or not, in dressing, diapering, bathing, feeding, burping him, etc., will inevitably leave memory traces in the nature of commands.

These physical primordia of prohibitions and commands are not easily recognizable in the ultimate organization which is the superego. Verbal communication, because of the extraordinary advantages and facilities it offers, has appropriated the field of information and communication practically to the exclusion of all other media. That is surely evident from the way in which so-called visual education is extolled as a wonderful new discovery, to the point that special university departments are created for it. The psychoanalyst is not free from this bias and mostly pays attention to the functioning of the superego when it is manifested in a verbal form, like in the self-reproach of melancholia, in "the small inner voice," in the dictates of conscience, etc.

Including this physical primordium into the concept of the adult superego poses tantalizing problems and at the same time opens up new avenues of psychoanalytic research. It might for instance lead to a better understanding of psychosomatic disease. More obviously, hysteria comes to mind, where it is perhaps licit to assume that the variety of hysterical paralyses, which result from a conflict between the ego and the id, hark back to that age when the conflict between parent and infant led to the physical restraint of the latter.

We cannot neglect either a related series of the infant's experiences even more widely varied than those just mentioned. I am referring to the early libidinization of organs and organ systems, which can take place in the course of the birth process (see Greenacre, 1941, 1945). Equally significant are later experiences in the course of the first year of life resulting from surgical, medical, or parental intervention, the last particularly evident in folk customs (Greenacre, 1944). The consequences were considered mainly in terms of erotization. This can then result either in the use of the libidinized organs or organ systems for pleasure gain or in a secondary elaboration leading to inhibitions in the particular sector in one form or another.

This field offers vast possibilities for investigation. The question arises, for instance, why this archaic primordium of the superego becomes effective in hysteria, whereas in the more deeply regressed obsessive compulsive syndrome, in paranoia, in the cyclothymias, it is the auditory, that is, the verbal and ideational aspect of the superego which determines the clinical picture and the symptoms. Our knowledge is obviously insufficient. We will have to await further clarification from the clinical approach on the one hand, from direct observation and the experimental approach on the other.

The Fate of the Aggressive Drive

Returning to our considerations about role-playing games, their function in the formation of the ego ideal was always tacitly accepted. The 15- to 18-month-old little girl, who preens herself before a mirror, as she has seen mother do, is just as familiar to us as the little boy, who, at the same age, puts on father's hat, takes father's cane and strides up and down the room, makes his voice deep and says, "Daddy, Daddy!" The role of the libidinal drive is self-evident in these actions. It is the attempt to *be* as the love object *is*.

The role of the aggressive drive is somewhat less evident. One of its roles, as we have seen from our exploration on the beginnings of communication, consists in enabling the child to achieve a form of semantic communication through identification with the aggressor, through a dynamic process. Needless to say, this semantic communication is destined to assume an extraordinary importance, not only for the individual, but also for the species.

I believe that the role of the aggressive drive in the process of achieving semantic communication has been recognized up to now only implicitly; since both drives are involved in all human activities, the aggressive drive had to be present at the inception of communication also. I have discussed elsewhere (Spitz, 1957) the important role played by the conflict between the aggressive and libidinal drives in the emergence of semantic communication. Recently, Dr. John Benjamin, in a personal communication, called my attention to the fact that there probably is a relationship between the stage of nondifferentiation and Abraham's (1924) oral sucking level on one hand, between the stage of the eight months anxiety (that is, the beginning of true object relation), and Abraham's oral biting level on the other.

One obvious relationship between the stage of nondifferentiation and Abraham's oral sucking level immediately comes to mind. Both belong to the same period of the infant's life, to the first three months. Both operate on a level of perceptive discrimination which is similar in that it is not yet differentiated. This lack of perceptive discrimination corresponds to the absence of differentiation in the psyche at this stage; we may even say, for the first few weeks of life, to the lack of the differentiation of the psyche from the soma. The differentiation develops gradually in the course of the subsequent weeks and months. I have discussed elsewhere (Spitz, 1955c) that the perceptive organ which initiates this perceptive development is the oral cavity, a finding that is in good agreement with Abraham's propositions on the oral sucking level.

Conditions are not as clear-cut regarding the relations between the stage of the eight months anxiety and Abraham's oral biting level. At this period of life, a substantial measure of differentiation has been achieved, not only in the sector of perception, but also in the organization of the infant's psyche, and in the instincts and their functioning, as well as in the manner in which the ego has become able to deal with them, etc. For a more detailed account, the reader is referred to my book *No and Yes* (Spitz, 1957).

One of the problems arising at this stage is the way in which the infant deals with the aggressive drive. There cannot be any doubt that at the oral biting level, the aggressive drive will find its outlet in a number of destructive, hitting, tearing, and particularly biting and chewing activities. Experimental psychologists have remarked on the predominance of these activities in the second half of the first year, when the child seems bent on reducing everything he can reach into its smallest component parts. At the same time, however, the aggressive drive is placed into the service of sensory discrimination, and it may not be too fanciful to point out that here also, in the visual field, one percept is being dissociated and distinguished from the other. That becomes particularly evident in the child's capacity to discriminate between the love object and a stranger, a capacity which will lead to the eight months anxiety.

From a variety of infant observations I will select two extremely dissimilar ones, which seem to me to illustrate the dissecting tendencies of the oral biting stage particularly well. It should be remembered that the oral biting stage will blend imperceptibly with the anal stage and that, to me at least, it remains an open question whether anal sadism is not ultimately derived from the oral biting component. One of these examples is an observation made by Charlotte Bühler (1928). She used a variety of materials to investigate the creative activity of the child. Among the materials she offered the children, the experiment with plasticine is of particular interest to us. Charlotte Bühler found that, when the child tried to create a shape from this material, he would use one of two diametrically opposed methods. One of these consisted in molding a large lump of the material into the intended shape. The other consisted in forming discrete units of the material and putting them together into the intended shape. This method she called "synthetic." The outstanding example of the synthetic approach is that of a little girl who had just reached her third year and who wanted to form a ring out of plasticine. She detached pieces from the material and put them together until the ring shape was achieved. No earlier observations of this infantile creative activity are available.

An adult trying to make a ring from plasticine might form a sausage and bend it till the ends touch. Or he might make a flat disc and punch a hole in it. This child formed pellets and put them together to achieve a ring. From my own observations we may assume that this pellet-forming and putting-together activity starts very much earlier.

As I have published elsewhere, coprophagic children play with their stool, forming pellets out of it, rolling them, and using them both as a toy and to put into their mouths already in the age range of 8 to 15 months (Spitz, 1949).

In presenting these two examples, we have already crossed into the territory of the way in which the aggressive drive is dealt with in the course of the oral biting and anal level. The destructive activities tend to be replaced, or rather to be transformed into a series of constructive games. The hollow blocks which, up to then, had served only for hitting against each other, are gradually held carefully against each other, as if to measure their respective proportions and relations; and finally one hollow block is placed into the other one. The hollow sticks, which had first only been used to hit anything in sight, then for hitting each other, become interesting because of their potentiality of being hollow. Fingers are stuck into the opening; and finally one stick ends up in the other, with a triumphant expression of the child at this achievement.

It would be rewarding to observe the detail of this transition, to find out whether it has to do with the giving up of the biting and chewing activity on all objects available, the giving up of stuffing everything into the mouth. Can we surmise, for instance, that the stuffing into the mouth will be carried over by the aggressive drive to the hollow block, to the hollow stick, and that the child endows these objects with a make-believe personality, when he puts one block into the other one, one stick into the other one?

And what, we may ask ourselves, is the role of neutralization in this process? I cannot include its exploration into the present study and will limit myself to the statement that, in my opinion, the prerequisite of neutralization is the availability of a certain measure of ego organization. This organizational level of the ego is only reached after the eight-months anxiety appears. As explained elsewhere (Spitz, 1959), the eight months anxiety can be considered to be the indicator of a subsequent unfolding of numerous functions in the autonomous and nonautonomous sectors of the ego, some of which will be placed into the service of the domestication of the drives.

Origins of Identification

From the child's gradually increasing understanding of the meaning of the prohibition the defense mechanism of identification with the aggressor will emerge. We may ask why the child should identify with the adult as a result of unpleasant experiences. Freud (1920) had discussed this question at length. He gives the example of the child into whose throat the doctor looked or on whom the doctor performed a minor operation; such a child will make this frightening experience the subject of his next game. Freud explains that the identification with the doctor offers a gain in pleasure. As the child goes from the passivity of the experience to the activity of the game, he inflicts on his play-partner the unpleasure which he experienced, taking his revenge on the person of this substitute. And Freud stresses that all the games of the child are influenced by the wish to be grown-up and to be able to do what the grown-ups do. We would add to this that these games are attempts at mastering the traumatic experience. The child puts himself in the role of his aggressor and inflicts on others what has been done to him.

One may well wonder, whether the boy who dons father's hat, the girl who preens herself before the mirror, the child who plays "nurse," handing out diapers—whether these children are not doing the same. Of course, they have chosen activities that seem removed from the traumatic experience. The activities chosen are not aggressive, or at least not hostile, but they are characteristic of the aggressor-frustrator. We can perhaps say that all these identificatory imitations have one quality in common, that of mastery.

Reducing these activities to the common denominator of "mastery" does shed some light on their origin. They originate from the child's insurgence against his infantile helplessness. They are an attempt to overcome the passivity of the narcissistic stage, to take over the functions of the external ego, of the mother.

We will describe two cases in which this is impressively illustrated.[1]

Case Pr 4 (0:7 + 16). The mother, holding the child in her lap, is feeding the child from the bottle and introduces the nipple into his mouth. The child accepts it, sucks, *and at the same time pushes his fingers into the mother's mouth*. The mother understandingly permits him to play this reciprocal role and facilitates it.

At this age level we observe something which is typical of such early identifications. The child does not identify with the essential purpose of the mother's action, namely the feeding. He identifies with one element of this process, namely with the "sticking into the mouth." It will not come as a surprise to the psychoanalyst that this early identification takes place only in the sector of oral activity.

Case Pr 9 (1:1 + 3). This child is six months older and more advanced in every respect, also in regard to what he identifies with. The child is sitting at a small table next to the mother. The mother is feeding the child a diversity of foods with the help of a spoon. Pr 9 has developed a minor feeding difficulty. He places the feeding situation into the service of his object relations, particularly when being offered solids. There are no problems with his drinking milk from a cup, but when he is offered cake, noodles, etc., he is more interested in offering these to his mother than in eating them himself. We see him first putting a piece of cake into his mother's mouth and then some noodles. Pr 9's mother also behaves understandingly and munches the child's offering.

We note that this older child is already able to disregard the inessentials of the activity. He does not attempt to use the spoon, nor does he try to stick just anything into the mother's mouth, be it his finger or a toy. He is not playing a make-believe game. He selects a piece of food, which is the essential of the activity, he has grasped the meaning of feeding. The mother's contented munching of the food proffered by her son manifestly increases his willingness to eat, an observation with which any mother is familiar.

INTERCHANGE OF PHYSICAL ACTIONS, A PRIMORDIUM OF THE EGO IDEAL

I see in the interchange of physical actions, which are used meaningfully and are obviously emotionally cathected,the primordia from which the ego ideal will be shaped. In its turn, the ego ideal ultimately will form a part of the superego and represent the individual's aspirations.

Nunberg's concept of the role of the ego ideal in the formation of the superego differs slightly from mine. As I do, he considers the ego ideal's

[1] The cases are drawn from our film records: Karl, Pr 4, 0:7 + 16, reel 170; and Knut, Pr 9, 1:1 + 3, reels 214/215/216/217. [These films may be found in the René Spitz Film Archives. See Part 7. Ed.]

origin to be predominantly maternal and pregenital. From what I have outlined above, it can be seen that I place the earliest origins of the ego ideal specifically in the first half of the first year. That is not to say that the major part of the ego ideal will not be acquired subsequently, but one would presume that the process which governs the earliest modes of conforming with the parental wishes will make itself felt in the acquisition of later additions to the ego ideal.

The process of which I am speaking is a physical one. It consists in the parental facilitation or inhibition of infantile movements. One may speculate whether this is not one of the sources of gesture imitation. It is only *one* of the sources—and we believe not the essential one at that; for imitation seems to be anchored much more importantly and much more archaically in phylogenesis.

It is evident from this that we do not necessarily follow Nunberg in his assumption that the ego ideal is only formed through renouncing instinct gratification out of fear of losing the object. That appears to us to be a later addition to the original archaic process.

We also differ from Nunberg's opinion that the predominantly paternal superego can be observed first in the genital stage. As I will show further on, I consider Anna Freud's finding that identification with the aggressor is a preliminary phase of the superego of the greatest importance. This particular defense mechanism can be demonstrated as one of the primordia of the superego at the beginning of the second year. At this time it is quite unlikely that it should be of paternal origin. Again, we may assume that additions will expand this primordium at a later date, making it meaningful in the oedipal situation.

THE THREE EARLIEST PRIMORDIA

The three primordia of which I have spoken appear to be of a very different dignity. Imposing physical action on the child, whether to inhibit his initiative or to facilitate his striving, is a far cry from the psychological. Yet it must have a counterpart in the infant's psychic apparatus, such as it is at this stage. It inevitably provokes frustration or gratification, and will subsequently lead to the development of the psychological correlates to the physical compliance or resistance of the child. One step further are the child's attempts at mastery by means of identification with parental actions—one hesitates to call them identification proper; Berta Bornstein has spoken of identification with the gesture, which is unquestionably a step on the road to identification proper. The third of the primordia is, however, already a genuine defense mechanism, identification with the aggressor. All three, despite their essential differences, appear to be steps leading from compliance with parental wishes via imitation to the wish to identify with the love object.

Looking back, we find that we have explored three of the primordia of the superego. The chronologically earliest, most archaic of them, is the physical intervention of the parent, both in the sense of arresting physically the child's activity and in the sense of imposing upon him a physical action. The second is represented by those parental actions which become endowed with positive meaning for the child and with which he identifies in his attempts at mastery. They will form the primordia of the ego ideal. The third and most advanced involves identification with the aggressor on the ideational level, resulting among other things in the achievement of communication. All three have in common the wish to identify with the love object at all cost.

FURTHER DISCUSSION OF THE ORIGINS OF IDENTIFICATION

From my observations of infants, I have gained the impression that at this age, between 6 and 18 months, the wish to identify is so strong and plays such a major role in object relations, as well as in the need for mastery, that the child identifies indiscriminately with any behavior of the love object he is able to appropriate. It is as if the mechanism of identification at its inception would go through a phase of nondifferentiation. It is indulged in by the child for identification's sake, as it were. It is used for object relations, as well as for mastery, for defense as well as for attack. Perhaps this indiscriminate way of appropriating *everything* that is available from the love object—things, gestures, inflections, actions, attitudes, etc.—explains the origin of identi- fication with the aggressor.

We believe that a very general law of development can contribute to our understanding of the sudden mushrooming of both imitation and identification in this particular phase of infancy. I am referring to the findings of McGraw (1935), according to which any behavior has an initial phase in which its beginning can be recognized, a second phase in which it proliferates so that the activity itself becomes the incentive for repetition, and a third phase in which the exaggeration of this particular behavior or movement becomes checked or inhibited by the emergence of other and newer ones. In our opinion, this law applies not only to behavior patterns, but also to the ac- quisition of new psychological functions and, in our case, to a mechanism of defense.

In the phase around the first year of life a major part of the child's object relation takes the form of identification. It goes without saying that these identifications will be selective ones, and we will come back to the question of the principle of their selection. The child's increased use of identification at this stage corresponds to the phase of proliferation in the McGraw series. In a later phase the tendency to identify at all cost will recede and will be replaced by other psychic processes.

If the child identifies for identification's sake on the one hand, in his efforts at mastery and in his rejection of passivity on the other, with anything the love object does, then he will identify also with that which causes him unpleasure. Once the pattern is laid down and has followed through a certain period of development, it will become established, because it turns out to be a useful one in many aspects in the process of adaptation.

SELECTION OF CONTENT IN IDENTIFICATION

However, it appears desirable to be more specific about what the child takes over when he identifies with the aggressor. He tries to appropriate everything from the love object in innumerable other identifications in which the love object is not aggressive. Yet each individual child obviously makes a selection of his own among the vast number of items which he could take over. To my knowledge, the conditions which govern the selection of what the child identifies with have never been studied. One of the principles governing the selection is obviously derived from the personal emotional history of each individual child.

But I also believe that there exist more general principles for this process and that some of them become evident in the 15-month-old in the specific instance of identification with the aggressor's head-shaking "No." One such general principle refers to the question what the 15-month-old *is able* to take over from the love object by virtue of the limitations of his own psychic organization. These limitations will determine the way he can deal with what is made available to him by the love object.

The elements which the 15-month-old can assimilate in identifying will have to be age adequate; it is the child's mental capacity at a given age which will act as a screen in his selection of what he identifies with.

The principle of selection is of course of greatest importance for the choice of the elements from the surround, or rather from the parental object, which can at any given time enter into the child's actual experience. For they will form the matrix from which at a later stage the superego will be molded. At the stage of which we are speaking now, we have seen that it is probable that one of the early constituents of the ulterior superego is furnished by the mechanism of identification with the frustrator. We will therefore proceed to investigate what the child can appropriate with the help of this identification.

Among the variety of psychological and physical components which constitute the love object's frustrating action, we can distinguish three constant ones. They are: (1) the object's behavior; (2) the object's mental processes (this includes the contents of which the behavior is an expression); (3) the affects which underlie and accompany this behavior. The child deals differently with each of these.

1. The 15-month-old's psychic equipment enables him readily to perceive and to distinguish diacritically the love object's physical behavior, the head-shaking. Accordingly, in his identification, he will appropriate this component fairly exactly. After having appropriated it and performed the identification with the aggressor, he will become able to endow it with semantic meaning and to turn it *against* the parental figure, but also against himself.

2. On the other hand, the adult's mental processes and the possible rational reasons for his "No" are completely beyond the 15-month-old's capacities of understanding. He cannot understand whether the adult prohibits something because the child's safety may be in danger or because the child does something the parent has forbidden. At this age, the child does not yet think in rational categories, and ignores the laws of cause and effect. For this reason, as well as because of his lack of insight into the processes going on in him and other persons, he is not capable of empathy in the commonly accepted sense of the term.

THE GLOBAL PERCEPTION OF AFFECTS

3. The situation is again different in regard to the third component, namely the affects underlying the adult's frustrating behavior. From my observations it appears that in the second year of life the child still has only a global perception of his partner's affects. This level of perception of affects is comparable to the global *sensory* perception of the three-month-old. Just as the three-month-old will develop diacritic discrimination of the detail of sensory percepts only later in the course of the first year, the older child will, much more slowly and over many years, develop a discrimination of the various affects perceived in others and of their reasons.

As regards the second year of life I am inclined to assume that the child distinguishes in the adult partner two affects only. I will call them the affect "for me" and the affect "against me." In our usual somewhat dramatizing terms, the child feels either that the love object loves him or that the love object hates him.

This lack of discrimination in the child can be clearly demonstrated in motion pictures. Case Pr 2 shows impressively how little the child understands the motivation underlying the adult's actions.

Case Pr 2 (0:11 + 24). In this case the observer is playing a game with the child and offers him a toy. After the child has taken possession of the toy and played with it, the observer takes the toy away again and puts it in his pocket, so that a large part of the toy remains visible. When the child reaches for the toy, the observer wags his finger, shakes his head and says, "No, no." Notwithstanding the smiling friendly expression of the observer, Pr 2 hastily draws back his hand, and sits with downcast eyes and an expression of embarrassment and shame as if he had done something terrible.

This child at the age of 11 months and 24 days clearly understands the prohibition. At the same time he misinterprets the prohibiting adult's affect in a global manner: "You are not *for* me; therefore you are *against* me." Three or four months later we may expect him to be able to take over the prohibiting gestures from the adult.

If we now consider the child's selection in his identification with the aggressor in the "No" gesture, we can say that the child takes over from the adult the diacritically perceived sensory data of the head-shaking gesture, and/or the "No" word. But the affects still will be perceived only globally, as "against." The affect "against," together with the gesture, will be taken over in the identification with the aggressor when the child experiences unpleasure because of a demand or a prohibition of the adult. If on this occasion the experiencing of unpleasure and of the affect "against" generates a thought process in the child, it will be all his own and certainly not taken from the aggressor.

The identification with the aggressor in the "No" gesture therefore remains limited to the imitation of the physical action, and to the appropriation of the global quality of the affect; the two are then turned against the aggressor. Simultaneously, thought processes are triggered in the child. All three together—imitation, turning of the affects against the adult, thought process—represent energy transformation on a large scale. This energy transformation is a step forward in the domestication of the drives, as a result of the ever growing closeness of object relations. In this transformation of energies the motor expression of the affect "against" has been subjected to the control of the ego and modified, with far-reaching consequences.

From the viewpoint of thought process also a significant development has been initiated when the child indicates a decision in the form of refusal through head-shaking. The use of this gesture is the manifest evidence of a judgment at which the child has arrived. When the child expresses this particular judgment, he also discloses that he has acquired the capacity to perform the mental operation of negation. This step in turn inevitably will lead to the formation of the abstract concept underlying the negative, the first abstract concept to appear in mentation.

STRUCTURAL CHANGES

Our present concern, however, is with the structural changes which have occurred. When the child turns the "No" against the parent, he shifts from the passivity of obeying the prohibition to the activity of imposing a negative. With this, a new avenue has been opened for the discharge of aggression coming from the id. Up to this point the possibilities for discharge of aggression were limited to fight or flight—to repression at best. From now on discussion has entered the scene. Communication opens up an avenue of discharge so new that it represents the major turning point in phylogenesis: it is the humanization of man.

From the viewpoint of the ego the changes are numerous and evident. The dynamics inherent in the identificatory process were set in motion under the pressure of repetitive frustration and through the child's efforts to overcome them. Thanks to the shifts of cathexis which I have indicated before, the ego has now acquired a method of dealing with the environment, with the drives, and with the self which hitherto had not been available. Within the system of the ego, two functions have visibly been established. One is the function of abstraction, with all its ulterior consequences for the process of mentation and for the achievement of verbal communication. The other is a new mechanism of defense, that of identification with the aggressor, which at a much later stage will be used in the formation of the superego.

This is also a major step in the child's progress from initial helplessness and complete dependency to an ever-increasing autonomy. The application of the capacity of judgment in his dealings with the surround, on one hand, in his dealings with himself on the other, leads to a progressive objectivation of mental processes. Moreover, the radius of object relations has been expanded. Previously, physical resistance was used in unpleasure situations. Now refusal can be expressed without involving action. With this, as stated before, the period of discussion and also the period of stubbornness can begin.

Finally, the superego: needless to say, in all this no trace of a superego or anything which resembles it can be detected. However, I believe that when the defense mechanism of identification with the aggressor is integrated into the ego, a prerequisite has been established for what Freud has called a "differentiating grade in the ego." I feel justified in positing that the establishment of the defense mechanism of identification with the aggressor, indicated by the semantic use of the head-shaking "No" gesture, is a necessary, though not a sufficient, prerequisite for the later formation of the superego.

It also has to be distinguished from Anna Freud's preliminary phase of the superego, not only in regard to the age at which it is manifested, but also in regard to its structure. In the preliminary phase described by Anna Freud, the five-year-old, after internalizing the parent's criticism, externalizes his offense and projects his guilt. He manifests this by becoming indignant at the grown-up's wrong-doing.

Not so in the 15-month-old. He does not internalize criticism, he internalizes prohibition and the global affect "against." He does not externalize an offense, at least not a specific one. One might say that he externalizes the global offense of being "against." I greatly doubt whether guilt is involved at all in this projection; I do not feel justified in ascribing guilt feelings to children at this age, even though a number of children I have observed present under these circumstances what one can only call a "guilty" facial expression.

I have two reasons to be reluctant to ascribe the specific term "guilt" to this facial expression: (1) we do not know what the child feels; (2) it is more than likely that, at this age, this expression also corresponds to a more global feeling. This more global feeling involves guilt as well as shame and embarrassment and mortification and fear and probably other shades of feeling. We will have to create a special name for this global feeling. It will be differentiated later into a variety of shadings, of which guilt will be one.

Glover (1950) expresses similar views in discussing the three stages of psychic stress. In the second, the intermediate stage, when the ego is organized up to a certain point and imposes specific defense mechanisms, it is still subject more to anxiety than to guilt. This seems to me to be a good description of the period which follows the eight months anxiety and which includes the emergence of the defense mechanism of identification with the aggressor (manifested in the acquisition of the head-shaking "No"). I would assume that turning this gesture against the self marks the inception of a differentiating grade in the ego. I would further assume that, on the one hand, the intrapsychic conflict between the libidinal and the aggressive drives, simultaneously directed toward the love object in this achievement, will ultimately lead to the development of guilt feelings in the course of the second year. On the other hand, the necessary condition for the development of guilt feelings is the differentiating grade in the ego, which makes it possible to turn one part of the ego against the self.

I do not feel that it is useful to speak of this differentiation in terms of an archaic superego. We are not yet dealing here with an organization within the ego, it is rather an *ad hoc* mode of functioning of the ego, which is put into operation when the circumstances warrant it. As shown in the role-playing games of the child, the operation of this function is tried out playfully, and its potentialities will be gradually explored in extremely varied imaginary as well as in actual situations. It is one of the primordia destined to go into the ultimate organization of the superego, which contains many other such primordia—I need only mention Ferenczi's sphincter morality.

THE THREE PRIMORDIA

We have explored three of these primordia in the sequence in which they follow each other chronologically. The first is the very archaic experience of inhibited and facilitated physical action. This is followed by something which, for lack of a better term, we have to call identification with the love object. Actually, physical imitation has as much a part in producing these behavior patterns as does identification. They are placed in the service of mastery and will ultimately participate in the formation of the ego ideal. Somewhat later, in the beginning of the second year, the third primordium, the above-mentioned identification with the aggressor, will appear.

As yet, the role of the earliest, the archaic primordium in the formation of the superego is insufficiently understood. Much clearer is the role of the identifications which go into the formation of the ego ideal. The prototypes from which the ego ideal is derived, the parents, are ever-present physically in the child's actual life. The ego ideal ultimately will come into conflict with the oedipal disillusionment, and will at that time undergo a severe reappraisal. A devaluation of the actual prototypes begins in the course of this reappraisal. The ideal derived from them, however, will be introjected, forming that part of the superego which sets unattainable goals for the individual. It acts as a spur and a reproach. It will be confronted by the child with reality achievements which forever must fall short of this ideal. For this ideal is a global one, detached from the physical and moral inadequacies of the devaluated parent, and it remains divorced from reality.

The chronologically latest of the three primordia, the mechanism of identification with the aggressor, will form a most important component of the superego. Not only can it be turned against the libidinal object and serve for the discharge of aggression, it can also be turned against the self, against the id, and against the ego. This makes it suitable to form that differentiating grade in the ego which is the necessary prerequisite of the superego, providing a line of demarcation between the superego and the ego. In alliance with the ego ideal it will impose on the ego, in the form of judgment, in the form of prohibitions and commands, both the aspirations and the avoidances of the ego ideal.

In my investigation of the origin of communication, I have also explored the origin of the affirmative, of the semantic signal for "Yes." It is a later acquisition than the "No" and I do not doubt that it will play an important role in the formation and in the organization of the ego ideal and consequently in that of the superego. The investigation of this role presents some difficulties. As Anna Freud (1936, pp. 9–10) remarked, we only become aware of the boundaries of the superego, when it is in opposition to the ego. The affirmative does not offer as easy an access to the study of the superego as the negative. Its exploration therefore will have to be left to the future.

CONCLUSIONS AND OUTLOOK

I realize that the roles which I have assigned to these three primordia in the formation of the superego can only be tentative ones. These roles are in the nature of approximations. Any abnormality in the development of the infant, in his object relations, in his identifications, will inevitably distort the role played by one or the other of the primordia and perhaps even eliminate it from the superego formation. We will then get a distorted or partially defective superego.

This is an assumption which points up the significance of our understanding of these steps in the child's development for purposes of prevention. It is self-evident that an appropriate amount of prohibition and of frustration in the proper form at this age, between 9 and 18 months, is the *sine qua non* for the normal development of the child, for the establishment of the basis for the later development of his superego. We will, however, have to investigate the forms in which the prohibitions are desirable, the amounts of prohibition or frustration needed, and the timing of such frustrations.

It is equally self-evident that the prototypes for the identifications which go into the formation of the ego ideal must be made available to the infant. And furthermore, that restraint as well as facilitation of muscular activity in the earliest months of infancy and throughout the first year of life cannot be left to an inanimate enclosure, whether this consists in the straitjacket of a blanket tightly wrapped around the child's arms and body, or in the bars of his cot. These restraints have to be imposed by a responsive human being, just as the facilitations have to be offered by someone capable of empathy.

Finally, we come to the therapeutic aspect of what we have discussed. It seemed rather obvious to me that the ever-increasing number of imitations and identifications of the growing child are indicators of his progress toward the formation of the ego ideal; that the timely development of the head-shaking "No" gesture is the indicator that the child has acquired the mechanism of the identification with the aggressor. This knowledge should be used for diagnostic purposes. Furthermore, continued research should make it possible to develop an instrument, with the help of which we can evaluate where too little and where too much prohibition or frustration has been imposed, as well as information on how to facilitate imitation and identification. Such an instrument will enable us to introduce correctives where the above-mentioned diagnostic signs indicate it.

Aggression and Adaptation

Lorenz (1963) described how indispensable intraspecies aggression is for the preservation of the species and for its evolution. On the other hand, aggression is a constant threat to society. It must be made inoffensive; in phylogenesis this takes place through *ritualization* of the derivatives of the aggressive drive, of hostility. It has to be diverted from its original goal, reoriented, and placed in the service of *communication* between the sexes. I stress again that in the animal this metamorphosis occurs in the course of phylogenesis. It will not be easy for the psychoanalyst to guard against the impression that this phylogenetic modification of the meaning of animal behavior appears to have parallels in human psychopathology.

One thinks of Lorenz's description of the crane's behavior when courting a female, and of his reoriented make-believe attack against a substitute object, a piece of wood, a rock. I am reminded of the ritual of an obsessive-compulsive patient, whom I met on the grounds of a psychiatric institution and who on seeing me from afar greeted me always with exquisite politeness, taking his hat off. But he *was* an obsessive-compulsive; and, before he could grasp his hat, he had to snap his fingers two or three times loudly. It was not difficult to uncover in the course of his analysis that the ritual of finger-snapping was the replacement, the ritualization of a murderous gesture. It was an unconscious memory that made the finger-snapping submissive gesture of greeting into the hard-earned camouflage of his murderous feelings of hate against an almighty person in the past. Against a person, before whom he always "forgot" to lift a hat: the finger-snapping reminded him of the severely punished "forgetting," of the ruler, with which the teacher hit him over the fingers. One might say that he snapped his fingers so as to prevent taking me by the throat.

Are we justified in drawing such parallels? I think that we are, as long as we remain conscious of the differences. In the case of the crane, ritualization was crystallized out of the struggle between hate, fear, and the sexual drive

Reprinted from *The Journal of Nervous and Mental Disease*, 149:81–90, 1969. Copyright © 1969 by The Williams & Wilkins Co. Reproduced by permission.

[This paper was part of a collection in honor of Lawrence Kubie. Five paragraphs of introduction giving tribute to Kubie and to Konrad Lorenz have been eliminated in the interests of space. The historian will want to refer to the original publication for a full sense of Spitz's introduction. Ed.]

through successive processing along uncounted generations in the course of phylogenesis. In the case of our obsessive-compulsive, it is also the struggle between hate and fear. But it is not processed in the course of phylogenesis; it is dealt with during ontogenesis, in the unconscious, where this struggle leads to the bizarre finger-snapping ritual. In the case of this patient we see how compromise produces the substitute action in the course of ontogenesis. The power which enforces the substitute action, the reorientation of the instinct, is not the pressure of natural selection; the obsessional ritual is imposed on the ego by the pressure of the superego.

The conclusion at which we have arrived is not very spectacular. In nature, morphological innovation, morphological creativity, is practically unlimited. The creation of new *forms,* each more improbable than the previous, has no end. But where it is a question of the creation of new *methods,* the picture changes; nature disposes only of relatively few methods; and when a method has been elaborated and has worked in one case, it will be applied again and again and again, be it reasonable and applicable to another given case or not.

Lorenz gives the example of the wings of the Argus pheasant, which are completely inappropriate from the viewpoint of that bird. Another case is that of the "clan hate" of rat families. It appears licit to posit that, when ritualization itself becomes the principle which governs natural selection, this leads to consequences which ultimately will endanger the survival of the species itself.

I think that there are comparable elements in the ceremonial of the obsessive-compulsive. Obsessive-compulsive ritualization also inhibits discharge of aggression in the form of hostile action. But it has no rational survival value. No wonder, obsessive-compulsive ritual has not developed as a result of the pressure of natural selection, but in consequence of individual response to intersystemic pressure. Nevertheless, this ritualization provides for the individual, for the obsessive-compulsive, a compromise between his aggression and his superego; it becomes for him—and only for him and not for the species—a *modus vivendi.*

I would like to correct certain points in Lorenz's ideas. He places ritualization in the category of instincts, and I would like to apply here a correction in terms of drive theory. I wish, therefore, to advance the proposition that ritualization is to be considered as a phylogenetically developed biological model (one of the numerous biological prototypes) for later psychological elaboration. As such it will represent a pattern, phylogenetically initiated. This phylogenetically developed pattern of the mastery of aggression with the help of ritualization can serve as a model for the psychological development of a defense mechanism of the ego in man for mastering conflicts between instincts and the superego.

I consider certain of these phylogenetically developed behavior patterns of the nonhuman animal kingdom as potential physiological prototypes for certain defense mechanisms of the ego in man (Spitz, 1961). They are not to be equated with these—the resemblance is misleading—but they do provide models for methods, which perhaps lie in readiness for the needs of the human psyche. Formulated less rigidly, such phylogenetically acquired models of animal behavior are placed into the service of the ontogenetic needs of the human psychic organization. Since in man the creation of the drive-regulating, organized, and drive-directing devices occur in the course of ontogenesis, we may ask ourself what may have led to this new, infinitely more flexible and remarkable, innovation.

We are in debt to Lorenz, his associates, and his followers for the explication of the evolutionary development of the regulation through that psychological unit which Lorenz calls "the parliament of instincts." The analyst will prefer to speak of partial drives, which, in the course of individual development, are gathered under the primate of genitality and are regulated by the operation of the pleasure principle and the reality principle. This cannot be equated completely with Lorenz's parliament of instinct. The partial drives which we distinguish are not identical with the behavioral patterns which Lorenz calls instinct, nor does he really spell out the regulatory principle of the great parliament.

This may be due to a conceptual difference: our partial drives have not been defined primarily from the viewpoint of behavior, but from the viewpoint of affect. Their derivatives, of course, can be observed and described in the form of behavior—and for some of them Freud did exactly that. When Lorenz derives his concept of instinct from nonverbal behavior only, that is obviously due to the fact that he works with subjects with which verbal communication about feelings, motives, and affects is not possible. It must remain, therefore, an open question, whether and how far there can be found anything in common between our formulation of partial drives and Lorenz's concept of the parliament of instincts—or whether we speak about radically different matters.

One of our tasks for the clarification of this problem would be a systematic research of the partial drives, their structure, their relation to each other, their classification, and the exploration of their natural history. We probably know more than Lorenz about the partial drives of sexuality; he probably is way ahead of us in the exploration of the role of aggression in the parliament of instincts. A comparison of the two conceptual systems will only become possible when these gaps are filled in from both sides, particularly in the field of regulation and evolutionary development.

For our present purpose it is essential to remember that these regulations are developed in the animal through the pressure of natural selection in the course of phylogenesis. This leads to relatively rigid behavior patterns in the animal. These either are ready for application already at birth or are latent as anlages, becoming operative later in the course of development. They are tuned to the average expectable environmental conditions of the given species. However, during the lifetime of the single individual they make adaptation to major environmental changes either impossible or very difficult.

In man the situation is different. His long dependency on the parents and his practically complete lack of inborn behavior patterns give him a nearly unlimited opportunity to learn and acquire parental and social traditions in the course of ontogenesis. That endows man with a vastly more flexible capacity to adapt to changing environmental conditions. But what causes rapid changes of environmental conditions?

Apart from changes in climate, like glaciation, which take place in the course of geological time spans, apart from natural disasters, which are either unique and unpredictable, or are repeated at relatively regular intervals in the identical manner, like floods, innundations, etc., and apart from changes in the conditions of food production, like drought, which take place relatively slowly, there remains one factor, which is subject to rapid change. That factor is the social structure within which the human child grows up.

Here is the spot, I think, where the role of aggression in stimulating adaptation might have operated decisively in the course of the evolution from animal to man. I must add possibly; for, of course we do not know this, but it appears as if the ever more complicated levels of organization of society coincide in time with the development of progressively more efficient tools and more efficient arms for implementing hostility. Beginning with the primitive "hand ax" (fist hatchet), we have a list of increasingly complicated proximity weapons. The given social organization, which in the beginning was just as primitive as the fist hatchet, seems to increase in complexity in temporal parallel to the progressing effectiveness of the weapons. We may surmise that it was the weapon which preceded and enforced the changes in the given social forms existing at the time. Thrown weapons, like throw-stick and sling, effective at a distance, probably did more to make other forms of social structure possible than did proximity weapons like the fist hatchet. It is likely that, as further consequences of this changed social organization, it was comprised of more individuals, and the change in social form and the greater numbers of individuals required changes in interindividual relations also.

This form of change does not exist in the nonhuman animal; neither weapon nor social organization change in the course of one generation or even of many generations. "For the shark has sharp teeth, dear," and so has the wolf; the elk has his horns and his hoofs; the lion has his claws. All this does not change, and the form of society, the *code*, the form of behavior to the other individual of the same species does not change either. But, in man we see both weapon and social organization subject to constant and seemingly parallel change, beginning with our most distant human ancestors.

At this point, when adaptation to a rapidly changing environment became necessary during ontogenesis, evolution began to discard that form of psychological organization which Lorenz called the "big parliament of instincts." Traces of this changed direction of evolution are perceptible already in the behavior of the large primates. Now a structuring of the psychic apparatus takes place. We owe to Freud's genius that model of the psychic apparatus which permits us to conceptualize the functioning of these structures, their interaction, their dynamics, their role of mediation between drive and surround in the form of a coherent system. Freud (1913) wrote a brilliant and penetrating essay, an attempt to reconstruct the history of this psychic structuration, in *Totem and Taboo*. It is a welcome confirmation of my propositions that he stressed in this book the resemblance between the rites of primitive (preliterate) societies and the ceremonial of obsessive-compulsive neurosis.

Furthermore, we actually have a reconstruction of the life of primitive man in *Totem and Taboo,* a drama in which the chief actor is the society-creating, progress-stimulating power of aggression. Reoriented aggression against individuals of the same species (in the case of *Totem and Taboo,* the group of the sons against the father) becomes the creative principle. Ten years after the publication of this book, Freud introduced that model of psychic structure of which I spoke above: it is the personality model consisting of the three psychic structures of id, ego, and superego.

In the original German, Lorenz gave his book *On Aggression* the subtitle *On the Natural History of Aggression.* He knows, of course, and we know, that this natural history comprises much more than aggression alone. It touches, for instance, on the natural history of the development of thought process.

In our approach to the development of the thought process, we remain always aware of the fact that processes taking place in the unconscious obey the laws of association by contiguity, as Breuer and Freud (1895) stated already in *Studies of Hysteria*. I advanced the proposition that the conditioned reflex is a bridge leading from the unconscious to the conscious, from the essential drive to a selective reaction to the signal. It is also a conspicuous example of association according to contiguity. Furthermore, we can observe in the phenomenon of the conditioned reflex the operation of a law or principle, which I consider to belong to the transition from the unconscious to the conscious, the so-called "law of effect." According to this law, formulated by Thorndike (1913), an organism learns more quickly those reactions that are accompanied or followed by satisfactions. Conversely, it learns slowly or not at all those that result in an annoying state of affairs. The law of effect leads to the acquisition of a causally oriented behavior; in the course of phylogenesis this develops into a causally operating thought process.

Let us consider briefly the earlier prototypes of causal behavior. Among these we have mentioned above the conditioned reflex and the innate releasing mechanism (IRM). Both are physiological prototypes of the thought process. From a formal viewpoint the IRM functions like a conditioned reflex. A stimulus is offered to the subject. This triggers an instinctual action, which does not have *this particular* stimulus *as such* as its instinctual goal.

The IRM differs from the conditioned reflex only in the fact that in the latter, the stimulus is laid down in the psychic apparatus during the lifetime of the subject, whereas in the case of the IRM certain conditions of the stimulus are laid down already phylogenetically and transmitted through the genome. While in the conditioned reflex there is complete liberty in selecting the attributes of the stimulus, in the IRM one of these attributes mostly consists of the reflex-specific developmental phase of the subject during which the stimulus is offered. But just as in the conditioned reflex, the conditioned stimulus is in no way necessarily connected with the aim of the instinct. In the case of the IRM we have an inborn, often ritualized behavior, of which Lorenz showed that it is the result of displaced, reoriented aggression. What distinguishes, therefore, the inborn ritual from the conditioned reflex is that in this case, the conditioned stimulus or rather the conditions which trigger its beginning to function are transmitted in the genome; they are hereditary. One would be inclined to assume that they are laid down in the central nervous system.

What distinguishes even more the IRM from the conditioned reflex is that in the former the role of the affect is much more conspicuous. Anything can be conditioned; only something vitally important can become an element of the inborn releasing mechanism and only this will be ritualized. The vitally important functions (*e.g.,* the following function, the sexual function, the displaced attack) are all connected with affects of individual life which have survival value for the individual or the species. And this affect will be used, under the pressure of natural selection, for the creation of the inborn, of the ritualized behavior.

Again, the psychoanalyst is reminded of Freud's (1933) formulation regarding affects. He remarked: ". . . affects are also reproductions of very early, perhaps even pre-individual experiences of vital importance; and I should be inclined to regard them as universal, typical and innate hysterical attacks, as compared to the recently and individually acquired attacks which occur in hysterical neuroses and whose origin and significance as mnemic symbols have been revealed by analysis."[1]

We can see from the examples given by Lorenz that, for such a mechanism to become hereditary, it has to make use of the conditioned reflex. But over and beyond this it acquires a rigidity which is not characteristic of the conditioned reflex. The ritual, the inborn releasing mechanism, does not become extinct in the sense of the conditioned reflex. Either these rituals will not deteriorate at all, or, if they are not triggered during the critical period, they will atrophy and cannot be triggered anymore. The conditioned reflex is quite different; it requires reinforcement—without reinforcement it becomes extinct, but can be reconditioned again.

Two factors are probably responsible for this difference: first, the conditioned reflex is acquired during the lifetime of the individual, while the inborn releasing mechanism is acquired in the course of phylogenesis. Even more essential and very probable is that the inborn releasing mechanism is created by a vitally important affect and that the reliable functioning of this mechanism is placed from there under the pressure of natural selection.

A conditioned reflex is its complete opposite. Anything can be conditioned if sufficiently repeated. I have recently heard of an experiment with 2,000 repetitions. The affect plays no role in this process or only a small one.

As mentioned above, we may assume that association through contiguity is connected with the establishment of any conditioned reflex. Perhaps this is a primitive form of the functioning of the nervous system in the sensory sector. This association can take place without the intervention of the consciousness. The question remains of how this would lead to the development of causality, to the development of the consciously perceived: if *B* follows under all circumstances after *A*, then *A* is the cause of *B*, and from there would follow the next step: if I want to produce *B*, then I must achieve *A*.

At this point I will advance a further proposition: what happens when an IRM is triggered? A process is set into motion accompanied by a very considerable, a powerful affect. In the course of this process the aim is the gratification of the straightforward drive (instinct) through the achievement of the unconditioned stimulus. It is not very likely that these conditions make for the implementing of intellectual performances in the nature of perceiving causal sequences, and the laying down of the memory traces of these sequences is very likely.

---

[1] [Spitz is here providing his own translation from the 1931 German edition, "Neue Folge der Volesungen zur Einfuhrungin die Psychoanalyse," in *Gesammelte Werke*, London: Imago Publishing Co., 1946. He appears to be referring to a passage on p. 81 of the *Standard Edition* reference (1933). It would appear, however, that he is also including points made in an earlier passage (1916–1917, pp. 395–396). Ed.]

It appears probable to me that intellectual performance is the result of a detour function: a detour which takes place through the slow, endlessly repeated learning conditioning, cathected with relatively small quantities of affect, which takes place in the course of the life of the individual and not in the course of the existence of the species. It is pretty generally accepted that neither large quantities of violent affect nor too easy gratification of the instincts is conducive to the operation and carrying out of thought processes. Also, that anger is a bad counselor is proverbial, and just as correct as the admonition of the teachers of antiquity: *Plenus venter non studet libenter.*

The development as well as the unfolding and operation of the thought process obviously presupposes the possibility of processing and reorienting aggression. To explore and put into action this reorientation, the organism needs time—time to split the affect into manageable quantities by linking it to a variety of memory traces to which it will be attached. Time to perform the function of relating these fractioned affective charges and their traces with each other, performing the task of anticipation.Time to relate the anticipated constructs to the given reality situation—in other words, time for introducing the reality principle, with the purpose of a better solution of the given situation by postponing immediate gratification of the drive. Time to compare, to weigh, to evaluate, and to decide. And it is in this introduction of the time function into the psychic process, in contrast to the timeless (or rather minimal time-consuming) stimulus-reflex response, that the thought process differs from the time-abolishing computer.

It is the reality principle, the capacity to postpone drive gratification, which places at the disposal of the human infant this necessary minimum of time. It is this postponement which makes possible the fractioning of the drive, the processing of the drive in the most varied manners, and among others to provide discharge of sizable fractions of the drive with the help of substitute objects.

Unprocessed elementary aggression is reduced through this processing to a manageable entity that is proportionate to the goal of the drive, without jeopardizing the achieving of this goal. On the contrary, various redirected fractions of the aggressive drive are modified in such a manner that in their new form they insure a more reliable reaching of the goal of the drive. Lorenz showed this in phylogenesis in the animal, for instance, in the ritualized reorientation of peace-insuring ceremonial. I have made an attempt to show this in the human thought process in the case of the head-shaking "No."

We may, then, view the thought process, the development of thinking activity, perhaps as the latest of the great adaptive achievements of evolution. It is one more example of the effectiveness of the aggressive drive in stimulating evolution and adaption.

Lorenz's book enriches our thinking in many other directions. One of these is the way Lorenz is able to present to us the uninterrupted continuity of evolution. Another is that it stimulates us to ask ourselves questions in regard to certain aspects of our own discipline. One is tempted to formulate a few of these questions, to ask where the step to the ego is situated on the evolutionary scale, where one is justified to speak of internalization.

I would like to ask how the animal psyche is structured, when it becomes able to differentiate between "young" and "small." We learn from Lorenz that there exists in the animal kingdom a somewhat labile prohibition against damaging the young of one's own species: we know also that some of the highly developed mammals very often extend this consideration to the young of other species. But I wonder what prompted my Siamese cat to the following behavior. She lay sleeping on a chair and my two-year-old, overlively and active grandson approached her with a gleam in his eye and before my horrified eyes hit her in the belly with all his strength, at the same time stretching out his head to look closely what the result would be. I was too far to intervene and expected that the cat would sink her claws into his face. She did wake with a start, but hesitated one instant—and licked the hand of this unknown child.

A two-year-old child is not "a small, helpless animal" in proportion to a cat, but a giant. How did she know that, notwithstanding the difference in size, it still was a silly "animal young"? It seems to me that the explanation of the prohibition of aggression against the younger animal cannot be derived alone from the care of the young of one's own species.

One may also ask oneself at what point the humanization of man began. With speech, which makes the transmission of experience in ontogenesis possible? I attempted in a book (Spitz, 1957) to explore the archaic beginnings of speech in individual ontogenesis and to apply to them my own propositions. It became evident that for us also it is a question of reorienting aggression which leads eventually to a gesture—or should I say, to a ritual? A ritual, namely the head-shaking "No," comparable to the "flagging" of seagulls. A ritual which makes it possible to use discussion instead of physical aggression?

In the last five decades we have been able to follow the origins, the archaic forms, the prototypes, and the precursors of human thought process into ever-earlier stages of individual development. It appears to me that we are also proceeding now to explore the hominization of our species into ever earlier geological periods. Today we are reaching to the Olduwai; Lorenz, in his book on aggression and its role in adaptation, shows a direction which goes far beyond that.

In my own thinking I have assigned a role to aggression which I compare to the carrier waves of radio transmission (Spitz, 1953). I concluded at that time that without the aggressive drive the development of the individual, of his psychic apparatus, the unfolding of his attributes and capacities, would be impossible. I have not had to change this view since then. It is, then, not surprising that I share fully the opinion of Lorenz on the significance, the vital importance of aggression for life itself and its evolution. Under the circumstances I can only come to the conclusion that we as psychiatrists and psychoanalysts have also the obligation to take on the task, and for us it is an uneasy one, of exploring the devices which will make it possible for man to domesticate aggression, to find how to reorient it, how to place it in the service of the survival of the species and its development. For we are all aware of the danger that aggression might develop in the wrong direction, in that direction which leads to annihilation of the species.

And here we rejoin again the work of Lawrence Kubie. When I think of his "A Research Project in Community Mental Hygiene: A Fantasy" (1952), I dream of unleashing his gift of creative imagination and replacing it in the service of a fantasy on a major scale, a fantasy on the problem mankind is facing and will face in the future: How can we redirect aggression on a more than individual, on a global scale?

Elsewhere (Spitz, 1957), I have attempted to reconstruct the inception of hominization of the infant which is marked by the acquisition of verbal communication. It seems licit to apply the biogenetic law of Haeckel also to psychological evolution. Therefore, we may assume that the beginnings of semantic communication in the infant's ontogenesis are a recapitulation of that fateful turning point in phylogenesis, the birth of communication in man. For the birth of verbal communication marks the hominization of the species. It introduces into the interindividual relations the possibility of substituting discussion for hostile aggression. It makes flexible the rigid ritual which up to then served to reorient aggression.

Perhaps it is the limitless flexibility of this miraculous invention that was fateful. For we seem to have exhausted the effectiveness of that miraculous invention in the course of the millennia. Verbal communication is losing its effectiveness; it appears to be breaking down and to be fulfilling its task of redirecting and neutralizing aggression haltingly. We seem to be drifting toward a holocaust, unless the species again succeeds in producing a miraculous invention leading to a new turning point of equal cosmic significance as was that of the invention of verbal communication.

I will end these musings which are drifting into wish-fulfilling dreams. But having envisioned, perhaps as a myth in the prehistoric path, the *hominization* of man, may I also dream of the *humanization* of mankind and hope that Larry will unleash his imagination, making us the present of his fantasy of the next turning point?

PART 5

INFANT PSYCHIATRY

Editor's Introduction

The case studies from "The Smiling Response" are included in this section on infant psychiatry for several reasons. First, they illustrate that any assessment of troubled infants must pay attention to positive affect and its variations as well as to negative affect and depression. Second, they illustrate the early approach of Spitz and Wolf who, in 1946, were already taking note of the importance of assessing social reciprocity in the infant. This observation led to an emphasis on the relationship between infants and mothers, a theme which later tended to become overshadowed by Spitz's concerns with extreme environments and by his emphasis on maternal causes of infant deviance. Third, although brief, these case descriptions are of interest in their own right and offer some surprises for today's clinician. An example is the use of separation and reunion with the mother in assessment; in one case Spitz attributes importance to the observation that a 1½-year-old shows anger at mother's approach. As noted earlier, the use of brief maternal separation and reunion sequences is now becoming a standard part of infant assessment in the "strange situation" (Ainsworth et al., 1978) and its variants (Harmon and Morgan, 1975; Gaensbauer, Mrazek, and Emde, 1979).

In his 1950 paper on "Psychiatric Therapy in Infancy," Spitz offers some treatment principles gleaned from his experience up to that point. He emphasizes the role of environmental change, with regard to provision of both love objects and inanimate objects and discusses the importance of locomotion and peer relations in treating infantile depression. Spitz had not yet formulated his genetic field theory (1959), and he would later revise his view that psychological development is a smooth, uninterrupted process. (The fact that there are many discontinuities in development and in its psychopathology is now well documented. See Clarke and Clarke, 1977; Rutter, 1979). Spitz also later revised his statement that for an infant to recover from depression resulting from a separation, reunion with mother was necessary within three months (see "Anaclitic Depression," this volume, and the editorial commentary related to it).

Today's reader may not be familiar with the Hetzer-Wolf Baby Tests. These developmental tests were among several that sought to systematically document the unfolding of behavioral milestones. Also known as the "Viennese Tests," they were especially rich in social-emotional items. They are now superceded by the Bayley Scales of Infant Development (Bayley, 1969), which incorporate many items from the Hetzer-Wolf tests and other baby tests in use throughout the 1930s, 1940s, and 1950s. The Bayley Scales are well standardized and can be used psychometrically. It is worthwhile noting that the use of the Bayley Scales in research is so widespread, particularly in the United States, that the tests may have achieved the status of a "marker variable"—a basis for comparing results of research done with different samples and for different purposes (Bell and Hertz, 1976).

Spitz's 1951 paper, "Psychogenic Diseases in Infancy," contains his scheme for nosology according to "psychotoxic" and "deficiency" diseases of mothering. This scheme sounds grossly unidirectional and possibly even naive by today's standards; however, it is important to realize that Spitz was starting with the obvious importance of the environment in his understanding of how problems develop. In a later paper (Spitz, 1971) Spitz emphasized two additional categories of disease, namely, major infantile problems (such as blindness and deafness) and "mismatching" problems, both of which sound more interactional. Indeed, in that paper he also comes to the view that infant disorders are best viewed as problems of adaptation. Today's readers should also note that psychotic mothers (or fathers) need not produce abnormal or deviant infants; many do quite well with this phase of parenting (for discussion of contemporary studies of psychotic parents see Anthony and Benedek, 1970).

Some Case Studies from "The Smiling Response"

with Katherine M. Wolf

NEGATIVE REACTION: THE INFANT FIXATES THE GROWN-UP'S FACE, BUT
DOES NOT RECIPROCATE THE SMILE

This reaction can obviously only occur after directed reaction to visual stimuli
has been acquired. This is the only reaction which could be considered truly
negative. In such a case the infant concentrates his gaze on the smiling adult's
face, often even frowning while carefully watching the adult's facial activity;
it may sometimes have a puzzled expression, but it will not return the adult's
smile. This negative reaction is also of diagnostic significance, but as we
shall see, its significance differs from that of an absence of reaction due to
absence of perceptive development.

Cedric at the age of 0;3 + 4 had a general developmental quotient of 147,
which means that he was developmentally advanced 1½ months beyond his
chronological age (Figure 1). An exception to this advancement is found in
his social relations. There he is retarded below his chronological age. He had
failed to perform the test for the third month in the social sector, which
consists in reciprocating the grown-up's smile. He manifested the behavior
described previously. He looked very attentively at the smiling grown-up's
face, frowned but did not smile. This retardation in the social field was still
apparent when we tested Cedric again at the age of 0;4 + 4, 0;5 + 16, 0;6 + 8,
and 0;7 + 13 (Figure 2).

The chart of his development on each of these occasions is so startlingly
similar to the previous ones that they could be superimposed upon each other:
relative retardation in the social sector, unusual advancement in every other
sector of the personality. A quotation from the protocol taken at 0;6 + 8 is
very characteristic:

Cedric's reaction to the grown-up is that of interest and objective observation. The

Reprinted from "The Smiling Response: A Contribution to the Ontogenesis of Social Relations," *Genetic Psychology Monographs,* 34:57–125, 1946.

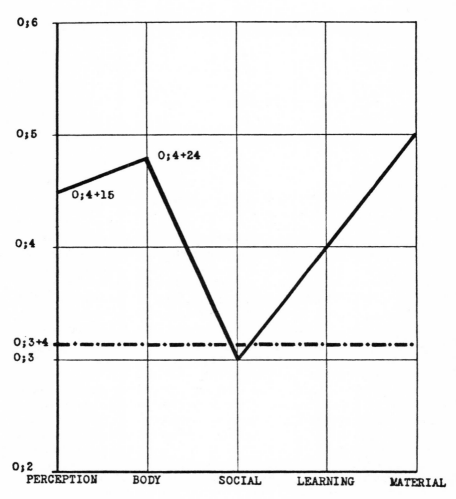

Developmental age: 0;4 + 18   Developmental quotient: 147

FIGURE 1. CEDRIC, MALE, WHITE, 0;3 + 4

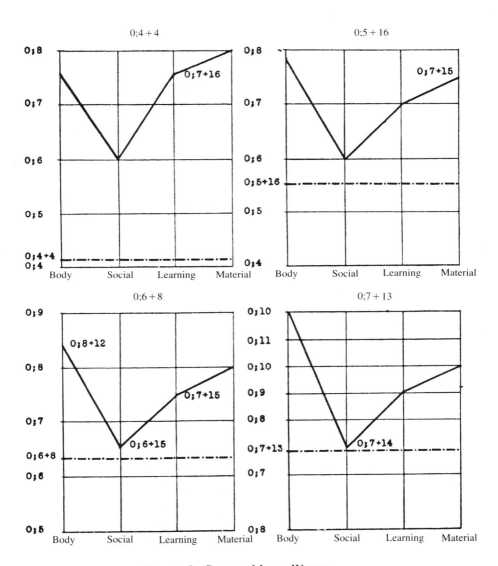

FIGURE 2. CEDRIC, MALE, WHITE

grown-up is an object to look at and to study; his reaction to this stimulus does not differ from that to other stimuli, except that for him the grown-ups are the means to get play objects, the things he wishes to have. He has no real social reaction. It had been previously stated by the mother that the grandfather was the only person in Cedric's world who had been able to induce him to smile. Even now his smile, which occurs very rarely, is extremely superficial.

The child was observed by us until the age of 1½ years; at the age of 1 year he had learned to smile and to be afraid of the grown-up, but his social reaction remained extremely retarded. We quote from the protocol taken at 1 year:

> Cedric is intellectually very advanced and completely asocial. He now expresses a longing for social contact but it is one-sided. He is not capable of any organized games, he always takes, but never gives.

Reciprocity on a primitive level appears in the normal child at 8 months. A higher level of reciprocity with adults is normally achieved soon after the twelfth month; but since his general developmental level is that of a 14-month-old child Cedric's absence of an understanding of give and take in social relations is a striking phenomenon.

The environmental background of Cedric provides an explanation for his unusual emotional behavior. Cedric's parents are intellectuals who have absorbed everything currently in vogue pertaining to the way good parents should behave with their children. On the other hand, both of them simmer with hostility, repressed and sometimes not so repressed. The mother's hostility is unconscious but ever present, overlaid with a slightly acid, syrupy veneer of sugary small talk. One of its overt manifestations is her solicitous, somewhat anxious attitude. The father's hostility is overt and more explosive, partly due to his character, partly to the fact that he has to concentrate it into briefer periods of contact with the child. When we saw him, he came in, blustering, and began immediately to perform exhibitionistic stunts with the child, picking it up and swinging it around on his shoulder with a lighted cigarette in his mouth; he narrowly missed burning the child, upsetting the mother greatly, and showed no insight into the inappropriateness of his behavior. The grown-ups in this child's environment were much more eager to use him for their own exhibitionistic and narcissistic purposes than as a love object. Under the circumstances it was not surprising to find Cedric at the age of 1;6 + 0 playing with the two experimenters happily, though without particular friendliness in the absence of his mother, and exhibiting a tense and hostile expression on his face and uttering screams of rage and anger at the mother's approach.

The other child who refused to return the smile of the grown-up between the third and the sixth month shows environmental factors similar to Cedric's. We conclude that the absence of the smiling response is definitely not a sign of retardation, because it is compatible with greatly advanced behavior in every other sector. It is characterized by a tenseness in the expression of the child, and we suspect that its diagnostic significance is one of psychiatric involvement in the emotional field, though we are not prepared to say at this moment how far this psychiatric involvement goes, or what its nature is.

LACK OF INTEREST IN THE STIMULATION OFFERED BY THE ADULT'S FACE

These cases are rare. It is hardly possible to get contact with these children by offering them a smiling face. They react to it either not at all, by looking at something else, or they take a brief look at the adult's face and just look away from it indifferently. It is still harder to get their attention a second time. The contact is just as fleeting and no smile is evoked. This is a reaction which we have found in some children suffering from hospitalism (Spitz, 1946b). We believe that this is a deeper disturbance than the previously described one. Emotional contact with such children is nearly impossible. Those are the ones who present the factors described by Pichon (1936) as *agénésie affective*. They have never reached the developmental level of an emotional reaction either to an instinctual or to a social situation. Their emotional reactions are in response to their own narcissistic experience, and take place in accordance with the pleasure-pain principle. Even this statement is possibly an exaggeration. They do not show pleasure at anything, their emotional behavior is actually along the lines we have described for the newborn. Environmental stimuli either leave them indifferent and quiescent, continuing to be absorbed in their own concerns; or they are disturbed by them and react with more or less violent emotional manifestations such as screaming. It would perhaps be more correct to say that they function in accordance with the pain-quiescence principle.

SCREAMING INSTEAD OF SMILING

These children show a rather puzzling picture. When the observer approaches them while they lie quietly and pleasantly in their bed, often playing with a toy, they mostly react with a look which in an adult would be called one of suspicion. If then the experimenter bends over the child and speaks to it smilingly, it either looks at the experimenter with a distinct expression of mistrust, which in a few seconds turns into crying, or it immediately starts to scream violently. It is perfectly obvious that the experimenter is experienced by these children as a very disagreeable stimulus. The moment the experimenter steps out of the visual radius of the child it quiets down and sinks back either into pleasant contemplation or contented playing. That these children wish the experimenter to be removed immediately is unmistakable.[1]

The case of Evamar is a particularly instructive one. The mother of this child is detained in prison and the child was raised from birth in the prison nursery. The conditions prevailing in this nursery are unusually good ones as compared to institutions in general (Spitz, 1946b). Evamar is a well-developed infant with a developmental quotient of 117. An investigation of her background disclosed that the mother has an intense passive homosexual attachment to another prison inmate. The latter was a girl with a violent, domineering, rebellious personality who was constantly instigating her prison mates to revolt while treating them alternately with caresses and blows. We will call her the ringleader. As a result of this emotionally upsetting relationship Evamar's mother behaved in a resentful, noncooperative manner, was bitter, and rejected all advice in regard to her child. This background was investigated because we are trying to find the reason for Evamar's unusual response to the smiling stimulation. When approached by the experimenter at the age of 0;4 + 13, she screamed instead of producing the normal smiling response.

0;4 + 20: The reaction was not changed. At this point the head matron of the nursery undertook a psychotherapeutic intervention, consisting, on one hand, in a brief discussion of her attitudes with Evamar's mother and, on the other, in an environmental manipulation, consisting in the removal of the domineering, rebellious ringleader to another building of the prison.

0;4 + 26: The child suddenly showed a perfectly normal smiling reaction to the observer's face.

0;5 + 4: The same reaction was observed and filmed.

A fortnight passed; the disciplinary measure inflicted on the ringleader was lifted and she returned to the nursery part of the prison.

0;5 + 18: The smiling reaction disappeared. Evamar screamed violently at the approach of the examiner and quieted down when the examiner withdrew. It was learned from the matron that the mother had again taken up her relationship with the ringleader to the extent of participating in an attempted riot, which was nipped in the bud.

The matron again discussed the situation therapeutically with Evamar's mother, who became penitent and showed attachment to the matron to the extent of bringing her baby to show how well she was treating it.

0;5 + 25: The child was again examined and showed a reaction on beholding

---

[1] The behavior of these cases is reminiscent of some speculations of the English school of psychoanalysts on the role of screaming in the infant (Searl, 1933, pp. 193-205).

the experimenter's face which was neither screaming nor a full-fledged smile. It was rather a sort of vacillation between a smile and an expression akin to anxiety, but which on the whole was nearer to smiling.

Films were made of some of these reactions. It is obvious even to the most casual observer that this child was emotionally disturbed and that her emotional disturbance paralleled closely the ups and downs of her mother's emotional vagaries. In this particular case this need not further surprise us, since one of the ringleader's peculiarities was that she asserted her domination over the mothers by forcing them alternately to neglect their own children and look after her child, allowing them, if the fancy took her, to show kindness again to their own children. Small wonder that Evamar found herself confronted with insoluble emotional problems.

A protocol taken four weeks later shows the factors operative in the child's behavior with particular clarity.

0;6 + 23: The child was approached by one male experimenter and two female experimenters. She immediately started to cry. The child could not be reassured and, therefore, the three of us left the room; the crying subsided.

Two minutes later: The male experimenter returned alone. The child, still crying a little, was quite ready to take up contact with the male experimenter and responded with a smile as long as he remained alone. When two female prison inmates appeared in the doorway, the child started to scream again violently.

The male experimenter now left the room. The mother took the child to the diapering room. After quite a while the child quieted down.

Ten minutes later: The male experimenter returned and in the presence of the child's mother elicited the child's smile without difficulty. The experiment was interrupted.

Two minutes later: The two female experimenters were then sent in and approached the child with smiling faces. The child immediately reacted with screaming. The experiment was interrupted.

Two minutes later: One female experimenter was sent in to the child. Again the reaction was crying but the screaming was not as violent as when two female experimenters had approached the bed.

Five minutes later: The now quiet child was again approached by the male experimenter whom the child greeted with a smile.

Ten minutes later: The female experimenter was sent in to the completely quiet child. The child immediately started to cry and the more the female experimenter tried to reassure her, the more the child cried.

A few words of explanation are in order. The striking difference between the child's reaction to the male experimenter as contrasted with that to the female experimenter is understandable since in this nursery the children did not see any other men. The upsetting experiences of the child were connected with its mother and the ringleader, not with males. We must assume that the child, who had been seeing my face from week to week in connection with agreeable experiences such as social contact, reassurance, petting, and toys, was at the age of 6½ months, able to differentiate it from female faces with which emotionally disturbing experiences had been connected.[2]

It appears, furthermore, that this child was not only able to differentiate the measure of gratification offered by the male as contrasted with the female, but that it was even capable of realizing that two females, i.e., his mother plus the ringleader, are more painful than one. This is manifested in the much more violent rejection of two female experimenters than one female experimenter.

We believe that in the course of its first few months the infant has linked the perceptive experience, "another human being," with all experiences endowed with emotional significance in the course of its life. This "other human being" is the mother. She was identified in the beginning with relief from suffering and with coenesthetic security. She became further identified in the course of development with a visual Gestalt to which the child reacted with the smiling response. Why then are there children whose reaction to the human face remains negative during the critical period?

The answer is to be found in the background of the children who showed an emotional disturbance in their relationship to their mother. Again, it should be stressed that emotional disturbance is a loose term. Not every child suffering from an emotionally disturbed mother-child relationship lacks the smiling response. We do not know enough as yet to circumscribe more exactly the factors necessary for this result. We only know that every child who does not smile in the second trimester of its life has a disturbed emotional relationship with its mother, though not every child with an emotionally disturbed mother-child relationship lacks the smiling response. And we know of one factor which appears to be operative in each of these cases: hostility on the side of the mother towards her child is always present, well repressed behind a surface of syrupy sweetness in our cases. We have been able to demonstrate this factor in some of our films in the movements of the mothers. We believe that these movements, perhaps by producing the sensation of lack of security, transmit the emotional attitude of the mother to the infant, via the sense of vibration and deep sensibility.

---

[2] The early appearance of this discriminatory capacity concords with my frequently stated opinion that painful experiences during the first year are, within limits, the basis for the acquisition of mastery and developmental advance. This child had its fill in regard to painful experiences in the social sector and we do not think it surprising, therefore, that it should manifest an advance in this sector.

We can, therefore, assume that the pattern of the positive response to the smiling stimulus is established by the child's experience with the central figure of its early life, the only other human person, one might say, with whom the child has any contact, namely his mother. This confirms statements of Gesell, Bühler, etc.: the mother's face is seen in innumerable emotionally charged situations, both during feeding as well as in every other situation of child care, and it is always seen *en face*.

Psychiatric Therapy in Infancy

Psychiatrists rarely think of applying their science to the first year of life. The reason for this is that our present dynamic approach in psychiatry is based on the verbal behavior of our patients, even though nonverbal behavior is not only taken into consideration, but forms an important part of the clinical picture and even of the methods of approach to psychiatric disease.

Nevertheless, a moment's reflection will show that the verbal behavior of the patient—the patient's verbal interpretations of his conditions, emotions, sensations, experiences, wishes, urges, etc.—is the principal source on which we draw in our understanding as much as in our description and in our treatment of psychiatric conditions in adults.

In the infant this source fails us completely. It fails us so completely that we hardly even have a way of knowing when the infant is suffering. It is certainly one of the great handicaps of pediatrics that the manifestations of displeasure observed in the infant may or may not be in a one-to-one correlation with any detectable cause of these manifestations. Accordingly, we have a wealth of such statements as: "The infant screams because it has gas pains," leading to a quasi-religious ritual of "bubbling" indulged in in the British Isles; "Screaming is a necessary exercise for the infant," frequently leading to a shocking disregard of the infant's needs; "Baby is wet," and so on. All these statements may be quite correct at times; but mostly they betray simply our ignorance of what goes on in the infant.

From the psychiatric point of view this situation puts the infant on the level at which we think about animals. Psychiatric disturbance is not considered a possibility; if it is considered at all, it is considered in terms of congenital or inherited somatic malformation or deficiency of the central nervous system. The era of organicism in psychiatry is still very close to us and it seems to us that the preverbal stage of infancy is the last stronghold of this school.

Of course, logically, there is no reason for assuming that psychiatric disturbance is only possible when language has been acquired. There is no jump between the preverbal stage and the later phases. The development of the psyche is a smooth, uninterrupted process in which each step is predicated on the preceding one. This is a fact which was most self-evident to academic

Reprinted from *The American Journal of Orthopsychiatry,* 20:623–633, 1950. Copyright © 1950 the American Orthopsychiatric Association, Inc. Reproduced by permission.

psychologists who followed up development genetically. Theoretically at least, psychoanalytic thinking based itself on this proposition. In psychoanalytic writing, this resulted mostly in applying findings made on older children, adolescents, and adults to the more elementary general phenomena of infant life.

Our approach to the problem was a different one. We reasoned that, as the psychoanalytic technique of verbal exploration is not feasible with infants, we would have to use the approach of experimental psychology. The problems to be investigated and the principles according to which experimental psychological methods could be applied were based on the propositions furnished by psychoanalytic theory.

It was in an endeavor to elaborate this idea that our research was started 12 years ago. In its course, with the help of methods described elsewhere, we have established certain norms of development which can be correlated to extensive experimental psychological research done by others as well as by us. Our own material on the subject covers long-term observations of 366 infants. In the course of these observations we have not only been able to establish a first approach to the criteria of normal psychological development at different age levels of infancy, but we have also been able to distinguish certain nosological entities which we are inclined to classify as "psychiatric disturbances of infancy." Of these we will speak later. We will first have to discuss the fundamental differences which we have slowly come to perceive between the human being in the preverbal stage and the human being after the acquisition of language.

These differences are both of a quantitative and a qualitative nature; they apply to the most varied sectors of personality. In our approach we have used the Hetzer-Wolf Baby Tests (1928) which enable us to differentiate between six sectors of the infantile personality: (1) perceptive mastery, (2) body mastery, (3) social relations, (4) mastery of memory and imitation, (5) manipulative ability, and (6) intelligence.

Brief reflection shows that in all these sectors there is an enormous gap between the capacities of the child and those of the adult. As regards the last-mentioned one, intelligence, everybody realizes that it has to develop. But the same applies to manipulative ability, to memory, to mastery of social relations, to bodily activities, and to perception. All are undeveloped at birth and take a long time to reach a level where their functioning is in any way comparable to that of adults.

These are facts which can be, and have been, demonstrated by experimental psychological methods. The infant has a quantitatively and qualitatively differentiated function from that of the individual at a later stage of life; it follows that the infant's experience of his environment, perceptive and otherwise, will be profoundly different from that of the older individual.

This holds true also of that sector of the personality with which psychiatry is most intimately concerned, namely, the emotions. Emotions in the infant are not easily evaluated or classified. What we can observe is apt to be confusing; one fact stands out: at birth, like every other function of the infant, the emotions are undifferentiated and unorganized. A slow process of development in the course of the first year differentiates emotions first into two great classes, the "positive" and the "negative" emotions. From these then progressively the emotions of fear, anxiety, anger, rage, jealousy, cupidity, love, affection, etc., are differentiated in the course of the first year, leading in the next few years to progressively finer subdivision (Bridges, 1932; Spitz, 1947).

In terms of psychoanalytic theory, we can say that the infant at birth does not possess an ego, that is, a central steering organization. Starting around the third month, a rudimentary beginning of an ego will be delimited from the rest of the personality. In the course of the first year it will develop progressively; but even at the end of the first year it will be far from completely organized. This is a task which will take many more years.

In the first year of life the different part organizations of the ego will still be largely undifferentiated. We have already referred to the ego organizations which can be observed during the first year: we described them as the six sectors of the personality. Even these six sectors, however, are still quite undifferentiated; they merge not only with each other, but also with their somatic counterparts in a much more intimate manner than in the adult. The result of this lack of differentiation is that traumata, be they psychic or somatic, will be received by an organism which can respond to them mainly in a generalized, unspecific manner. Furthermore, the consequence of the qualitative difference between the functioning of the infant and the adult is that traumata which to the adult may represent little or nothing can be extremely serious in the infant. On the other hand, the infant may not even perceive experiences which for the adult are seriously traumatic.

The traumata to which the infant is exposed in different areas of his personality are related to emergencies of survival. Such emergencies of survival refer to the infant's needs; these can be classified into somatic needs and emotional needs.

The somatic needs are easily understood. They refer to the infant's humoral balance, to his thermic balance, to his hygiene, his bodily integrity, his nutrition. There are surely others; for instance, it is our belief that a minimum of stimulation is one of the somatic needs of the infant, though it remains a moot question whether this is not equally an emotional need.

The question whether to gratify or not to gratify the emotional needs of the infant has had many, and often antithetical, answers. The most striking interference with emotional needs was the Watsonian idea of treating the infant more or less as a machine for intake and excretion, with no emotional interchange. This approach, which, we are convinced, has surely done much harm in the course of the last 30 years, is going out of fashion now. It has been recognized that the infant does have emotional needs.

It should further be stressed that the emotional needs of the infant are much greater than those of the adult; they vary according to the age level which is under consideration. The survival value of their gratification is in direct proportion with the infant's biological helplessness, with his lack of specific responses and his lack of performed behavior patterns. Accordingly, the infant's emotional needs will be greatest in the beginning and will diminish progressively in the course of the first year.

This is a statement which appears to be contradicted by everyday experience. The contradiction, however, is only apparent, for the issue is beclouded by the special conditions under which the newborn lives. At birth the infant spends close to 89 percent of the 24 hours of the day in sleeping or dozing; and even at three months he spends 69 percent of the day thus (C. Bühler, 1937b, p. 5). The remaining time is to a large extent taken up by providing the infant with the food, hygiene, etc., which must be forthcoming if he is not to die in short order. During these ministrations it is almost impossible to exclude a large amount of emotional interchange between the nursing person and the infant.

Accordingly, infants in their first three months will rarely suffer from a lack of emotional interchange. This should not mislead us into the assumption that their emotional needs are small—we should recognize that nature has insured that the newborn gets the necessary minimum in this respect, just as nature has provided him with an admirable protection against the hazards of extrauterine life. This protection, which decreases slowly in the course of the first few months, is the infant's extraordinarily high threshold for environmental stimuli, on the one hand, and the long period of sleep which fills his days on the other. But after this first period wakefulness increases and perception becomes more acute. In the second, third, and fourth trimester of the first year the emotional gratification offered during the period of bodily care becomes inadequate. Thus it would seem as if the quantity of emotional gratification required by the child at this time is greater than in the beginning. Actually it is only the much longer waking periods, without an increase in obligatory handling of the child, which increase the overall requirements.

Toward the end of the first year a further change is brought into the picture of the child's emotional needs. The first steps into the outside world are taken. The child ceases to be the passive recipient of emotional gratification that he was up to the acquisition of locomotion. He sallies forth, actively to demand assuagement of his emotional demands. This activity, this independence, has to be encouraged by a decrease of the emotional manifestations of the environment which by now would become cloying to the child.

In this process of development, the six sectors of the personality, as well as the emotional sphere, are so closely interrelated as to be indistinguishable from each other. They represent the progressive coordination of one part of the child's personality into a steering organization for the whole, into the ego, as it is called by Freud. Thus is an ego structure laid down in the course of the first year.

It is here that the problem with which we are dealing is situated. For psychiatric diseases, by and large, are diseases of the ego, or of the relations of the ego to the other spheres, be they the superego, the id, or the environment. Therefore, when we speak of psychiatric disease in infancy, we are making the assumption that some disturbances have occurred in some part of the rudimentary ego or that some deficiency in the factors necessary for its development is present. In the latter sense those child analysts who think of psychiatric diseases in infancy in terms of development are correct.

Any therapeutic measures for such disturbances will have to compensate for the possible deficiencies in the very limited world of the infant. These deficiencies may be in the nature of the lack of necessary factors; they may be in the nature of too much of certain factors; and they may be, and mostly are, in the nature of an imbalance between the factors needed.

In considering such therapeutic measures, we must once again return to the picture we have drawn of the infant. The outstanding factors in this picture were a lack of differentiation, a lack of organization, a lack of discrimination. This discriminative inadequacy results in a generalization both in the afferent and in the efferent sectors of the psychic apparatus. This generalization is conclusively shown by a number of psychological experiments the description of which would lead us too far afield. It is manifested by the infant's reaction to total situations rather than to single stimuli. But the generalization is not limited to the infant's psyche; as already mentioned, experiences in the somatic sector show an overflow into the psychic sector and vice versa.

Imbalance in the psychic sector of the infant's personality will occur through the infant's perceptions, visual, auditory, tactile, etc. We believe that an important sense organ of the infant is to be found in deep sensibility, the functioning of which has as yet been insufficiently explored. These modes of perception will provide us with the approaches for the psychiatric treatment of the infant; they are, after all, also our avenue of approach in the treatment of the adult. The difference in our approach will be that we cannot use verbal methods of communication; no agreement between infant and adult on signals and cues is possible except on a very elementary level.

We possess, however, another avenue, more elementary, to the treatment of psychiatric disturbances in infancy. As already stated, psychiatric disturbances will be the consequence of deficiency in the gratification of the infant's needs, be these needs somatic or emotional. By deficiencies we do not necessarily mean the absence of gratifications; imbalance in the gratification of the need pattern, or the surfeit of one or the other need, may be just as pathogenic. With this in mind, we realize that one approach to therapy will consist in the removal of environmental obstacles which represent an impediment in the gratification of the infant's urges or drives; or the approach will consist in the proper adjustment of those environmental stimuli which are responsible for an overstimulation of one or several of these urges and drives.

Having thus defined the field in which any therapeutic measure of infant psychiatry can be undertaken, we will review the clinical pictures which we have thus far been able to isolate in our observations on psychiatric disturbances in infancy, and we will discuss specific measures of treatment.

1. *Marasmus*. This is a condition in which the infant's psychic development is first arrested, and then shows a regression of a specific type leading in a large percentage of the cases to mental impairment or death.

2. *Anaclitic depression*. The picture is that of a depression with a quite striking symptomatology including weeping, unappeasable screaming at the approach of strangers, withdrawal, eating disturbances, and sleeping disturbances as well as developmental arrest.

3. *Motor restlessness*. This is the picture of children in the first year of life whose main activity consists in rocking in the knee-elbow position.

4. *Coprophagia*. We have given this name to the syndrome because of its most outstanding presenting symptom. The children subject to this condition, besides rejecting all toys except their own feces, show a deeply disturbed expression which often goes to the point of paranoid suspiciousness.

5. *Eczema*. This condition could be considered a purely somatic one were it not for the fact that the mental development of infants subject to eczema shows a circumscribed specific difference from the mental development of children who are not affected by this disease. The outstanding characteristics of the picture are a reflex irritability already present at birth, a conspicuous retardation in the capacity for negative responses in the field of social perceptive discrimination, and an equally conspicuous retardation in the field of imitation and learning. The whole picture is one of severe disturbance in the formation of object relations on the basis of identification.

6. *The "three months colic."* This is a condition on which we have relatively little material and information, but which is acknowledged by pediatricians as a disturbance of psychogenic origin.

On the basis of the concept of the infant's psychic structure and its peculiarities described above, a certain number of etiological factors can be isolated as underlying these conditions either singly or in various combinations. The factors we have isolated are as follows:

1. *Emotional starvation of the infant.* This condition can be subdivided into several components which will influence the resulting clinical picture. In the first place, emotional starvation can occur in degrees varying as to severity, from the emotional neglect to which children in foster homes and particularly in broken homes may be subjected, to extremes like those described by Kingsley Davis (1940, 1947). A second component in the picture of emotional starvation is also quantitative. This is the length of time during which the infant is subjected to emotional deprivation. A third and equally important component is the developmental period of the child's life at which emotional starvation is inflicted. According to the way in which these components are varied the resulting picture will vary also. All the results, however, can be considered as emotional deficiency diseases falling within the framework of infant psychiatry.

2. *Withholding of age-adequate stimulation.* This also can be classified as a deficiency disease and is usually a concomitant of emotional starvation. We have yet to see a case in which age-adequate stimulation was withheld without concomitant emotional deprivation.

3. *Maternal hostility to the infant.* This can be classified under two aspects: overt hostility and repressed hostility. The latter may take the form of either overprotection or rejection. Both headings have to be subjected to closer terminological definition, as various forms of maternal behavior can be observed in each of them.

With these we have the prerequisites for our discussion of the possible therapeutic approaches to psychiatric conditions in infancy. We have suggested four such approaches: (1) prophylactic measures; (2) restitutive measures; (3) substitutive measures; (4) modifying measures.

1. *Prophylaxis.* It is strange that in psychiatry the concept of prevention plays such a subordinate role. The term "preventive psychiatry" is one which hitherto has hardly been used in our science, notwithstanding the fact that we are more and more aware of the preventive nature of many of our measures in the fields of social work, child guidance, etc. It is regrettable that the preventive measures in these fields have been concentrated until now mainly on remedying psychiatric disease which had already become manifest. The measures therefore were preventive only insofar as they prevented the solid establishment and the dangerous sequels which would develop from a process already begun.

Our concept of preventive psychiatry is different from this. We do not believe, of course, that preventive psychiatry will obviate any and all outbreaks of psychiatric conditions. We believe that certain environmental factors in infancy will lead to psychiatric disease, either immediately or by establishing a predisposition in the individual which favors its later outbreak. The prophylactic measures we have in mind can best be compared with dental prophylaxis which has the purpose of removing environmental conditions leading to dental caries. Equally, psychiatric prophylaxis will make suggestions regarding the avoidance of factors which have been shown to lead to psychiatric disease.

Our prophylactic suggestions are of the simplest and like so much of psychiatry correspond to the dictates of common sense. They are:

a. During the first year of life, depriving infants of emotional interchange for prolonged periods should be strenuously avoided. Infants should under no circumstances be deprived of their love object during the second half of the first year for a period of more than three months without an adequate substitute. The practice of pediatric hospitals of forbidding parents to visit their sick infants in the hospital or, as is the case with some hospitals, of permitting parents to visit only when the infants are a sleep, cannot be condemned too severely.

b. Depriving infants in their first year of life of toys, that is, of age-adequate stimuli, with the usual hygienic motivation, should be strenuously avoided. The toys provided should be age adequate. They should not be chosen from the point of view of grown-ups who fancy a "cute" toy. They should be chosen as an incentive for the child to develop his activities toward the age level immediately following the one at which he is at the given moment. For example, up to six months rattles are adequate toys. After six months hollow blocks should be added. Toys fancied by adults are frequently a source of anxiety to children. We have observed, for instance, that dolls frequently provoke the most violent anxiety, even panic, on the part of certain children in the second half of the first year.

c. Providing the infant with age-adequate stimulation includes also the necessity to provide, beginning at the latest at six months, the fullest opportunity for locomotion. Both hospitals and other institutions for the housing of infants disregard this need flagrantly. It is one which is important from other aspects, too, which we will discuss under therapy.

2. *Restitution*. When infants have been deprived either of their love object or of age-adequate stimulation during the first year, and a disturbance develops, a reliable cure for this disturbance will be achieved if the love object and the stimuli are restored within a maximum of three months.

3. *Substitution*. In a number of cases neither prophylaxis nor restitution is possible. The love object, the mother, may die, or may suffer prolonged illness and hospitalization, etc. In such cases it is imperative to attempt the

substitution of another love object for the original one. In this process utmost flexibility must be observed. In the course of the substitution the infant should be encouraged as far as possible to choose his preferred love object and to manifest his likes and dislikes and should be closely observed for such manifestations. If the substitute is disliked, a replacement should be provided. It is a great advantage if at this point the infant has already achieved locomotion, whether erect or on all fours. If that is the case, locomotion should be encouraged as much as possible. This enables the infant, on the one hand, to divert a portion of his libidinal drive into the field of motor activity. On the other hand, it enables the infant to use this activity in first selecting his love object, or in manifesting his preference and then approaching his new love object whenever he feels like it.

It is gratifying to note that our findings on the emotional needs of infants during their first year have recently been confirmed for the first time by experimental psychological studies on animals. Our findings on infants have sometimes encountered opposition on the part of laymen or physicians who insist that the damage we observed in emotionally severely deprived infants must be due either to some physical impairment or to a congenital inadequacy in their inherited or inborn equipment. These persons were unable to accept the destructive nature of emotional starvation. Of course one cannot counter such objections by experiments—they are inadmissible on infants. Our results were arrived at by careful observation of infants in existing life situations or institutions and by systematic analysis of the different factors involved. It is doubly gratifying to find that in his observations on the conditioned reflex Henry Liddell has been able to demonstrate on goats during their infancy phenomena exactly similar to those we have observed in infants. In the case of animals such experiments are possible and the factors involved can be rigidly controlled.

We mention this in connection with substitutive therapy, because it is in this field that another measure, that of putting infants who have lost their love object together with other infants, is confirmed by the animal experimenter. Indeed the animal experimenter, in this case Dr. Jules H. Masserman, has quite independently introduced this measure in the treatment of experimental neurosis in cats.

In institutions and hospitals for infants, such a measure is considered "unhygienic" and is usually rejected. It is for this reason that we have regularly found the sickest children in the isolated cubicles of the most "hygienic" institutions. In contrast children on the common wards of less "hygienic" institutions were a much healthier, lustier lot.

It should be repeated here again that children deprived of their love objects must be provided with age-adequate toys. We do not mean that children deprived of their love object, or any other children for that matter, should be showered with expensive toys of the most varied kinds. Measured by adult standards, variety in itself is neither perceived nor appreciated by the child of this age, except in its grossest degrees. Nor do we wish to imply that the infant's love object can be replaced by toys. But the least we can do for a child who has been deprived of his mother is to provide for his most obvious needs as she would have done.

It should be noted that all coprophagic children and most deprived children tend to throw every object they can out of their cribs, including sheets, pillows, articles of dress, and even mattresses. One toy at least should therefore be suspended above the child in such a manner that, though he can reach it, he cannot throw it out.

Within the field of therapy proper, there are a number of other measures which suggest themselves but on the effectiveness of which we have thus far relatively little information. Such measures consist of the forcing of stimulation in the case of children who have been deprived of their love object. The first of these stimulations is the handling of the child, the offering of tactile stimulation and of stimulation of the sense of equilibrium. We have observed surprising results in deprived children whom the nurses had been instructed routinely to take in their laps and fondle for appreciable periods. This has been confirmed by personal communications from Dr. Harry Bakwin of Bellevue.

Another field of stimulation is the auditory one and experiments should be made in offering deprived children auditory perceptions. We have observed the avid eagerness with which deprived children react to the human voice even when they do not see the person. It seems, on the other hand, self-evident that if we want a child to learn to talk, then that can take place only with the help of a person who will talk with the child. A quantitative proof of this statement can be found in our publication "Hospitalism: A Follow-up Report" (Spitz, 1946b); children in an institution where they were not offered these auditory stimulations were almost without exception unable to talk by the age of four years. We would therefore wish to introduce into the life of deprived children periods at which routinely somebody would talk and sing to them.

Visual stimulation, by and large, is the one of which least need be said. But we cannot conclude the discussion of these stimuli without mentioning that hospitals as a matter of course offer visual stimulation at its lowest through their arid, whitewashed, colorless and "hygienic" equipment. This could easily be remedied. We want also to call the attention of all those interested in child welfare to a practice common to hospital nurses, namely, that of hanging sheets over the bedrails to get the children to sleep and to be quiet.

In one such institution we found that the sheets sometimes remained there all day, limiting the child to a view of a little part of the ceiling. That we cannot speak of normal development under such circumstances need hardly be said.

4. *Modification*. We have up to this point spoken mainly of measures to be taken in the case of deficiency diseases of the infant's psyche. In the cases in which the child's love object, the mother, offers inappropriate stimulation, whether it be too much stimulation or unbalanced stimulation, an environmental manipulation will have to take place. This environmental manipulation can take two forms: (1) removing a fundamentally inappropriate mother and replacing her by a substitute; (b) modifying the personality of the mother with the help of psychotherapy.

After all we have said about the undesirability of depriving children of their love object, the suggestion that the mother should be removed may strike the reader as contradictory. However, there are a certain number of exceptions in which this is the best course. It will frequently be so when the mother is psychotic. As an example we may mention a case which has been described in one of our publications—the case of a manic-depressive mother observed by us who regularly performed cunnilingus on her child. The result was an extremely severe disturbance of the child, who obviously would have fared better even with a poor substitute (Spitz, 1946a, 1949).

We shall not discuss the modification of the mother's attitude through psychotherapy. Suffice it to say that the psychotherapy to be applied, which may go from counseling to long-term psychoanalysis, will be as varied as the cases in question. It is a field in which excellent results have been observed by us.

To summarize: The sum total of our findings on psychotherapy in the preverbal stage is that this has to consist in an environmental manipulation, both in regard to love objects and inanimate objects. The needs of the child are simple and an intelligent observation of the child's environment will readily disclose which of these needs is unsatisfied. For its satisfaction no elaborate measures, but only those of the simplest type, need be taken.

The Psychogenic Diseases in Infancy: An Attempt at Their Etiologic Classification

I. INTRODUCTION

In the following we will attempt to enumerate the psychogenic manifestations we have been able to observe in the course of the first year of life, which impressed us as deviating from the picture offered by the normal infant. We consider these manifestations as abnormal because, on the one hand, they are to be found only in a relatively small minority of children at that particular age. On the other hand, one and all seem to be the result of a damaging process taking place in the infant. In each of these manifestations we have been able to establish a psychogenic factor, without excluding that in some of them other factors, e.g., congenital ones, may be present. We will attempt to formulate these different manifestations as distinct nosological pictures, and then to classify them according to certain principles to be discussed further on.

Any study of psychogenic conditions in infancy will have to begin by making a clear distinction between adult and infant psychiatry. The reason for this lies in the structural and environmental differences involved. The infant does not possess the same personality structure as the adult, while at the same time the infant's environment also is vastly dissimilar from that of the grownup.

To begin with the personality: The adult personality is a structured, well-defined organization which provides certain individual attitudes representing personal initiatives in a circular interaction with the environment. The infant at birth, on the contrary, though he has individuality, has no comparable personality organization, develops no personal initiatives, and his interaction with the environment is a physiological one. The newborn is not conscious: no organization is demonstrable in its psychic apparatus. It is only toward the second half of the first year that a central steering organization, the ego, is gradually developed. During the whole period of which we are speaking, i.e., the first year of life, this ego remains rudimentary. It would be completely inadequate for self-preservation were it not complemented by an external

Reprinted from *The Psychoanalytic Study of the Child*, Vol. 6. New York: International Universities Press, 1951, pp. 255–275.

helper, a substitute ego as it were, to whom the major part of the executive, defensive, and perceptive functions are delegated. This delegate, who complements the infant's ego, is its mother or her substitute. We can speak of her as the infant's external ego; like the adult's internal ego, the infant's external ego controls the pathways leading to motility during the first year of infancy.

The second variable, the environment, consists in the case of the adult of a multiplicity of factors, inanimate and animate, of numerous individuals and groups. These and other dynamic constellations of varying dignity provide constantly shifting patterns of force which impinge on and interact with the adult's organized personality. Environment for the infant consists, crudely speaking, of one single individual: the mother or her substitute. And even this one individual is not experienced by the infant as a separate object, but is fused with the infant's need and gratification pattern. Consequently, in contrast to the adult, the normally reared infant lives during its first year in what we may call "a closed system." A psychiatric investigation of infancy will, therefore, have to examine the structure of this "closed system." As the system is a simple one and consists only of two components, the mother and the child, it is the relationship within this "dyad" which has to be investigated. We are well aware that in reality the total situation, i.e., the interrelations of roles within the household or the institution in which the child is reared, form his universe; yet this universe is mediated to him by the one who fulfills his needs, i.e., the mother or the nurse. Therefore, the personality of the mother on the one hand, the personality of the child on the other, will have to be brought into relation with each other.

The reason for these differences between adult and infant lies in the fact that the psychic system is not yet differentiated from the somatic system in the infant. What we might call psyche at this stage is so completely merged with the physical person that I would like to coin for it the term *somato-psyche*. Subsequently the psychic and somatic systems will be progressively delimited from each other. Step by step, in the course of the first six months a psychological steering organization will be segregated from the somato-psyche. This steering organization serves the needs of defense and of mastery. It is characterized by its organization, its structure, and by the quality of consciousness. This organized, structured and conscious steering organization is the nucleus of what we call the ego, a body ego in the beginning. It is thus delimited from the remaining unconscious part of the somato-psyche, which we will designate as the id.

The differentiation of the ego from the id takes place under the pressure of the need for survival. The physical demands on the individual made by the physical environment force it to develop the adaptive mechanism of defense and mastery which form the first ego organization. Hartmann (1939) has defined this part of the ego as the conflict-free sphere.

This process of differentiation is followed by an integration. I have elaborated upon this alternation of differentiation and integration in the course of psychological development in a paper read at a meeting of the Vienna Society for Psychoanalysis in 1936.

The differentiation of ego and id takes place progressively in the course of the second half of the first year, and is accompanied by the usual transitional hazards which characterize every phase of differentiation. In the course of the second and third year a further development of ego functions will follow. The new ego functions transcend the conflict-free sphere of the ego. A new process of differentiation begins, this time under the pressure of psychological needs, and produces a further set of mastery and defense organizations. The psychological needs in question are in the nature of demands made upon the individual by its human environment and are centered predominantly on the anal level. This psychological need pressure will gather momentum in the years to follow and eventually will lead to the formation of a further organization, that of the superego. This process, however, does not concern us in the present paper.

These successive processes of differentiation are the evidence of the progressive segregation of a psychic apparatus out of the somato-psyche. This segregation has to start from the inchoate beginnings of the infant, during which responses are manifested more or less indiscriminately, reminding one of overflow phenomena; it is difficult to assign the earliest responses to either the somatic or the psychological field, as they occur mostly in such a manner as to express the characteristics of both psyche and soma. Much of what we discuss in our present article will be of this nature, for it takes place during the first year, in the course of which the boundaries between these two systems are being established progressively. It is hardly necessary to stress that we do not believe that a rigid separation between soma and psyche can ever be postulated in the course of human life; but the functions assigned to the two systems are differentiated more and more clearly in the course of development.

II. Etiological Factors and Their Classification

We have stressed in our introductory remarks that the number of factors operative during the first year of life is limited. This has facilitated our work so that the modest amount of information we have gathered in the course of our research already enables us to make a preliminary attempt at an etiological classification of psychogenic diseases in infancy. We will eliminate the consideration of congenital disease which does not belong in our province. Like

the question of congenital disease, we also will eliminate from our considerations the possible consequences of physical infirmity. With this eliminated,
the factors which can operate in producing a psychological influence in infancy
are more or less reduced to the sole mother-child relation. Our first proposition
then will be that if the mother-child relation is normal, there should not be
any disturbance in the infant's psychological development, barring physical
interference in the nature of lack of food, sickness, etc. As for a satisfactory
mother-child relation, we will define it as being satisfactory both to mother
and child.

Limiting the action of psychological influences in infancy to the mother-
child relationship contains implicitly our second proposition that harmful
psychological influences are the result of unsatisfactory mother-child relations. Such harmful influences fall into two possible classes: (1) the wrong
kind of mother-child relations; (2) an insufficient amount of mother-child
relations.

The wrong kind of mother-child relation can develop in various ways. We
have found a number of specific psychogenic conditions which can be related
to specific inappropriate forms of mother-child relations. In such cases the
mother's personality acts as a disease-provoking agent, a psychological toxin,
as it were. We will, therefore, call this first group the *psychotoxic diseases
of infancy*.

Inappropriate maternal attitudes found in psychotoxic diseases of infancy
can be classified and divided into six subgroups:

1. Overt primal rejection.
2. Primary anxious overpermissiveness.
3. Hostility in the garb of anxiety.
4. Rapid oscillation between pampering and aggressive hostility.
5. Cyclical alternation of long duration in the mother's mood.
6. Hostility, consciously compensated.

The sequence in which the different etiologies are listed is mainly one of their
chronological occurrence in the first year of life.

Our own detailed investigations on large numbers of infants cover the
conditions of points 3, 4, 5, and 6. The first two conditions were included
in view of their general familiarity to the observer of infants. They have not
been investigated specifically by us, though we possess a number of individual
observations on these conditions.

The second main group, the restriction of the mother-child relations, can
be compared in its structure to a class of diseases well known to internal
medicine, namely, the deficiency diseases. We will, therefore, call our second
main group *emotional deficiency* diseases. According to our present findings,
this group can be divided into two subgroups, which reflect the measure of

the deficiency inflicted on the infant: (1) partial deprivation; (2) total deprivation.

It need hardly be stressed that total deprivation of the child of relations with its mother or her substitute refers only to emotional interchange. It is self-evident that a minimum of physical care consisting in food, hygiene, warmth, etc., has to be insured to any infant if it is to survive at all.

In Table 1 we present the psychogenic diseases in infancy which up to this time we have been able to segregate as distinctive nosological entities. In the left-hand column of the table we give the diseases, in the right-hand column the maternal attitudes we have found to be significantly related to the manifestations of the particular diseases.

TABLE 1. ETIOLOGICAL CLASSIFICATION OF PSYCHOGENIC DISEASE IN INFANCY ACCORDING TO MATERNAL ATTITUDES

Infant's disease	Etiological factor provided by maternal attitude
Psychotoxic diseases	
Coma in newborn (Ribble, 1938)	Overt primal rejection
Three months colic	Primary anxious overpermissiveness
Infantile neuro-dermatitis	Hostility in the garb of anxiety
Hypermotility (rocking)	Oscillating between pampering and hostility
Fecal play	Cyclical moodswings
Aggressive hyperthymic (Bowlby, 1944)	Hostility consciously compensated
Deficiency diseases	
Anaclitic depression	Partial emotional deprivation
Marasmus	Complete emotional deprivation

III. THE INDIVIDUAL SYNDROMES

A. PSYCHOTOXIC DISEASES

1. Overt Primal Rejection

The maternal attitude of overt primal rejection consists in the mother's global rejection of maternity and concurrently of the child. It is manifested often during pregnancy, but always beginning with the delivery. In an article published in 1938, Margaret Ribble described the reactions of newborn infants to rejecting mothers. In extreme cases the babies became stuporous, fell into a comatose sleep with Cheyne-Stokes respiration, extreme pallor, and diminished sensitivity. These infants had to be treated as in states of shock, by saline clysis, intravenous glucose and blood transfusion. After recovering they had to be taught to suck by stimulation of the mouth. If the situation was not dealt with immediately, it threatened the life of the neonate.

I have had the opportunity to observe such cases and to take a motion picture of one of them. The case history follows:

> *Case No. Mat. 55.* The mother of the child is a 16-year-old, unusually good-looking girl, unmarried. She was employed as a servant and seduced by the son of her employer. Allegedly only one intercourse took place, resulting in impregnation. The child was undesired, the pregnancy accompanied by very severe feelings of guilt, as the girl was a devout Catholic. The delivery took place in a maternity hospital and was uneventful. The first attempt to nurse, after 24 hours, was unsuccessful and so were the following ones. The mother, allegedly, had no milk. We found no difficulty in producing milk by manual pressure. Neither was there any difficulty in feeding the infant from the bottle. The observation of the mother showed her to behave during nursing as if her infant was completely alien to her and not a living being at all. Her actual behavior was one of withdrawing from the baby, with a rigid and tense attitude of body, hands, and face. The nipples, though not inverted, were not protruding and nursing did not appear to provoke turgor.
>
> This state of affairs continued for five days. In the final attempts, one of which was filmed, the baby was seen to sink back into the stuporous, semi-comatose condition described by Ribble (1938). Energetic methods had to be applied, including tube feeding and saline clysis, to bring the baby out of this condition.
>
> In the meantime, an attempt at indoctrination of the mother was made in view of her youth and background. The method used was not interpretative, but authoritarian, starting with exact instructions and exercises in how to treat her nipples to produce turgor and making nursing possible. After this indoctrination, and from the fifth day on, the nursing went on relatively successfully and the child recovered, at least for the subsequent six days during which I could observe it.

It remains, of course, an open question as to what the subsequent course of an infant's development will be when the mother's rejection is as manifest from the beginning as it was in this case. We have the suspicion that even when the threat to life involved in this primal reaction is successfully overcome, other though less severe psychosomatic consequences will appear, and that certain cases of vomiting of infants during the first three months of life probably also belong in this category, as illustrated by the following case history:

> *Case No. WF 3.* This child was breast-fed by its mother in the beginning. The

mother then refused to continue and formula was introduced. Both during breast-feeding and formula feeding the mother was full of complaints and recriminations. Breast-feeding was, she said, unsatisfactory because the child vomited; but the formula was not right either, because the child vomited also. After three weeks the mother contracted influenza and was separated from the child. The formula was fed to the child by a substitute. The vomiting ceased immediately. Six weeks later the mother returned. The vomiting started again within 48 hours.

If we were to formulate the impression we have gained from such observations, our statements would have to remain extremely general and tentative. It is evident that, at present, we do not have sufficient observational material at our disposal; nor do we have an adequate hypothesis regarding the kind of maternal personality structure which results in this form of global rejection. We are, therefore, unable to formulate a theoretical assumption covering these cases.

As the child grows, maternal rejection will, of necessity, take on a different form and lead to a different result. The infantile personality will become progressively more diversified with increasing age; the maternal hostility will clash with this more developed infantile personality; individual and varied maternal hostility patterns will evolve. In contrast to this, maternal rejection of an objectless nature, so to speak, not directed at an individual child, but at the fact of having a child in general, will be encountered in the pure form only during the very first weeks and perhaps months of the baby's life. It is to be assumed that the attitude of these mothers—i.e., of generalized hostility toward maternity—is related to their individual history, their relations to the originator of the pregnancy, their individual way of solving their oedipal conflict and their castration anxiety. In the course of a few months the further relations with the baby will play their part, and a secondary elaboration of the generalized hostility into specific forms will take place.

We will call the original, and at that time still unstructured, rejection of maternity seen in these cases *overt primal rejection*. It impinges on an infant who has not even begun to develop any method of defense or adjustment. For at birth the infant is in the earliest narcissistic stage, in the act of developing the earliest patterns of orality, which will progressively be structured into what is known in psychoanalysis as the oral stage. In this earliest stage the contacts of the infant with the environment have just been shifted from the umbilical cord to the mouth and to intake. It is not surprising then that the symptoms manifested in the cases we have described are in the nature of a paralysis of intake during the very first days of life, in the nature of a rejection through vomiting at a somewhat later stage.

2. Primary Anxious Overpermissiveness

The maternal attitude of primary anxious overpermissiveness consists in a special form of overprotection during the first trimester of life. David Levy

(1943) introduced the term of "maternal overprotection." This term has been used rather indiscriminately by various authors to cover a wide range of behavior patterns and attitudes without too much regard for underlying motivations. In the following we will try to differentiate various forms of overprotection with the help of investigations directed at the maternal motivations underlying the individual forms, and we will attempt to correlate them with specific clinical pictures of the infant. For the first of these forms I have coined the term of "primary anxious overpermissiveness"; its consequences in the child we believe to be the so-called "three-months colic."

The "three-months colic" is a condition, well known in pediatric circles, with the following clinical picture: After the third week, and up to the third month, the infants begin to scream in the afternoon. They can be temporarily reassured by feeding. They appear to be subject to colicky pains. Changing of formula, or introducing formula instead of breast-feeding, is of no avail. Various measures have been tried, all without success. The stools of these infants show nothing pathological, though at times diarrhea may be present. The pains may go on for several hours and then subside, only to start again the next day. The time of the day may vary. Around three months the condition has the tendency to disappear as inexplicably as it had appeared, to the great relief of mother and pediatrician.

I was struck by an interesting observation of Spanish and South American pediatricians on this subject. They also were familiar with the "three-months colic" which they call "dispepsia transitoria."[1] But first Alarcon and later Soto (1937) observed that the "three-months colic" is unknown in institutionalized children.

This is an observation which we can fully confirm from our own experience. In none of the institutions which we observed was "three-months colic" a problem. It was least so in the institutions where the infant had no maternal care whatsoever. It appeared most frequently in the institution we called "Nursery," in which the mother-child relations were at their best. Even there it was rather rare. In the relatively small number of infants in private families we observed, however, it was not infrequent.

Soto's explanation of the absence of "three-months colic" in institutions is that the children here are not "pampered," as he puts it; he describes institutions where the nurses look after the physical needs of the children, but the children do not get toys, and there is just "no nonsense." In contrast with this, he says, children in private families are "extremely pampered."

The observation appears to have merit. It is a pity that Soto ignores the other consequences of institutionalization which are infinitely more serious

---

[1] A similar condition has been described by Finkelstein under the name of "Spastische Diathese" and ascribed by Weill to lack of tolerance of mother's milk on the part of the infant.

than "three-months colic." If, however, we translate his conclusions into our current conceptual framework, he appears to assume "maternal overprotection" of some kind as the causative factor in the "three-months colic."

This is a finding which lends itself to demonstrate the misleading nature of such overall application of the term "overprotection." Indeed, Alarcon's and Soto's findings will have to be confronted with a series of observations made recently by Milton I. Levine and Anita I. Bell (1950). They found in a series of 28 infants who had developed "three-months colic," observed over a period of three years, that in 90 percent of the cases the condition disappeared when the infants were given a pacifier.

However, "giving a pacifier" is certainly a measure which would be classified as "overprotective." How can we reconcile Alarcon's and Soto's findings with those of Levine and Bell? Certain aspects of the Levine-Bell patients duplicate closely the Alarcon-Soto assumptions. Thus, all the 28 children were raised in private families and not in institutions; but over and beyond this, with very few exceptions, the Levine-Bell babies were on a self-demand schedule. The assumption that the mothers of the babies were particularly permissive is, therefore, justified.

On the other hand, Levine and Bell state that in almost every instance the infants in question were hypertonic. Their work does not inform us whether the hypertonicity was observable already at birth and consequently represents a congenital factor. If so, we may advance a two-factor hypothesis in which the infants' congenital hypertonicity would represent a bodily compliance, to which the mothers' overpermissiveness would have to be added to result in the "three-months colic." We might even go further and presume that such overpermissive mothers are perhaps more prone to develop anxiety when confronted with unpleasure manifestations of the child; that they can only deal with such unpleasure manifestations by increasing their permissiveness still more, and that thus a vicious circle will develop in which the child's cry, which in reality expresses the need for tension release, is answered by a proffering of food which increases the tension and produces further colic. This vicious circle is then interrupted when the pacifier is introduced; for the pacifier lends itself to reduce tension without interfering with metabolic processes.

A clarification of the sequence would be desirable, for it is perfectly possible that (even without the congenital hypertonicity) the mother's anxiety in itself could produce the vicious circle, and that the hypertonicity will result from this vicious circle without necessarily being congenital. The decision which of the two assumptions is the more probable one can only be made through a detailed investigation of a significant number of children.

The assumption that the pacifier acts as a release of tension and consequently as a cure for the "three-months colic," is in accordance with David Levy's findings. He showed that sucking frustration, an oral frustration which increases tension, leads to increased finger-sucking.

However, not only oral frustrations and tensions, but, as we stated, any kind of tension finds its release primarily through an activity of the oral zone in the first trimester of life. K. Jensen (1932) demonstrated manometrically that newborn infants who were exposed to a series of stimuli (among which heat, cold, pinching of toe, pulling of hair, sudden dropping, etc.) reacted in a statistically significant number of cases with a sucking response. Therefore, the assumption that the pacifier acts as a release of tension and consequently as a cure for the "three-months colic," appears perfectly plausible.

3. Hostility Garbed as Manifest Anxiety

The maternal attitude in this clinical picture consisted in manifest anxiety, mostly in regard to the child. It became soon clear that this manifest anxiety corresponded to the presence of unusually large amounts of unconscious repressed hostility.

A study was made by the author of this paper, jointly with Katherine M. Wolf, on 220 children. We followed them in the environment called Nursery (Spitz, 1945b) and observed 28 children who developed skin affections during the first year of life. Of these, 24 were studied thoroughly, and the diagnosis of eczema was made in 22 cases by the pediatrician.

The mothers' unconscious hostility became evident in the frequency with which they barely avoided inflicting serious damage on their babies, such as feeding them an open safety pin in the cereal, dropping the baby several times on its head, consistent intolerable overheating of the baby's cubicle, knotting the baby's bib so tightly that the baby became blue in the face and barely escaped strangulation, etc. The same mothers showed a curious inhibition: they were afraid to touch their children or they refused to touch them, which is hardly surprising in view of the combination of repressed hostility and overt anxiety. This fear showed itself particularly vividly in some of these mothers who were always trying to get others to diaper, wash, or feed their children. This fear was also manifest in some of the statements protocolled by us, like, e.g.: "A baby is such a delicate thing, the least false movement might harm it."

We investigated the personality of the children with the help of tests and developmental profiles (Hetzer and Wolf, 1928). As described elsewhere (Spitz, 1948), these tests provide quantifiable measures for the personality sectors of perception, body mastery, social relations, memory, manipulative ability, and intelligence as well as an overall developmental quotient. In the group suffering from eczema, a characteristic retardation was observable in the sector of learning (memory and imitation). Less conspicuous, but mostly present also was a consistent retardation in the sector of social relations.

A detailed discussion of the findings regarding this eczema group is in preparation (1951a). We may, however, mention some of the conclusions we have reached in this study in regard to the dynamics we have assumed to be present.

In the case of the eczema child, we have an anxiety-ridden mother who avoids touching her baby because of her more or less repressed aggression. If the mother avoids touching her baby, she makes it impossible for her child to identify with her, and that at an age at which the baby is still in the stage of primary narcissism, when the child's ego is incomplete, and when the mother assumes the functions of the ego. In the process of psychological development in the course of the first year the child acquires its ego with the help of numberless identifications with its mother which are made possible through the sensory experiences offered by her. Among the most important of these, if not *the* most important are the tactile experiences which include both superficial and deep sensitivity.

When this external ego, represented by the mother, withdraws psychologically because of anxiety, the child cannot develop its own ego with the help of identifications with her. This is specifically true in the second half of the first year when it has begun to delimit itself from the mother through the formation of secondary identifications. The anxiety-ridden mother, as part ego, offers no opportunity for secondary identification in bodily activities of a manipulative and imitative kind. Therefore, the infant's libidinal and aggressive drives which normally would be discharged in the course of the handling of the mother and converted into identifications, remain undischarged. It seems that they are discharged in the form of a skin reaction. The comparison may seem farfetched, but one is reminded of the discharge phenomena taking place in adults in the peptic ulcer syndrome.

4. Oscillating Between Pampering and Hostility

We have found that a maternal attitude oscillating *rapidly* between pampering and hostility appears to lead frequently to a disturbance of motility in the child. In the following we will encounter several other such disturbances of the motor system. From the descriptive point of view these disturbances can be divided into two principal groups, namely hypermotility and hypomotility. In both groups further distinctions can be made in regard to quantitative increase or decrease of motility on the one hand, in regard to normal and pathological motor patterns on the other.

Within the group of hypermotility there is one form which appears in large numbers, particularly in the institutional environment. This is the well-known rocking behavior of infants. In itself, this behavior can hardly be called a pathological pattern, for it is manifested occasionally in a transitory way by most children. In the cases observed by us, it differed, however, by becoming the principal activity of the children affected, by substituting for most of their other normal activities, by its frequent, striking violence which appears out of proportion with the physical resources of the child, and by the fact that it seems actually to involve a much larger amount of motor behavior than is seen in the average normal child of the same age. Its phenomenology consists in rocking movements, mostly in the knee-elbow position, not infrequently in the supine position at earlier ages, and not infrequently either in the standing position at later ages.

We studied this condition with the collaboration of Katherine M. Wolf in a group of 170 children and discussed our observations and our conclusions in our article "Autoerotism" (Spitz, 1949).

Clinically the children show, apart from hypermotility, a characteristic retardation in the social and in the manipulative sectors of their personality. We concluded that rapidly changing maternal attitudes, oscillating between overpampering and extreme hostility, will impair the formation of object relations of all kinds in the psychic sphere, while resulting in hypermotility, manifested as rocking, in the physical sphere.

5. Cyclical Mood Swings of the Mother

The maternal attitude toward the child remained stable for a number of months, after which it would change into its opposite and again persist for a number of months.

For the purpose of this study (Spitz, 1949) we observed 153 children and their mothers. In 16 of these children we found fecal play and coprophagia in the fourth quarter of the first year. On investigation, the mother-child relation turned out to be highly significant. We found that the bulk of psychosis in these 153 mothers was concentrated on those whose children manifested fecal play.

The clinical symptoms of depression with long-term mood swings were evident in the mothers of the coprophagic children. The mothers' attitude toward the children would be oversolicitous for many months and then suddenly change to extreme hostility with rejection. In our publication we offer a dynamic proposition as to the reason why such an attitude should result in coprophagia, that is in the oral introjection of an "object," during the transitional period from the oral to the anal phase.

6. Maternal Hostility, Consciously Compensated

The term is self-explanatory. The parents of these children are more eager to use them for their own exhibitionistic and narcissistic purposes than as a love object. They realize that their behavior toward the child is not appropriate and consciously overcompensate it with sub-acid syrupy sweetness.

We have observed only a few cases of this type, of which we have described one (Spitz, 1946d). The data and follow-up studies on these cases are not sufficient to permit more than a tentative assumption. We believe that children confronted with this maternal attitude stay retarded in the social sector of their personality during the first year of life, while at the same time they are advanced in all other sectors. They present a picture in the second year in which hostility is predominant.

Our tentative assumption is that in the course of their later development they will present the picture of the aggressive hyperthymic, described by John Bowlby (1946).

B. DEFICIENCY DISEASES

1. Partial Emotional Deprivation

In a study made with the assistance of Katherine M. Wolf (Spitz, 1948) on a total of 170 children, we observed 34 children who after a minimum of six months' satisfactory relations with their mothers were deprived of them for longer or shorter periods; the substitute offered for the mother during that period proved unsatisfactory. These children showed a clinical picture which was progressive from month to month in proportion to the length of separation: First month: increased demandingness and weepiness. Second month: tendency to scream, loss of weight, arrest of developmental progress. Third month: refusal of contact, pathognomonic position (lying prone with averted face), insomnia, further loss of weight, intercurrent ailments, restriction of motility becomes generalized, facial expression rigid. After the third month: rigidity of facial expression becomes stabilized, weepiness subsides, retardation and lethargy.

If within a critical period of three to five months the mother is returned to the child or an adequate substitute provided, the condition improves with surprising rapidity.

We have called this condition anaclitic depression because of the similarity it shows with the clinical picture of depression in adults, although we consider the dynamic structure a fundamentally different one in the infant.

2. Total Deprivation

Whereas in partial deprivation the existence of good mother-child relations prior to the deprivation is a prerequisite, this is immaterial in total deprivation. Regardless of the mother-child relations existing prior to total deprivation, its consequences will lead to the severest of the emotional deficiency diseases we have observed until now.

For the purposes of this study (Spitz, 1945b) we observed 91 children in a foundling home situated outside of the United States where the children were raised by their mothers during the first three to four months of their lives. During this period they showed the picture and developmental level of average normal children of the same country. After three to four months they were separated; they were adequately cared for in every bodily respect, but as one nurse had to care for 8 children officially, and actually for up to 12, they were emotionally starved.

After the separation from their mothers, these children went rapidly through the stages we have described for partial deprivation. Then the picture for motor retardation became fully evident. The children became completely passive, lying in their cots in a supine position. They did not even reach the stage where they could turn around sufficiently to perform a withdrawal by lying prone. The face became vacuous, eye coordination defective, the expression often imbecile. When motility returned after a while, spasmus nutans in some, and bizarre finger movements in all were manifested, reminiscent of decerebrate or catatonic movements. The developmental level regressed by the end of the second year to 45 percent of the normal; sitting, standing, walking, talking were not achieved even by the age of four.

The progressive deterioration and the increased infection-liability lead in a distressingly high percentage of these children to marasmus and death. Of the 91 children followed by us for two years in Foundling Home, 37 percent died. In contrast, in another institution, Nursery, where the children were cared for by their mothers, not a single death occurred among 220 children observed during a four-year period. It appears that emotional starvation leads to progressive deterioration, which is in direct proportion to the duration of the deprivation which the child has undergone.

IV. CONCLUSIONS

The discussion of the single diseases tabulated in Table 1 shows that our classification at this stage is a crude attempt to orient ourselves in the field of psychogenic disorders in infancy. We have used for this purpose the criteria of etiology. At the present stage of our knowledge this approach cannot provide as diversified or detailed a picture as would a symptomatological approach. It would be possible, for instance, to divide the psychogenic affections in infancy according to the systems which they involve predominantly, like the motor, the intestinal, the circulatory, the respiratory, or other systems.

I believe, however, that such an approach would be both difficult and confusing. As discussed in the first part of the paper, in infancy the boundary lines between the different systems, both psychic and somatic, are fluid. We will always find more than one system involved in each of the conditions and, as can be seen for instance in the picture of the emotional deficiency diseases, in the progressive course of the ailment one system after another becomes involved. I believe also that it would be much more difficult to establish nosological entities with the help of symptomatic criteria than with the help of an etiological classification.

As in all research of this nature, our understanding of the fact that more than one or two nosological entities were involved came only very gradually. This was developed in the successive investigations we have published, each of which attempts to study in finer detail both the symptomatology and the etiology of the infant's disturbances. It is clear that in the future the tools of investigation will be perfected and refined, the approaches modified, new ones developed. These improvements will result in a far greater differentiation of nosological pictures and more exact specification of their etiology. The crudeness of our approach at this point presents the advantage of giving a general orientation as to the directions in which future and better solutions can be attempted, and more satisfactory criteria developed.

The etiological approach offers another advantage. It provides already at this point cues in regard to prevention and therapy. In our own work we have at times made use of these suggestions. We have published a paper on some of the fundamental aspects of psychiatric therapy in infancy (Spitz, 1950d).

I am well aware that the most important part of this work still remains to be done. We must provide the link between these early disturbances and the psychiatric and somatic conditions which will develop in later life. As yet no clinical connection has been established with the pioneer work of Anna Freud, August Aichhorn, Bruno Bettelheim, John Bowlby, Beata Rank, Berta Bornstein, Lauretta Bender, and all the others who have investigated the psychiatric disturbances of the preschool child. Future research projects will take into account that it is of decisive importance that psychiatric disease in infancy is observable in *statu nascendi* and under controlled conditions. We can expect, in the not too distant future, much enlightenment from the continued observation of the later development of children in whom we were able to diagnose early psychiatric abnormality. This should provide us with information on the etiology of later psychiatric and medical problems of childhood, adolescence and adulthood as well as with valuable pointers in the field of preventive psychiatry.

V. SUMMARY

1. The differences between the organization of the infant's personality and environment and that of the adult are discussed.

2. In view of these differences the possible etiological factors operative in psychogenic diseases in infancy are considered and reduced to the sole mother-child relation.

3. Variations of this etiological factor are reduced to the wrong kind of mother-child relation conducive to psychotoxic diseases on the one hand, to the insufficient amount of mother-child relation conducive to emotional deficiency diseases on the other.

4. A classification of nosological pictures in infancy on the basis of these criteria is presented.

PART 6

CLINICAL PSYCHOANALYSIS

Editor's Introduction

Spitz was active as a psychoanalytic practitioner and teacher as well as an infant researcher. Although he published much less in clinical psychoanalysis than he did in infant research, the two papers included in this section have been widely used in the training of psychoanalysts. In them, Spitz speaks of developmental principles in both the transference and the countertransference. These principles are inherent in the analytic situation and have their roots in early mother-child interaction. It is interesting to note that when placed together, these papers highlight the special features of the dialogue as it exists in the analytic relationship. The discussion of the analyst's "diatrophic" attitude in particular conveys what is conducive to the formation of a working alliance.

These papers do not deal with a reconstructed past but rather with early modes of functioning. The analytic relationship, later in development, allows for the recapitulation of certain aspects of an earlier relationship. The issue of whether there can be a veridical reconstruction of the infantile past does not enter into these discussions. Spitz would also be among the first to point out that more could be learned from the differences between the early relationships and the later analytic relationship than from their similarities.

Transference: The Analytical Setting and Its Prototype

In the following presentation I shall limit my remarks to some aspects of transference and shall concentrate on the theory of its origins. Among the numerous authors who have written on the subject in recent years, I shall single out three for the purposes of the present discussion. They are Ida Macalpine (1950), Daniel Lagache (1952, 1953, 1954), and Phyllis Greenacre (1954).

Lagache begins his study with an epistemological investigation of the concept of transference. With great lucidity he establishes two dichotomies: the first is that between transference manifestations proper and transference neurosis. The second is between what he calls the "dynamic" causes versus the "mechanistic" (or "spontaneous") causes for the development of transference. This second dichotomy requires a somewhat more detailed description. The "dynamic" causes for the development of transference are the frustrating interpersonal relations imposed on the patient by the rules which govern the analytical situation. The "mechanistic" or "spontaneous" development of transference on the other hand is the consequence of the repetition compulsion. It is due to the narcissistic trauma to which the personality of the patient was originally subjected. Accordingly, the "spontaneous" development of transference will take place irrespective of the environmental factors.

It is evident that the "dynamic" concept of transference corresponds closely to transference proper and consequently to its therapeutic potentialities. The "mechanistic" concept by contrast covers transference neurosis and its significance as resistance. A bridge connects the two concepts: that is the dual function of the repetition compulsion. As Bibring (1943) and Hendrick (1942) demonstrated, it has not only a repetitive-reproductive function, but also a restitutive one.

Lagache postulates a dual function also for the fundamental rule: (1) It frustrates the repetition compulsion's urge to repeat *action* prohibited by the ego. (2) This prohibition of action has also a liberating function. It permits the ideation of prohibited actions in the form of thought and word. Thought

---

Reprinted from *The International Journal of Psycho-Analysis*, 37:380–385, 1956.

This paper was presented at a "Discussion of Problems of Transference," Nineteenth International Psycho-Analytical Congress, Geneva, July 24–28, 1955.

and word originally were inhibited by the patient because they lead to action. This liberation of ideation leads inevitably to thoughts about the analyst, that is to transference manifestations. As Nunberg has pointed out (1951), inhibited, "frozen" psychological content, when liberated from the domination of the unconscious, will come under the domination of the ego. That makes it possible for the ego to exert its restitutive tendencies on these contents.

The analyst's "passive" role and his interpretations are calculated to make available to the patient the impact of relived experience. At the same time the analyst safeguards for his own understanding the informative value of this reliving as long as it is acted out. This discussion of the concept of transference clarifies also some important problems of the management of transference. Acting out on the part of the analyst obviously becomes inadmissible. Modifications of the analytical situation may be permissible and desirable inasmuch as such modifications enable the patient to master excessive tensions which otherwise would overwhelm him. They should enable the patient to master these tensions as it were *refracta dosi*. Distinction of the various aspects of transference, its origins, its effect, and its management invalidates the idea that reducing the number and the duration of treatments is therapeutic. He explains that such reductions can only serve to diminish the analyst's control of the transference relationship, which is exactly the opposite of the aim we are striving for in psychoanalytic treatment.

Lagache's lucid and systematic analysis of the concept of transference and the conclusions he draws from this concept for its therapeutic management is one with which I fully agree. I am well aware of the importance and significance of the "mechanistic" aspect of transference, that is, with the role of the repetition compulsion in the phenomenon. In my present remarks I will however limit myself mainly to "dynamic" aspects, that is to the parts of the phenomenon induced by the analytical situation. Both Greenacre and Macalpine also are primarily concerned with this aspect.

Greenacre's paper shows an approach which is deceptively simple; solidly grounded in theory and observation, it is pragmatic and clinical, and presents the epitome of psychoanalytic common sense. Her statement that the matrix of transference comes largely from the original mother-infant quasi union of the first months of life practically covers the subject of which I will speak today. Her concept of the analyst acting as an extra function lent to the analysand in the transference situation corresponds closely to my proposition of the mother as the infant's external ego. Her views coincide with Macalpine's ideas when she states "the non-participation of the analyst in a personal way in the relationship creates a 'tilted' emotional relationship."

According to Macalpine, psychoanalytic therapy is unique among psychotherapies because the analysand is not transferred to. Strictly speaking, the analytic transference relationship therefore ought not to be referred to as a relationship *between* analysand and analyst, but should more precisely be referred to as the analysand's relation to his analyst. Psychoanalysis is the only psychotherapeutic method in which a one-sided, infantile regression is induced in a patient, analysed, worked through, and finally resolved.

Macalpine carefully described the elements in the psychoanalytic situation which, without any direct intervention of the analyst, provide a setting which makes a "new edition" of an early life situation not only possible but practically inevitable. Given transference readiness in the analysand, psychoanalytic technique creates an infantile setting, and many of the factors which are operative in this setting are enumerated by Macalpine. Among them I will focus on those which are germane to my present discussion.

The capacity of forming a transference relationship is based on the formation of earliest object relations. As Macalpine puts it: "To respond to the classical analytic technique, analysands must have *some* object relations intact." She holds that when the patient is exposed to this "early infantile setting," he will gradually, step by step, adapt to it by regression.

In the following, we will examine two factors of the transference readiness: (1) The infantile setting as such; (2) the stages in the formation of the object relations to which the adult may regress in the transference relation.

In dealing with the first point, I will base myself on the ideas I have elaborated in my recent publication, "La Genèse des Premières Relations Objectales" (Spitz, 1954). There I have made the attempt to follow the formation of object relations from their very inception at birth both in their generally known and in the less well studied aspects.

Freud stressed the helplessness of the infant at birth. It is this helplessness which forces on the human infant a line of development that leads necessarily to the formation of object relations and ultimately to social relations. We have to remember that the infant is not only structurally different from the adult in his personality but that his environment also is different. For the adult the environment consists of multiple and multiform factors, numerous individuals, groups, social climate and background, inanimate objects. An enormous variety of dynamic constellations operates between these factors, which become effective as shifting fields of energies that impinge on and are in interaction with the organized personality of the adult. The adult exerts his volition originating in his motivations, but at the same time he responds to the structure of the field of forces.

With a certain oversimplification, we may say that in the infant the effective environment consists in a single individual: the mother or her substitute. This is, one might say, a closed system. Even within this system the effective forces are different from what they would be in the case of the adult: the infant is, above all, the *passive* recipient; the mother is the active partner, the one who directs the relations, such as they are. The infant, in the beginning, communicates what goes on in him to the mother, not by coordinated communication, but by expressive manifestations. In due time these will progress to subjective manifestations of appeal for the mother's varied ministrations.

It is not difficult to see the similarity between the analytical setting and this description of the infant's condition. The main difference lies in the fact that for the infant this situation is determined by his physiological helplessness, that is by the laws of nature. In the analytical setting this relationship is created on one hand by the patient-doctor relation, on the other by the rules which we impose on the patient.

To begin with the patient-doctor relation: the patient comes to the analyst as one *seeking help* against a condition in which he finds himself helpless. Thereupon, by two inconspicuous expedients which in their simplicity carry the hallmark of genius, Freud created a surprising parallel to the infantile situation.

The two expedients are: (1) The couch on which the patient lies in the infantile situation, without seeing, but hearing the analyst, having to address his appeals and expressive manifestations into the emptiness of space like the infant and also, like the infant, aware of a role-changing Presence. (2) The other expedient is the fundamental rule: To say everything that comes into one's mind. In other terms, to turn the light of one's conscious perception on to what goes on *inside* of oneself and to relate this without selection or censorship. I am well aware that this is a rule more honored in its breach than in its observance; yet it corresponds closely to what the infant does when he manifests, without selection or inhibition, by movement or sound, by silence or agitation, the processes of his own organism of which he becomes aware. Like the infant the patient cannot become active, he is confined to the crib-couch. The analyst has the prerogative of intervention or of withholding intervention.

We might add a point not mentioned by Macalpine but not infrequently reported to me by patients: the feeling that he, the patient, is being humiliatingly *forced* to be a child, because reclining; and of the feeling that the analyst is a grown-up, because he is sitting up on a higher level, the level of the parent.

So much for the setting. I concur with Macalpine in her postulate that if there is transference readiness in the patient the setting becomes a stimulus, a cue, a particularly favorable configuration for the provocation of transference. In this setting regression is not only greatly facilitated but practically imposed.

Let us now examine the progressive stages in the development of the infant's object relations and see whether some of their particulars will not yield information regarding the patterns evident in transference relations. I have observed three major stages in the first year of life.

The *first* is the objectless stage of nondifferentiation. It reaches to the end of the third month. No ego is present; the I is not differentiated from the not-I, the self from the not-self; or percepts, sensations, etc., from each other. At this stage we cannot speak of memory traces being laid down in the sense in which we use this word in the adult. We can speak at best of mnemic traces of a somatic nature being established, in connection with coenaesthetic functioning. Instincts also, at least in their manifestation, are not clearly differentiated from each other, and something of the same nature appears to hold, at least in the first weeks, for the difference between sleeping and waking. Nothing in the nature of an object or of object relations appears to exist.

The *second* is the stage of the establishment of the first libidinal object. It reaches from the end of the third month to the end of the first year. Differentiation sets in, in all the fields just mentioned, in an ever-increasing measure. The infant turns from passive reception to an ever more active perception of his surroundings; the manifestations of the instincts become observable and distinguishable from each other. A circular process of action-reaction patterns develops between the infant and his environment, that is his mother. Memory traces of a visual nature can be demonstrated experimentally, and by the eighth month the establishment of univocal, directed, and affectively richly cathected object relations between the infant and his mother are evident. These lead to a rapid expansion of the infant's activity patterns by his own initiative on one hand, by his identification with the object on the other. Prominent among these action patterns by the end of the first year are the first attempts at acquiring verbal communication.

The *third* stage is the stage of the elaboration of object relation with the libidinal and other "objects." It reaches from the end of the first year into the second half of the second year. From the psychoanalytic point of view its major features are the acquisition of the symbolic function. This involves both the capacity of communicating through the abstractions which words represent; and the inception of the ability to perform mental operations based on the availability of these abstractions in the infant's mind. I refer the reader to the work done on this subject by Jean Piaget (1950).

In connection with this process the first precursor of the superego, in the form of a code of "do's" and "don'ts," of commands and prohibitions, is laid down; needless to say, not without a great deal of affective exchange of both libidinal and aggressive nature between the child and the object. The experimental psychologist would add to this epigrammatic description that the acquisition of mental operations with the help of abstracts enables the child to master the exquisitely human achievement of using tools and is indeed a tool function in itself. He would furthermore stress that the achievement of locomotion has expanded immeasurably the radius of the child's possible experiences, contacts and exchanges.

I need hardly state that for heuristic purposes I have indulged in an extreme simplification of the real state of affairs.

Let us now return to the analytical setting and see how it compares with the situation in early infancy. Ostensibly the patient is required to inform us verbally of what passes through his mind. We invite him to make use of the mental processes made possible through the acquisition of the symbol function, of verbal facilities. We also admonish him to overcome the mental censoring imposed and acquired by him in the course of his adjusting to society.

But, while requesting from the patient a behavior which corresponds to a quite high level of integration, both in the verbal and in the behavioral sector, we put him into the analytical setting, which forces him toward a much earlier stage of integration. Without stating this explicitly, the setting forces him to the earliest phase of the infant, to the nonobjectal phase.

Dr. Anna Freud calls my attention to a point on which I have not expressed myself with sufficient clarity. In her opinion, the objectless first stage does not return in the transference. It is rather that which determines the limits of transference.

I fully agree with her. When I stated that the analytical setting forces the patient to the nonobjectal phase, this was intended as an indication of a direction and not of an ultimate destination. Even in the second stage of the infant's development, the stage of the object's precursors, it is very unlikely that memory traces are laid down which could ever be made available to the patient. Memory traces which can be made available to the patient in the course of analysis, though mostly in exceptional cases, are laid down only in the third stage, when the symbolic function is acquired.

It is not the objectless phase which returns in the transference of the patient. It is the analytical setting which reproduces many of the elements of this phase. Through this reproduction the analytical setting pulls, funnel-like, the patient's transference in the direction of the objectless phase. In his endeavor to express the feelings he experiences in the process of this transference, the patient uses the ulterior elaborations which have been built upon the structured feeling tones of his earliest experiences. Some facets of this process have been discussed by Bertram Lewin (1946, 1948, 1953b), in his publications on the dream screen, by Otto Isakower (1938) in his paper "A Contribution to the Pathopsychology of Phenomena Associated with Falling Asleep," and by myself in my paper "The Primal Cavity" (Spitz, 1955c).

We frustrate the patient's visual participation of the object; tactile participation is precluded by the conditions of the analytical situation. We frustrate his auditory perception by responding sparingly and rarely to his manifestations. Like an infant, we place him into the reclining position and we also restrict his locomotion and his muscular activity by enjoining him against "acting out" and insisting that he *inform* us instead verbally of his urges. The parallel of the resulting feeling tone with that of infancy is striking. Even that less obvious rule of analysis, the prohibition of social contact between the analyst and the patient, makes the analyst and his private life as mysterious as that of the parents is for the child; and, we may add, as speculation-provoking.

The setting encourages a regression to a life period from which few or no memories have been preserved. The fundamental rule forces the patient to exteriorize, as best he may, the mental contents which refer to this early phase. Since he has no memories of them, but only traces of a nature which differs from our adult memory and of which we will speak anon, what he will produce are derivations and the later elaborations built on these foundations. The patient will progressively tell us of the various ulterior stages through which his early object relations have gone.

Our problem then becomes to diagnose the transference manifestations as such and to recognize them where they appear, to distinguish them from what has been called "ordinary behavior" or "the establishment of rapport" between two persons by the various writers on transference. We must then determine the diagnostic signs which enable us to distinguish transference from ordinary behavior.

Analytical writers on the subject have at times stressed that transference manifestations are characterized by their inappropriateness. This inappropriateness is on one hand a *quantitative,* and on the other a *qualitative* one.

Quantitatively, minimal, often imperceptible manifest cues trigger disproportionate, dramatic, sometimes cataclysmic behavior responses. This fact parallels in a particularly impressive manner a specific level of infantile integration. The phenomenon of transference consists of three elements. The first is a *manifest external physical cue*. This evokes a latent *structured feeling tone*. The combination of the two triggers the third, the transference behavior itself. The manifest elements which can evoke the feeling tone are infinitely variable. Thus it will have the same effect if the analyst remains silent to the patient's wildly exaggerated admiration of the royal house of England or whether the analyst attempts to point out to the patient that he has consciously suppressed telling him a dream. In both cases the patient's response is: "I feel that you have an unutterable contempt for me and that in your eyes I am lower than a worm."

The inappropriateness of the transference behavior follows from the minimalness of the manifest cues. The example given above shows that the manifest part of the cue is more or less accidental and adventitious. That becomes particularly evident when we are confronted with the various perceptive and apperceptive distortions of our patients.

Take the case of that female patient of mine who, after nearly a year's analysis with me, in connection with a dream, expressed the opinion that I was the owner of a head of rich, somewhat curly brown hair. Confronting her with the sorry reality made it easy to lead her to the insight that the proprietor of that tonsorial adornment was her father, and thus to achieve one little step in the clarification of her insight both in regard to the emotions she felt towards me and to those which she had originally felt towards her father.

But what do we mean when we speak of the structure of a feeling tone? It would be more precise to consider the cues for transference behavior structured emotional situations. It is here that the similarity of the adult in transference to the infant is particularly impressive. In the first three months of life the great majority of the cues which trigger behavior are emotional. But even in the second stage, that of the establishment of object relations, the emotional aspect, the emotional relations, and the feeling tone established between object and infant is incomparably more important than the variety of gross physical perception available to the baby. A most impressive parallel exists between the infant's behavior at a specific developmental stage and the behavior of the patient in transference. Any adult who offers the minimal cue of two eyes, a nose, and a forehead, combined with motion, to the infant between the third and the sixth month of life, becomes the representative of that infant's security, and of that low degree of object relations—I have called them precursors of object relations—of which the infant is capable at that age.

In parallel with this, the quasi invisibility of the analyst in the analytical setting, his being situated higher in space than the reclining patient, become the minimal cues which make the analyst the target of the composite emotion directed towards him. He will be endowed, as the case may be, with the face of the love object or that of the enemy, or the persecutor. The direction of the patient's emotions is predicated on their being funneled through the analytical setting, through that asymmetrical relationship so well described by Macalpine and called a "tilted" relationship by Greenacre.

While the quantitative aspect of the inappropriateness of transference manifestations is to be found in the minimalness of the *cues* which trigger them, the qualitative inappropriateness is also evident in the *occasions* on which these manifestations arise. Take for instance the patient who feels despised by the analyst; he disregards several obvious facts. The most evident of these is that value judgments of symptoms or their consequences do not enter into the frame of reference of the therapist, who operates with the criteria of health versus disease. We will forego a discussion of the variety of qualitative inappropriateness of the occasion on which transference manifestations occur. The inappropriateness of the occasion is after all only a manifest one. It is the expression of unconscious psychological contents severely condemned by the patient's superego. The inappropriateness of the occasion for transference manifestations is one of the symptoms of the conflict between his superego demands and his incapacity to conform to them. Until this conflict is resolved, the patient will continue in his qualitatively and quantitatively inappropriate behavior, that is inappropriate behavior on inappropriate occasions in response to minimal cues.

This phenomenon, however, is not limited to transference only. It applies also to other neurotic or psychotic behavior. In the neurotic and in the psychotic the inappropriate behavior stems primarily from the interaction between the pressure of the drives on one hand, the functioning of the defense mechanisms used by the individual dealing with them on the other; the environmental cues play a relatively unimportant part in provoking this behavior. In this respect the psychotic, and to a lesser extent, the neurotic, might be considered to function in an autarchic system. It is not the environment which provides them with cues for their behavior, it is they who seek for these cues in the environment, and if the cues are not available, they will manufacture them.

As we have mentioned in the beginning, in the transference the analytical setting provides the cue and the analyst lends an external ego function to the patient.

It is this funneling of the patient's emotions onto the analyst which makes transference possible and fosters it until eventually the transference neurosis evolves from it.

In contrast to it stands the ego-syntonic, reality-adapted, mature behavior, that which we call the ordinary behavior of the so-called normal person. In the therapy of the neurotic this is achieved through the resolving of the transference relation which derives its energies from the id; that is how we achieve the goal set by Freud: "Ego shall be where Id was."

Countertransference: Comments on Its Varying Role in the Analytic Situation

The subject of countertransference has been widely debated; the concept itself is still ill defined. Since Freud first coined the term,[1] despite frequent attempts at its definition both from the pragmatic and from the theoretical viewpoint, no final agreement has been reached on its formulation. We have made no effort to duplicate the excellent historical survey on countertransference by Orr (1954). Since Orr's review appeared, Benedek (1953, 1954) and Racker (1953) published further important papers on the subject. For the purposes of the present paper we will give a working definition covering the range of the phenomena of which we intend to speak. Furthermore, we will consider countertransference as something which takes place between two persons, the analyst and his patient.

We will define countertransference as one part of the analyst's relation to his patient; it is one of the determinants of the emotional climate of a given analytic relationship; it usually originates in the analyst; its manifestations are varied. The particular shape it takes is due to the way in which the given patient's personality, his behavior, and the manifestations of his transference act on and are responded to by the given analyst's personality. The response will begin with a dynamic process in the analyst's unconscious. This will translate itself into derivatives, expressed in the attitude of the analyst. When the patient becomes aware of the analyst's attitude, changes in the nature of the patient's transference take place. Thus a circular process between analyst and patient is set in motion which determines the analytic climate.

The analyst's countertransference may be manifested either in a sublimated form or in the form of id derivatives or as a crude expression of a drive. The function of countertransference in the given analytic relationship will be determined on one hand by the form in which it is manifested, on the other by its content. In the further course of this paper we will speak of some aspects of countertransference as well as of its genetic origin and we will attempt to investigate its metapsychology.

The interpersonal aspects of this definition of countertransference coincide

Reprinted from *Journal of the American Psychoanalytic Association*, 4:256–264, 1956.
[1] To my knowledge the term "countertransference" was used for the first time by Freud in his letter to Ferenczi dated October 6, 1910 (E. Jones, 1955, p. 83).

to a large extent with the one given by Annie Reich (1951). We have for the moment omitted making the distinction which she has clearly established between countertransference proper, and the more general concept of countertransference worked out by her and Fenichel (n.d.) in their discussion on this topic, and which includes the analyst using the analysis for acting-out purposes.

It follows from our definition of countertransference that we believe that it is constantly present in analytic work and that it is a normal phenomenon. As Adolph Stern (1924) remarked, countertransference in the analyst is exactly the same phenomenon as transference in the patient. Gitelson (1952) expressed the same idea when he suggested abolishing the term of countertransference and calling it instead "the analyst's transference to the patient."

One of the most important single contributions on the subject is Annie Reich's (1951) article; it has influenced much of my own thinking. She states, "Countertransference is a neccessary prerequisite of analysis. If it does not exist, the necessary talent and interest is lacking." In this statement she indicates clearly the constructive function of countertransference. She explains that the psychological interest of the analyst is based on a very complicated countertransference which is desexualized and sublimated in character. In contrast with this she cites pathological examples in which the analyst's conflict persists in its original form and in which the analytic situation is used by him for one of three purposes: (1) for the living out of the underlying impulses; (2) for defending against these impulses; (3) for proving that no damage has occurred in consequence of these impulses.

Racker (1953) and (1956), have introduced the concept of "countertransference neurosis." Racker defines it as an independent entity, as the pathological part of countertransference and the expression of neurosis. He states that the countertransference neurosis, like any other neurosis, and also like the transference neurosis, is centered in the Oedipus complex.

In view of the recent conceptualization of this particular aspect of countertransference when it becomes pathological, it seems worthwhile to discuss it in some detail, particularly since the question has been raised whether the countertransference neurosis might not have its uses in treatment, just as the transference neurosis has.

In countertransference neurosis, like in any other neurosis, affect is released. Only in countertransference neurosis it is the analyst who releases his own affects, not the patient. We will now examine the conditions under which countertransference affects are released by the analyst, and the influence this has on the patient.

We attribute a goodly part of the therapeutic effectiveness of the analytic treatment to the release of affect by the patient and to his affective reexperience of repressed memories. This results in a modification of his personality. That is not necessarily the patient's intention; his intention, when he releases affects, is to modify the relationship between himself and the analyst. This may involve foisting on the analyst a role which is not justified by the reality situation. But the analyst refuses to change either the relationship or his own role in the relationship; instead of this he attempts to understand the patient's affective behavior and to transmit this understanding to him.

One may then ask how analytic therapy can be benefited if the analyst releases affects as a consequence of a countertransference neurosis. If we pursue the analogy between the patient's releasing affects and the same process in the analyst, it would seem that such a release by the analyst is an attempt either to modify his relation to the patient or to modify the role he plays in this relation, or both. Eventually it would result in an effort of the analyst to modify the patient himself. As a therapeutic goal the latter might be acceptable. As a therapeutic method it is open to question. The method certainly is not in accordance with the principles of psychoanalysis and the goals of analytic training. The latter endeavors to replace in the analyst the need to release affects in the treatment situation by insight and understanding. This does not imply that affects should not arise in the analyst in response to his patient's productions, nor that he should be in any way rigid, inflexible or not subject to change. We will discuss further in what way the analyst's personality should be flexible and what use he should make of his affects.

Continuing our parallel between countertransference neurosis and any other neurosis, we are reminded that neurosis is characterized by its compelling nature—a fact also stressed by Racker. This does not apply to compulsion neurosis only. Any neurotic finds himself under the inner constraint to act in terms of his neurosis rather than in terms of reality. He is under an inner constraint to act out his neurosis. He is under the constraint of the repetition compulsion. He is not a free agent.

That is exactly the opposite of what we expect of the analyst, whose activity in the treatment situation should be only controlled by his ego. An analyst acting under the compulsion of id impulses in the treatment situation has relinquished his therapeutic role. The degree of freedom available to the analyst is well formulated in the witticism of a Viennese comedian, who described the normal person as somebody who *may* do anything, but does not *have* to do it.

We would then say that in the analytic procedure countertransference neurosis in the analyst is not only not useful but highly undesirable. What we expect of the analyst is that he achieve a countertransference sufficiently *sublimated,* so that he can make use of it in identifications of brief duration with his patient. This process has been aptly described by Kris (1952) in regard to the artist. He called it a "regression in the service of the ego." That is exactly what we expect of the analyst.

In my recent discussion of transference (1956b) I referred cursorily to its dynamics and to some of its economic aspects, while elaborating extensively its genetic aspect.

If we agree to consider countertransference as an analogue of transference in the patient, then it follows that its genetic history is the same as that of transference. In other terms, it is a new edition, a facsimile, of impulses and fantasies belonging to the past. The past to which they belong, as I have shown in the previously mentioned communication, is the earliest parent-child situation. In agreement with Greenacre (1954), Macalpine (1950), Lagache (1952), and others, I explained how the situation of the child's helplessness was recreated in the analytic setting and would inevitably result in the reproduction of fantasies originating in that situation.

Countertransference assigns a role to the analyst which is the obverse of that of the patient. The patient is helpless, while the analyst's role is to be helpful. The situational stimulus in the analytic setting which acts on the analyst is, therefore, the patient's helplessness. It evokes in the analyst fantasies derived from the ego ideal which he formed in identification with his parents.

We have postulated that the analytic setting places the patient into an anaclitic relationship. I may be permitted to suggest a distinctive term for the role of the analyst in this setting. *Anaclitic* means leaning onto; I recommend for the analyst's attitude the term *diatrophic,*[2] which means supporting.

The diatrophic attitude has its origin in a developmental stage of the infant which emerges toward the end of the anaclitic relationship. The diatrophic attitude is a facsimile of the fantasies which belong to the stage in which the young child forms his secondary identifications with the parental figures. I am referring here to those early make-believe games, to be seen in the first half of the second year, when the child feeds its teddy bear from a nursing bottle, copies the nurse in a nursery by distributing diapers to the other children, etc.

There is a basic countermovement in the unfolding and the fate of the anaclitic attitude on the one hand, of the diatrophic attitude on the other. The anaclitic relationship is based on an experience of which in the normal course of development the reality aspects recede progressively and are lost, leaving behind them only memories and wish-fulfillment fantasies. With advancing age, anaclitic relations are relegated more and more to the realm of fantasy or pathology.

---

[2] From the Greek—to maintain, to support throughout.

The diatrophic relation begins with an identification fantasy, but with progressive development will end up in the reality situation of the subject becoming himself a parent.

In the analytic setting, in the ideal case, both anaclitic and diatrophic relations have to operate on the level of fantasies, conscious and unconscious, triggered by the conditions of the setting itself. Neither of them should be translated into action. The patient, in acting out, attempts to achieve reality fulfillment. The aim of the rule of abstinence is to frustrate this fulfillment. The analyst becomes able to impose this frustration on the patient only if he himself does not act out the diatrophic attitude. He has to understand the origin of his diatrophic fantasies sufficiently to be able to accept as a matter of course that *the rule of abstinence operates for himself as much as it does for the patient.* This is a point touched upon also by Racker. I would say specifically that this unconditional acceptance of the rule of abstinence requires not only the working through of the analyst's oedipal and pregenital development, but also his becoming able to relinquish the archaic wish for magic omnipotence.

Acting out the diatrophic attitude, of course, is not the only pitfall of his own unconscious which the analyst faces. If we disregard the well-known and extensively discussed acting-out possibilities presented by unresolved problems of the analyst in connection with the partial drives of the pregenital phase and those connected with the conflicts of the oedipal phase, there still remains the temptation for him to succumb to an unconscious wish for an anaclitic relationship to his patient. Obviously the analytic setting does not make acting out the latter easy. But as acting out in a countertransference neurosis disregards reality, it does not preclude it either. Needless to say that to act out anaclitic wishes is as undesirable for the therapeutic process as the other forms of acting out; indeed, it is one of the more dangerous ones of these forms.

The early secondary identificatory fantasies which underlie the diatrophic attitude have a very great adaptive value for individual development. They have mostly been studied in their significance for pathology and little has been written about their importance in the formation of personality. They operate at first in the process which I have called the humanization of the infant. This begins with the acquisition of language and of the first elements of the "do's" and "don't's." Eventually these secondary identifications will serve the process of the socialization of the child. The formation and the subsequent liquidation of the Oedipus complex is but one of the stations on this road.

In the course of the child's development, the progressive elaboration of these identifications is insured on one hand by the pleasure gain of drive satisfaction; on the other, these identifications are infinitely valuable to the child by providing him with ever-increasing mastery over the environment and with the concomitant narcissistic gratification. Throughout life, successive and ever more intricate elaborations of the diatrophic attitude in identification with the parents establish a genetic sequence in its development. Various stages of these identifications will be used for the purpose of occasional regressions.

In the analyst, the diatrophic attitude offers two possibilities. If ego-controlled, his brief regression to the parent ideal can be made therapeutically effective for the patient. Such transient identifications with the parent ideal enable the analyst to empathize with the infantile aspects of the patient's behavior and to reinterpret them in terms of infantile experience. On the other hand, this same regression, if not controlled by the ego, may give the therapist the opportunity to find a gratification of repressed drives. Identifications with the patient, with his parents, or with the vicissitudes of their relations which permit the surfacing of the analyst's repressed drives should be considered as acting out on his part.

I have stated that I do not consider acting out desirable on the part of the analyst. Such acting out can be an occasional one, provoked by transference manifestations of the patient. Alternatively, it can take place in the framework of a real countertransference neurosis, as a consequence of the neurotic personality of the analyst. In either case, it can only be an obstacle in what we call the analyst's understanding of the patient.

As we have stressed, a great deal of the analyst's insight results from brief, temporary identification with the patient, that is, from ego-controlled regression on the part of the analyst. If the ego-controlled regression is replaced by acting out, then the analyst can no longer remain aware of the derivatives of his own unconscious and cannot make appropriate use of them in therapy. When the analyst acts out in response to the patient's provocation, an interchange of acting out between analyst and patient takes the place of an understanding of the patient's productions. Therefore, the analyst's acting out cannot lead to a therapeutic interpretation.

When acting out replaces interpretation, the results will sometimes be spectacular. Such results are comparable to the successes seen in cathartic therapy. The dynamics of the two are different. But the successes will be haphazard and transitory at best, and it is to be expected that the drawbacks of such methods will far outweigh their advantages.

Acting out, as stressed by Reich and Fenichel, is but one of the manifestations of countertransference. It is the most obvious and easily recognized one. There is much less unanimity on what constitutes the other forms. I believe that many of our disagreements on countertransference are caused by misunderstandings provoked through the careless use of the term in our writings. We are prone to speak of countertransference, which is an unconscious process, when what we really mean are its conscious derivatives. It is only with these that we can deal on the conscious level; taking cognizance of these dervatives enables us to perform what Glover (1927) called "the analytical toilet."

One of the reasons why the analytic candidate undertakes a training analysis is to enable him to recognize the underlying unconscious motivation of these conscious derivatives in himself. When he performs this task, he becomes able to fulfill the diatrophic role of the analyst: like the parent ideal, he can tolerate aggression as well as the pressure of the patient's libidinal demands without retaliating in kind. He can permit the patient's initiatives to unfold into directions, however different from his own ideals, as long as they do not endanger the patient. Analysis has to be carried out in abstinence, said Freud; I may add, abstinence of the patient and abstinence of the analyst. For the analyst this does not apply to countertransference as such, but to its acting out, as well as to those others of its forms which are not syntonic with the requirement of free-floating neutral attention.

Countertransference is a necessary prerequisite of analysis. Its proper use involves three steps:

1. The analyst becomes aware in himself of the derivatives of his unconscious as they arise in response to the patient's unconscious.

2. From these derivatives he infers the underlying unconscious processes in himself.

3. He now has to possess sufficient freedom to perform a transitory identification with those processes in the patient which had provoked his own responses.

This, then, would be my concept of the metapsychology of what we call "understanding the patient."

PART 7

THE RENÉ A. SPITZ FILM ARCHIVES

The Films of René A. Spitz

Robert N. Emde and Robert J. Harmon

Spitz made a habit of filming during his research and always had at least one movie camera as a constant companion. He used movies both for documentation of important findings and for special study in their own right, subjecting them to repeated viewing and frame-by-frame analysis. Accordingly, Spitz's film legacy includes a variety of films that can serve each of these purposes. His published films are available for documentation, and his archival films are now available for special scholarly study in the René Spitz Film Archives.

Published Films

Spitz's early observations are documented in a series of black and white 16 millimeter movie films. Because they so vividly portray the infancy deprivation syndromes as well as many of Spitz's conclusions about early development, they have been kept in circulation and are available through the New York University Film Library (26 Washington Place, New York, New York 10003).

Before listing these films and our summaries of them, a word of commentary about their use may be appropriate. The story is told that when Spitz first showed sections of *Grief: A Peril in Infancy,* to a group of New York physicians, a number became teary and expressed agony because of a compelling empathic response to the suffering infants. In recent years, we have found that a more common experience is for viewers seeing these films for the first time to become anxious. Furthermore, if the viewers are not prepared for what they see, they may struggle to avoid feelings of sadness by "making

Robert N. Emde, M. D., is Professor of Psychiatry and Director, Developmental Psychobiology Research Group, University of Colorado School of Medicine; Adjunct Professor of Psychology, University of Denver; and a member of the Faculty of the Denver Institute for Psychoanalysis.

Robert J. Harmon, M.D., is Assistant Professor Psychiatry, Division of Child Psychiatry, University of Colorado School of Medicine; Adjunct Assistant Professor of Psychology, University of Denver; and Adjunct Assistant Professor, Smith College School for Social Work, Northampton, Mass.

light'' of the films, by focusing on inappropriate details, or by not paying attention. We have, therefore, found it important to adhere to a few simple procedures when using Spitz's deprivation films for teaching and discussion. First, we prepare the audience for what they are about to see by describing it to them ahead of time. We include the information that it is likely to be unpleasant and may even note that viewers often struggle to avoid recognizing sadness. Second, we allow sufficient time after a film for open discussions using an experienced group leader. With preparation and discussion, the viewers see and appreciate much more in the films.

At times we have been questioned about the usefulness of demonstrating conditions such as hospitalism and anaclitic depression, particularly because of the anxiety and discomfort provoked by viewing. We have responded in terms of both the films' historical value and their applicability to current clinical practice. Although it is now unusual to see an infant as severely emotionally deprived as those suffering from the hospitalism syndrome of the films, a sizeable number of cases of anaclitic depression are still seen in most pediatric hospitals each year. Since the total loss of the mother is not the only elicitor of these deprivation syndromes, and since a relative change in the amount of caregiving available can also lead to it, those unfamiliar with the clinical picture may fail to recognize a child with this syndrome. A mothering figure may be present but emotionally unavailable to the child. Seeing this film sensitizes the viewer to the fact that depression does occur in infants and young children and shows how to recognize it.

The ten available published films are summarized below.

1. *Grief: A Peril in Infancy* Published 1947

This film illustrates the classic conditions of anaclitic depression and hospitalism. The grief responses of infants who lose their mothers at eight months of age are shown and contrasted with the responses of infants who were deprived of maternal care early in their life. The impressive recovery of the older infants after the mother has returned to care for them is also shown.

2. *Birth and the First 15 Minutes of Life* Published 1947

Two newborn infants are contrasted to demonstrate the presence of individual differences in behavior immediately following birth. The expulsion and delivery of one child is shown, while the second infant is observed moments after delivery.

3. *Somatic Consequences of Emotional Starvation in Infants*
Published 1948

This film contrasts the development of middle-class infants with that of infants raised in an institution. The institutionalized infants are those described in the "Hospitalism" paper (this volume), who were cared for by their mothers for 4 months and then cared for by a nurse who was responsible for ten infants. The development of the two groups of infants is contrasted at age 4 to 5 months, when few differences are seen, and then again at 13 to 14 months, when the devastating effects of the institutional care on the infants' development are underlined by the comparison with the home-reared infants.

4. *The Smiling Response (An Experimental Investigation into the Ontogenesis of Social Relations)*   Published 1948

This film illustrates the development of smiling during the first six months of life. The beginning of the social smile at around two months is shown, while other sequences demonstrate that infants will smile at strangers prior to six months of age. The film includes comparisons of smiling in response to people of different races and to a three-dimensional mask and demonstrates that a "gestalt" of the human face is the primary elicitor of smiling.

5. *Genesis of Emotions*   Published 1948

The development and differentiation of positive and negative emotions during the first 18 months of life are depicted in this film. Early affective changes include the development from negative excitement to interest in the human face and then to the smiling response. Various stimuli that elicit the smiling response are demonstrated. Negative emotions are shown, with the major focus on "stranger anxiety" at 8 to 10 months of age. The reactions to strangers range from a "wary" or "shy" response to extreme distress. Finally, early anger responses to frustration and pleasure at achieving mastery are illustrated. The film ends with an overview of early development, stressing the view that the infant differentiates both negative and positive affects in response to the human and inanimate environment.

6. *Grasping*   Published 1949

Grasping begins as a reflex. This film illustrates its development and adaptation to purposeful use over the first year of life.

7. *Psychogenic Diseases in Infancy*   Published 1952

Spitz felt that a series of clinical syndromes involving psychological factors appear during the first year of life. He divided these into two categories: psychotoxic disturbances, in which there were adaptive problems in the mother-child relationship; and emotional deficiency diseases, in which there was insufficient maternal care. The film portrays seven psychotoxic disturbances and the accompanying maternal attitudes. Two types of emotional deficiency diseases are illustrated—anaclitic depression and hospitalism (or marasmus).

8. *Motherlove*   Published 1952

This film begins with a day-old infant and his mother. It demonstrates the effects of adequate mothering over the first three years of life through the mother's sensitive handling of feeding and weaning and her ability to include her three-year-old first child in the care and feeding of a sibling. In contrast, children who had been separated from their mothers during the second half of the first year of life are shown. Their earlier happy behavior evolves into depression after separation. The film ends with a brief episode of the first child happily playing with a stranger, illustrating the positive effects of his excellent social relations with his mother.

9. *Shaping the Personality—The Role of Mother-Child Relations in Infancy*   Published 1952

This film illustrates the influences of a mother's behavior and her conscious and unconscious attitudes toward her child on the child's early development. Five breast-feeding mothers are shown and inferences about their feelings toward their infants are made. These infants are then shown at various times during the first two years of life while feeding and in play situations. The effects of varying maternal attitudes on each child's personality are then demonstrated, ranging from positive attachment to extensive psychiatric disturbance.

10. *Anxiety: Its Phenomenology in the First Year of Life* Published 1953

This film demonstrates the phenomenology of anxiety throughout the first year of life. Differentiation of pleasurable and unpleasurable responses at three months of age are shown as well as the development of "anxiety proper" after six months of age. Anxiety is then traced as it branches into normal and pathological forms and examples of each are shown.

THE RENÉ A. SPITZ FILM ARCHIVES

The René A. Spitz Film Archives were established at the University of Colorado Medical School under the auspices of the Denver Institute for Psychoanalysis as part of the Department of Psychiatry. The films were donated by Spitz as part of his legacy, and the archival collection is virtually complete. In addition to copies of Spitz's ten published films, the Archives contains the catalogued original films of his institutionalized infants and the films of Spitz's other developmental studies. There is also a group of brief documentary films, which he called his "story films," and which he used to illustrate his well-attended lectures of the 1950s and early 1960s. Most of these lectures are also on file, with designations in the manuscript pages indicating where the illustrative films were used.

The purpose of the Archives is to enable visiting scholars to study in depth these invaluable film records and to place them in the context of Spitz's writings (which are readily available in the Department of Psychiatry library, also named after Spitz). Appropriate viewing equipment, including that for single-frame and slow-motion analysis, is available in the film Archives room. Scholars wishing to visit the Archives and make use of the facilities should write the director of the Denver Institute for Psychoanalysis for information about arrangements. Films and reprints are not available for distribution through the Archives.

PART 8

SEVEN COMMENTARIES:
THE RELEVANCE OF SPITZ'S WORK
FOR TODAY'S WORLD

Editor's Introduction

The seven commentaries that appear in this section were solicited by the editor from leaders in the designated disciplines. These authorities were asked for their opinions about the contemporary relevance of Spitz's work. The order in which the commentaries appear reflects an attempt to present a meaningful flow of ideas.

Psychoanalysis

Herbert Gaskill

The publication of René A. Spitz's selected papers provides psychoanalysts and students of developmental psychology an opportunity to review his research strategy and his seminal contributions to the understanding of the formation of psychic structure. He completed what was possibly the first formal training analysis with Freud in 1910. His clinical activities never involved child analysis, although his research was primarily focused on "the early stages of personality organization"—"the primordia"—particularly in the first year of life (Spitz, 1958b, 1965b). Using a genetic approach, Spitz aimed at delineating the precursors to psychological functioning (1962) rather than making reconstructions based on psychopathological phenomena derived from clinical observations (1966). These studies sought to establish "norms and regularities," that is, broad generalizations, as well as the "process of differentiation and integration into higher psychological units." For nearly four decades, Spitz's many scientific papers demonstrated his meticulous and systematic studies of the infant's transition from a physiological to a psychological organism.

Spitz's research method involved the systematic collection of data obtained from longitudinal child observation studies in a variety of naturalistic settings. He recorded much of his observational data on film, allowing repeated observations of the data as well as permitting other investigators to review the same data. Consonant with Freud's scientific thinking, Spitz's approach was primarily from a Darwinian evolutionary viewpoint. Although he organized his theoretical thinking around psychoanalytic metapsychology (1966), his approach was multidisciplinary, drawing on ethology, embryology, animal experimentation, Gestalt psychology, phylogenesis, and the organismic point of view. He saw the formation of psychic structure as the "epigenetically unfolding anlage" (Spitz, 1959, p. 11) in interaction with the surround. He emphasized the need to distinguish phylogenetically transmitted behaviors from those due to interactions with the maternal object. He made a distinction

Herbert S. Gaskill, M.D., is Clinical Professor of Psychiatry, University of Colorado School of Medicine; and Director, Denver Institute for Psychoanalysis.

between psychological and biological development. In approaching the latter he was greatly influenced by Paul Weiss's (1939) concept of "organic development," which was "prefunctional and preadapted, cumulative, progressive, and autonomous" (Spitz, 1959, p. 13). In contrast to learning theorists (Watson, 1924; Hull, 1943) who posited psychological development as occurring on the basis of continued and progressive enrichment through antecedent learning experiences, Spitz explicated the discontinuities and uneven rates of mental development, which involved transformations and hierarchical levels of organization.

In *A Genetic Field Theory of Ego Development* (1959), Spitz delineated the appearance of specific affect behaviors—the smiling response (an innate releasing mechanism in Lorenz's [1950] term) and stranger anxiety (Spitz, 1950a)—which were nodal points indicating the uneven rates of development. He suggested that these affect behaviors were "organizers of the psyche" (1959, p. 33) similar to the organizers of embryology (Needham, 1931). Such nodal points, which involved the interaction of the innate and the experiential, reflected major developmental shifts with increasing differentiation and even greater organization. In this, Spitz was following Waddington (1940) as well as Werner (1948; Werner and Kaplan, 1963), in moving from nondifferentiation[1] to differentiation with a hierarchical organization of integration.

In "Autoerotism Re-examined" (1962), Spitz returned to an earlier theme, the impact of the quality of the mother-child relationship on the infant's developmental quotient. In this study Spitz reexamines an unanticipated finding—that the presence or absence of genital play depended on the nature of mother-child relationship—in the light of Harlow's findings on surrogate-raised monkeys. Harlow's surrogate wire "mother" monkeys could supply nutrition and contact comfort, but not "the circular exchange of affectively charged actions between mother and child" (Spitz, 1962). He suggested that the deficient factor in the affect-deprived monkeys was reciprocity. When reciprocity was lacking for either human or rhesus infants, the development of object relations, including mature sexual functioning, was seriously damaged. Transformations such as the development of object relations represented discontinuities involving creativity in development. The important theoretical and clinical contributions of Loewald (1960, 1978), based primarily on reconstructions from psychoanalytic clinical studies, are in many significant ways concordant with Spitz's formulations.

---

[1] "In my concept, nondifferentiation applies to the organization of the psyche as well as to its functioning" (Spitz, 1966, p. 126).

Child Psychiatry

Louis Sander

The selection of seven different areas for commentaries describing the relevance of Spitz's work for today's world indicates the multidimensionality that is Spitz's unique contribution to today's child psychiatry. Child psychiatry grew up over the same span of years in which Spitz's astute observations of infancy demanded the attention of psychiatry and psychoanalysis, largely because of this capacity to give his work a multidimensional relevance.

The domain of investigative research in early infancy also grew up over this period, taking off in part from some of Spitz's pioneering observations, but now illuminating the infant for us as an organism that possesses from the very outset a sophistication of function that even Spitz could not suspect. The research of this period has carried us far beyond those observations of his that helped generate our current explosion of investigation. This is exemplified especially in research on the micro-elements of interaction underlying infant-mother dialogue, on elementary components in the expression of affect, on early learning, and on smiling behavior or the stranger reaction. The detailed picture of today's neonate, consequently, might contradict many of Spitz's assertions, including the role he assigned to particular infant functions in the developmental process and their times of appearance or transformation; and today's research might not allow us to grant some of the assumptions underlying the logic by which Spitz related infant behavioral phenomena to the organization of personality.

Because of the excitement generated by such a stream of newer findings, we may be inclined to bypass the multidimensional relevance with which Spitz's perspective endowed his observations. But the enduring significance of Spitz's work lies in the model provided by his way of thinking about his observations—a model that can be grasped only as we review the diversity and breadth of his contributions in a collection such as this volume. Only from such an encounter can the reader grasp the undaunted interest, the imagination that played upon his experiences, and the integrative talent that

Louis Sander, M.D., is Professor of Psychiatry, Division of Child Psychiatry, University of Colorado Health Sciences Center, Denver.

conceived and proposed the new frameworks by which Spitz ordered his observations in relation to concepts at a variety of levels. His was truly a "holistic developmental psychophysiological approach" (1972).

The present-day child psychiatrist's perspective on both clinical challenges and the newer data of early development must indeed be "multidimensional." As Spitz noted, "At no later period of life do so many different levels of the personality meet for the first time as in infancy" (1972). The matrix for discovery must be, as it was for Spitz, the inspiration to continue the attempt to harmonize observation with biology, physiology, phylogenesis, embryology, metapsychology, or even more distant domains. Spitz described his thoughts as "adventures and experiments of the mind" (1972). When a professional discipline becomes solidly established as child psychiatry has, when it acquires its own tradition, a generally accepted curriculum for training, and a common ideational content, it becomes increasingly difficult for the professional to preserve the identity of the discipline and yet remain free and creative in formulating novel relationships or propositions at variance with tradition—as did Spitz.

An even greater opportunity for the integration of dimensions exists today for child psychiatry as the burgeoning interest in "infant psychiatry" opens a new universe of biological, developmental, and clinical information. In confronting issues of primary prevention and the *facilitation* of the development of the high-risk infant and caregiver, it becomes essential to continue to construct the bridges that engaged Spitz's interest. Key to the ordering of this information is Spitz's integrative perspective of "organization"—his view of developmental process as organizing process. Spitz's formulation of the principle of a central organizing process governing development (1972) makes clear that the organizer is "a new formula of regulation." It represents a more efficient *modus operandi* for regulating the relations of the child's constituents with each other in the increasingly complex context for adaptation, as well as the relations of the individual as a whole with the surround. These modifications of regulatory procedure are then incorporated into the child's equipment, becoming available from then on for further regulatory purposes. As Spitz (1972) summarizes:

> The substance, and quite often even the structure, of the constituent parts has not changed from one developmental level to the next. It is the method that changes, the manner in which the components are related to each other and at the same time to the total individual.

Two of Spitz's seminal ideas that relate to the infants' advancing "methods" of regulation are particularly relevant to today's growing understanding of the ontogenesis of personality. One concerns the attention he paid to formulating an ontogeny of awareness, especially the mechanisms accounting for a progression of steps in this ontogeny as they relate to the emergence and establishing of the self. The other concerns the role he gave to negation and the infant's taking of a contrary position as part of this same process. Today's child psychiatrists should be fully cognizant of all that Spitz has written on these subjects if he or she is to assimilate the new information from early developmental research, or "bridge" to issues of later personality organization, such as the self psychology that is currently being argued with such great interest within the psychoanalytic community.

The construction of new bridges is a never-ending necessity for an advancing, changing discipline such as child and infant psychiatry. It is too easy to assume that we already have the essential empirical underpinnings, adequate conceptual formulations, or satisfactory curricula for training. Encounter with the ferment of René Spitz's spirit and thought and the legacy he left of their expression provides us with a model of creative validity, essential for the continuing development of the child psychiatrist now and in the future.

Pediatrics

T. Berry Brazelton

For pediatricians, René Spitz's approach to the interaction between emotional and physical systems has become a critical base for examining the effects on children of separation, trauma, and the hospital experience. Spitz's early work engendered the later formulations of Bowlby and of Robertson which, in turn, have led to changes in hospital practices for children all over the world. Attention to the physical care of infants and children in hospitals is now balanced by attention to their emotional well-being. Parents are included in the care of their children, and child activity experts who are trained to use play as therapy for recuperating children are included on the hospital staff. Spitz's work has forced us to examine the deleterious effects of affective depression on recovering physical systems. We now recognize that preparing children for surgery and attention to their emotional well-being after surgery increases their chances of survival. It shortens their recovery period and mitigates both the aftereffects of hospitalization and the trauma of surgery. None of this had been recognized when Spitz wrote of the effects of hospitalization in 1945.

My hope is that, as a result of Spitz's challenges to us, the next 35 years will result in more important work on the psychosomatic interactions in children who must undergo the traumatizing effects of hospitalization, surgery, and separation from home. An increase in our understanding of the interaction between affective and physical systems in small children could lead to major advances in pediatrics. We are indebted to Spitz for his original and challenging descriptions of these interactions in children he observed.

Spitz's observations of infants, conducted with Katherine Wolf, led to his formulations of the functions of the ego in infancy. These set the stage for infant research as we now know it. His work led us to realize the importance of nurturance from the environment for an infant's cognitive, affective, and motor development; the importance of the infant's responsiveness to the en-

T. Berry Brazelton, M.D., is Associate Professor of Pediatrics, Harvard Medical School, Cambridge, Massachusetts; and Chief, Child Development Unit, Children's Hospital Medical Center, Boston.

vironment; and the importance of the dialogue between the infant and the parents. As an active, contributive interactant, the infant fosters parental interaction. Spitz showed that dyadic interaction was at the base of attachment and the communication of affective interchanges between parents and small children. As soon as we realized that there could be dialogue between infants and their care-givers, the importance of this dialogue to all the participants became clear. We began to look at the infant with new eyes.

Feedback from the infant began to be seen as critical in shaping the adults as parents. Parents learn as much about themselves in such an interactive framework as they do about the infant. We have identified four stages through which a parent must progress in the development of parenting during the infant's first four months in order to be ready to foster autonomy in the infant by the fifth month (which Mahler calls "hatching"). These four stages are identifiable within the dialogue between infant and parent (Brazelton and Als, 1979), and are characterized by teaching the infant how to (1) achieve and maintain motor and state organization; (2) maintain a state of alertness for interaction; (3) alternate periods of interaction with periods of rest in repetitive "games" (D. Stern, 1974); and (4) take the lead in social play and substitute object play. Learning about oneself as a parent parallels the learning about the infant that must take place in such a developing system. The infant's role in this system is to convey through nonverbal responses, "Now you're on track," or "Not that way, I can't take it." This important feedback shapes the parents' interaction with the infant.

As we understand the infant better, we see that internal feedback systems provide the infant with a kind of learning about him- or herself (ego development) in stages that parallel those in the parent. When the baby can receive external information, incorporate it, and respond to it appropriately, he or she is fueled by an internal recognition of having closed an important feedback loop. This then provides a "sense of competence" that leads him or her toward the next step of development—motor, cognitive, affective, and somatic. As the infant learns a new step in development, recognition of it stimulates further development. The important feedback systems that underlie the dyadic communication between parent and infant underlie the developing attachment process as well.

Understanding the nonverbal system of transmitting messages between parent and infant has become the goal for many of us in infant research. This writer first became aware of the power of this system during the development of the Neonatal Behavioral Assessment Scale (Brazelton, 1973). A nurturing adult was necessary to provide a containing envelope for a newborn so that he or she could react optimally to external stimuli (visual, auditory, tactile, and kinesthetic). When this envelope was provided, the newborn could react in complex ways that none of us had been aware of heretofore. The infant's expressive reactions to a voice, a rattle, or to the human face were available in the neonatal period. Not only did these reactions give us a new interpretation of the newborn's capacity for responses, but they also led us to the realization that the baby was signalling back to us that we were important to him or her. Eliciting this expressiveness became a goal for the adult interactant, and one could predict that the baby would inspire nurturant reactions in the adults around him or her. The infant's reactions became an important window into the infant's individualized way of functioning.

With the present understanding of the interaction between parent and infant in normal situations, we have begun to outline the limits of normal, healthy development in early infancy. Deviations in infants' reactions or in parents' capacity that place a dyad at risk can be identified early on; and the construction of paradigms for early intervention can be our next goal. René Spitz paved the way for a preventive approach—now identified as "infant psychiatry"—in which all disciplines concerned with children can participate. The field of developmental pediatrics owes an enormous debt to the early work outlined in this volume.

Infant Mental Health

Selma Fraiberg

The reciprocity between developmental research and applied research finds its ideal expression in the work of René Spitz and the emergence of a new field called "infant mental health." This field is the natural outgrowth of Spitz's own studies and of other research generated by his work.

The impact of Spitz's studies of maternal deprivation in the 1940s and 1950s is not diminished as we enter the 1980s; and, indeed, I predict that it will be still greater in the time to come, as the painful truths that Spitz unearthed are fully assimilated by our society and the professions that serve infants and their families. The younger generation no longer knows first hand that when Spitz's studies of hospitalism and anaclitic depression appeared in the 1940s they were greeted in psychological circles with disbelief that deprivation of mothering could produce enduring effects on an infant's psychological development. As other studies followed those of Spitz, the arguments have diminished, and we are left with the painful truth and a new wisdom that can be translated into programs of prevention and remediation.

For the mental health professional, the truth and the treatment lie in these two directions: prevention and remediation. The diseases of maternal deprivation are largely preventable at the source. If we fully acknowledge that the child deprived of a mother or a substitute mother is an endangered child, we must summon all the resources of our society to provide mother nurture for every child, to insure the stability of human bonds in the early months and years, and to insure continuity in the relationship between baby and mother or mother substitute. When social policy or law does not acknowledge the primacy of infant-parent relations for optimal development of every child, or functions through archaic practice to disrupt these bonds, the mental health professional must speak for children and their rights to bring about enlightened policies and practices that can in themselves prevent damage to countless numbers of children.

Selma Fraiberg was Professor of Child Psychoanalysis and Director, Infant-Parent Programs University of California at San Francisco.

[Selma Fraiberg died on December 19, 1981. Her own contributions to infant mental health were greatly admired and will be cherished for many generations. Ed.]

If we understand Spitz's studies as mental health professionals, even the calamity of mother-loss can be mitigated by providing good substitute mother care for the infant. In "Anaclitic Depression" (this volume), 50 of the 123 children who had lost their mothers in the institution studied did *not* develop anaclitic depression. These were the children who received substitute mother care from other inmates. Loss of the mother certainly registered on these infants at six months of age, but the mother substitute provided the conditions for recovery and reattachment. Enlightened policy and practices in our courts and in foster home agencies could go far toward preventing grave disorders in infants and young children. At the point of deciding about custody and removal of a child from his or her primary attachment figures, every professional must consider the gravity of the decision for the child and the family; and an assessment of the quality of the attachment must be central to this decision. When the decision to remove a child from his or her mother's care must be made, the plan for foster home placement must insure that new attachments can be formed through substitute mother care and that these new attachments will have continuity and stability throughout the years of childhood. Loss and repeated rupture of attachments through poor foster home care and serial placements will almost certainly erode or destroy the child's capacity for love and trust.

Similarly, if we understand that prolonged daily separations strain the tolerance of all babies and that even temporary loss of the mother generates anxiety in the young child, our social policies and programs of day care must undergo stern scrutiny. Those of us who are advocates for babies and their parents should challenge social policies that support, encourage, and in some cases mandate employment of the mother, making day care of infants a necessity. If a mother chooses to work, or if she must work to support her family, the quality of substitute care in a home or center must pass the most stringent standards for infant mental health. Every child who is separated from his or her mother in day care must have a mother substitute—a person who stands in for the mother, who is centrally important to the child during the nursery day, who provides nurture, comfort, stability and continuity in the absence of a mother, and whose personal caring and devotion to the baby augment the bonds of love between the baby and the mother.

Thus far, we have spoken about preventing emotional disorders in infancy through social programs and ideologies that promote and sustain the bonds between an infant and parents. What about the babies who already show the signs of emotional impoverishment and developmental disturbance as a result of impaired mother-infant relationships? Here, again, we encounter the echoes of René Spitz's work in the form of applied research in programs of intervention with infants and parents. A new subspecialty has developed among the health and mental health disciplines that serve children. Infant mental health specialists are appearing in increasing numbers throughout the country to bring the developmental and clinical knowledge of infant-parent relationships into treatment programs for babies and families who are suffering from impairment in their relationships.

Psychology

Joseph Campos

The reaction of the experimental child psychologist to the work of René Spitz has been undergoing a dramatic reappraisal. At one time it was easy to dismiss some of Spitz's key ideas, which seemed predicated on outmoded or discredited views of the human infant. For instance, much of Spitz's theorizing about the development of ego functions rested on assumptions about the lack of differentiation of the neonatal ego and the dominance of the infant by a barrier against sensations external to the self, resulting in the lack of perceptual organization of the infant's visual world. These assumptions were contradicted by empirical research that began to appear shortly after the publication of one of Spitz's major works, *The First Year of Life* (1965b), and that consistently documented the unsuspected visual, auditory, cognitive, and motoric capacities of the newborn and young infant (see Stone, Smith, and Murphy, 1973). In addition, Spitz's postulation of precocious representational memory of the mother as one of the major factors underlying stranger anxiety has never been confirmed. Nor has Spitz's notion (summarized in Fraiberg, 1969) of an earlier development for the representation of the mother than for objects received support when task factors are controlled for (Jackson, Campos, and Fischer, 1978). Furthermore, the major affective phenomena that Spitz proposed—the period of undifferentiated affect in the neonatal period, the emergence of the social smile, and the onset of separation and stranger anxiety—were vigorously challenged. These challenges came both from those who claimed that the neonate possessed many more emotional expressions than Spitz realized (Izard, 1977) and from those who accounted for emotional development as epiphenomena of simple cognitive processes like "effortful assimilation" to a schema, which produces smiling, or "failure to assimilate" something to a schema, which produces distress (Kagan, 1971; McCall and McGhee, 1977; Kagan, Kearsley, and Zelazo, 1978). It comes as no surprise, then, that just a few years ago, Spitz's theory seemed to offer the experimental child psychologist very little of heuristic value.

Joseph Campos, Ph.D., is Professor of Psychology and Head, Developmental Psychology Program, University of Denver; and Clinical Associate Professor of Psychiatry (Psychology), University of Colorado School of Medicine.

Now the reaction to Spitz's work is changing, and his ideas are beginning to assume a central role in the contemporary psychology of affect. This revival in interest is not so much the result of startling empirical confirmations of some of Spitz's predictions. Rather, it is in part a reflection of the woeful inadequacy of some of the ideas, such as discrepancy theory, that were supposed to be simpler alternatives to Spitz's, but that proved incapable of accounting for separation or stranger distress, let alone anaclitic depression and sadness. It is also partly accounted for by a major change in today's zeitgeist—a change that makes Spitz's theory much more congenial to academic psychology. Particularly through the influence of Spitz on theorists like Emde (Emde, Gaensbauer, and Harmon, 1976), and Sroufe (1979), a much deeper appreciation of the conceptual power of Spitz's ideas has come about.

Today, many psychologists consider affect to be an *organization construct,* an idea that has many ramifications, most of which are strongly related to Spitz's theories. One ramification is that affect cannot be operationalized solely by reference to single response measures, whether these responses are measured from the face, the voice, or the autonomic nervous system. Rather, what unifies these disparate responses and allows one to consider them as alternative expressions of the same state is the *function* that these affective constructs serve. Some of these functions involve *social regulation.* For instance, both weeping and a downcast facial expression separately communicate sadness to the perceiver and elicit tendencies toward approach, nurturance, and consolation. Another social function of affect is referencing—using the emotional reactions of another to facilitate one's own appraisal of an uncertain environmental event (Campos and Stenberg, 1981). Other functions of affects involve *internal regulation;* affect is now recognized as a major influence on perception, helping to segregate significant percepts from the ambient visual and auditory flux. Affect facilitates the process of storage, rehearsal, retention, and retrieval from memory, as Bower's (1981) recent work so cleverly shows. Affect also helps to regulate behavior, not only by energizing one's responses, but also by selecting those responses that "steer" the organism toward the appropriate goal specified by the affect. Moreover, now that experimental psychology has been freed of the binds of a rigid behaviorism, psychologists increasingly realize the importance of *consciousness* and *feeling* for the understanding of human motivation and social relationships.

In its new emphasis on emotions as social regulators, psychology has come a long way from the time when William James wrote ". . . emotional reaction usually *terminates in the subject's own body,* whilst the instinctive reaction is apt to go farther and enter into practical relations with the exciting object"

(James, 1890, p. 442, emphasis added). In its new emphasis on emotion as an internal regulator, experimental psychology has begun to abandon this long-prevalent view that affects are mere epiphenomena, or reflections of more basic and significant processes; now affect is given both initiating and feedback roles in cognition and motivation. Finally, by conceptualizing affect as a conscious feeling state, academic psychology has come once again full circle to the time when Wundt and Titchener argued that feeling was a separate domain from that of sensation, perception, and cognition and was not reducible to any of these.

The congruence of these trends with Spitz's view of affect is, I think, well summarized by him in the following passage from *The First Year of Life*:

> I do not propose to discuss the role of affects in psychic processes, in sensation, perception, thought, or action. It should be pointed out, however, that most academic psychologists sidestep these questions, as well as the whole problem of affectivity, by speaking of "motivation." Psychoanalytic theory, on the other hand, has insisted from the beginning that all psychic functions, be they sensations, perceptions, thought or action, are predicated on shifts of libidinal cathexis, which are perceived both by the individual and by the surround as affects and affective processes. In other words, affective manifestations are the indicators of cathectic shifts; these provide the motivation for activating the psychic functions of which we have spoken above. In infancy, affects play the same role for the purpose of communication as the secondary process plays in the grownup [Spitz, 1965b, p. 139].

Needless to say, it is thanks to theorists like Spitz that academic psychologists are no longer sidestepping these questions.

Developmental Psychobiology

I. Charles Kaufman

In discussing Spitz's work in relation to developmental psychobiology, it is necessary to define the latter since there is a current tendency among some psychiatrists to limit the meaning of psychobiology (and thus also of biology), to the biochemistry of the brain, including pharmacological alterations thereof. *Webster's New Collegiate Dictionary* defines "psychobiology" as "the study of mental life and behavior in relation to other biological processes." In this brief definition, four aspects are noteworthy: (1) all mental life and behavior are included, not just pathology; (2) all biological processes are included; (3) mental processes are among the biological processes; and (4) the conceptual essence of the term is the interrelatedness of mental and other biological processes, invoking the idea of organismic organization and implying notions of systems and levels. To go further and comprehend *developmental* psychobiology, the definition must include study of how this organized complexity arises and functions, both phylogenetically and ontogenetically.

Developmental psychobiology is a large domain, both in its own substance and in terms of related disciplines and areas of inquiry. It calls for permeable boundaries of thought and far-reaching integrations and syntheses of empirical data. It is guided by evolutionary theory and the concept of adaptation. Developmental psychobiologists look for developmental continuities, but also for biobehavioral shifts and their signposts. They truly appreciate that "psycho" is the middle of "biopsychosocial."

René Spitz, both by example and by precept, was the very model of a modern developmental psychobiologist. As a clinician, he was forever concerned with how people got to be the way they are, but as a scientist, he was not content to settle for reconstructions. He went after the primary data by studying children and infants in homes, in hospitals, and in other institutions, carefully observing the effects of different environments and rearing conditions. He studied the natural history of a variety of psychological phenomena

I. Charles Kaufman, M.D., is Chief, Psychiatry Service, Veterans Administration Medical Center, San Francisco; and Professor and Vice-Chairman, Department of Psychiatry, University of California, San Francisco.

and functions, always looking for precursors and prototypes in earlier psychological phenomena and in still earlier physiological phenomena. He emphasized the roles of both maturation and development, which he viewed, respectively, as the more biological versus the more psychological aspects of growth—although he never countenanced a simplistic nature/nurture dichotomy. His studies of the development of smiling and anxiety are exemplars of developmental psychobiological research of natural developmental phenomena, while his studies of hospitalism and anaclitic depression exemplify the use of "experiments in nature" to clarify developmental processes. He looked always to biological disciplines—embryology, genetics, physiology, biochemistry, ethology—both for data and for ways of thinking about psychological data. He was a general systems theorist before he knew there was such a theory. He understood the need to cross boundaries. His last major talk was called, fittingly, "Bridges."

More than anyone else, Spitz realized the special developmental significance of mother-infant interaction, whose character he metaphorically captured in the label, "dialogue." His evolutionary perspective and his biopsychosocial stance allowed him to see how developmental achievements (such as the functions of anticipation and signaling) as well as developmental milestones (such as the expressions of affect) arise and have meaning in the context of dialogue. By generalization, he was able to suggest that all psychological functions develop from biological propensities in the context of emerging object relations.

In the last years of his life, Spitz was a charter member of the Developmental Psychobiology Research Group in Denver. His accumulated wisdom was an invaluable resource, but he never ceased to surprise us with his inventive, multidisciplinary, and integrative thoughts and suggestions about both research endeavors and theoretical notions concerning developmental processes.

Some of the themes Spitz constantly pursued—evolution, adaptation, organization, hierarchy, increasing complexity and organizational shifts, dialogue and transaction, the centrality of object relations, affects as indicators, the biopsychosocial view—remain major themes in developmental psychobiology. The papers collected in this volume are of more than historical import. They continue to have relevance for clinicians and scientists, especially for developmental psychobiologists.

Child Abuse

Brandt Steele

Many facets of the work of René Spitz on the complex interactions between infants and their mothers are relevant to the problems of child abuse and neglect, which are manifestations of highly abnormal relations between caretaker and infant. Especially useful is Spitz's division of such deleterious interactions into two types—those characterized by "deficient" mothering and those involving "distorted" mother-infant interaction. Spitz pictured quite clearly both the physical and psychological damage done to the developing infant by these two forms of aberrant caretaking.

Although the settings and circumstances of Spitz's studies of infants in a nursery and a foundling home were different from our present studies of neglected infants in their own biological families or in foster care, Spitz's findings are pertinent to our more recent observations. In three classic papers—the two on "Hospitalism" (this volume) and the one on "Anaclitic Depression" (this volume)—he describes quite well the babies we now diagnose as "failure to thrive due to maternal deprivation." His descriptions of the severe marasmus, which often led to the death of infants in the foundling home, are applicable to those babies we see today whose mothers lack the ability to adequately nourish or otherwise care for their charges. He noted the prolonged effects of deficient mothering in the production of delayed development; in the spheres of physical growth, social interaction, and general behavior; and in the cognitive functions, especially that of speech. These are all characteristics commonly found in children who have been neglected or abused in various degree and combination. We also see in the neglected babies the picture of what Spitz described as anaclitic depression, and we see it persisting at least in minor degree through childhood and on into the adulthood of the formerly neglected and abused child.

Spitz noted that deprived infants had a pattern of abnormal response at the time when eight months' anxiety would be expected. Such babies had either

Brandt F. Steele, M.D., is Professor Emeritus of Psychiatry, University of Colorado School of Medicine, Denver; and former Acting Director, C. Henry Kempe National Center for the Prevention and Treatment of Child Abuse and Neglect, Denver.

unusually severe reactions to a stranger, evidenced by prolonged screaming, or showed very friendly responses to any adult. These two extreme and opposite patterns are commonly seen in abused children, not only in infancy but throughout childhood and even into adult life, manifested either by excessive isolation and suspicious attitudes toward other people or by quick, shallow attachments to almost anybody. Such patterns are prominent in the transference reactions during therapy of formerly abused children.

The effects of distorted mother-infant interaction were described by Spitz in his articles on "Psychogenic Diseases in Infancy" and in the chapter on "Psychotoxic Disturbances" in *The First Year of Life* (1965b). He writes of the enhancement of the infant's primary narcissism and the impossibility of establishing adequate object relations due to inconsistent, contradictory actions of the mother. More specifically, in his discussions of coprophagic children, Spitz describes mothers who were extremely rejecting and hostile, who burned or injured their children; and he felt that without supervision, some children of such mothers would have died. He did not conceptualize these actions as we do now as part of the child abuse syndrome, but he was well aware that hostile behavior on the part of the mother often led to significant evidence of depression in the child. He also noted the appearance of affective states in the child that were similar to those existing in the mother, describing it as "an infection" of the child with the mother's tendency. We have found this concept of "affective resonance" between mother and infant applicable in our understanding of abused and neglected children, particularly in the area of aggression. We feel that very early in life the infant, through this route of "resonance," begins to identify with aggression, long before he or she is able to identify with an aggressor, thus establishing a basis during earliest ego development for excessively aggressive behavior in later years. Spitz believed that the bleakness of life in the early years had long-lasting sequelae related to this early deprivation. He wrote, "Infants without love, they will end as adults full of hate" (Spitz, 1965b, p. 300). Recent studies have indicated that violent criminals and a great majority of juvenile delinquents have been formerly neglected or abused children (Steele, 1976, pp. 20–22), thus supporting Spitz's belief that affective deprivation in early life contributes to later violent behavior.

Other insights of Spitz's concerning psychic development in the earliest years provide a background of normality against which we can contrast the deviant development in abused, neglected children. His contribution in "On the Genesis of Superego Components" (this volume), is especially pertinent. In this article he describes the very early primordia of the superego derived from

tactile and visual impressions such as restraining the child physically on the one hand, the facial expression as well as the tone of voice which accompanies such prohibiting interference on the other. Similarly, imposing physical actions on the infant whether he likes it or not, in dressing, diapering, bathing, feeding, burping him, etc., will inevitably leave memory traces in the nature of commands. These physical primordia of prohibitions and commands are not easily recognizable in the ultimate organization which is the superego.

In the abused, neglected child we can see such prohibitions and commands carried out with exaggerated infliction of severe physical and emotional pain, and can also observe the consequences in the development of what is later quite recognizable as an overly punitive, self-denigrating, restrictive, pleasure inhibiting, and aggression-releasing superego. Closely related to this, we see among the adults who maltreat their children the extremely low self-esteem, excessive self-criticism, and chronic, low-grade anaclitic type of depression, which can be traced back to their own earliest years when they experienced neglect and abuse from their own caretakkers. Thus, we see in the child abuse and neglect syndromes clear examples of the long-term effects of the deficient and distorted types of mother-infant interactions so clearly described by Spitz many years ago.

REFERENCES

Abraham, K. (1912), Notes on the psychoanalytical investigation and treatment of manic-depressive insanity and allied conditions. In: *Selected Papers*. New York: Basic Books, 1953, pp. 137–156.

——— (1916), The first pregenital stage of the libido. In: *Selected Papers*. New York: Basic Books, 1953, pp. 248–279.

——— (1924), A short study of the development of the libido, viewed in the light of mental disorders. In: *Selected Papers*. New York: Basic Books, 1953, pp. 418–501.

Aichhorn, A. (1935), *Wayward Youth*. New York: Viking Press.

Ainsworth, M. D., Blehar, M. C., Waters, E., & Wall, S. (1978), *Patterns of Attachment*. Hillsdale, N.J.: Lawrence Erlbaum.

Alarcon, A. G. (n. d.), *Dispepsia Transitoria del Lactante*. Mexico.

Ambrose, J. A. (1961), The development of the smiling response in early infancy. In: *Determinants of Infant Behavior*, Vol. 1, ed. B. M. Foss. New York: Wiley, pp. 179–201.

Ament, W. (1899), *Die Entwicklung des Sprechens und Denkens beim Kinde*. Leipzig: Wunderlich.

Anderson, P. W. (1972), More is different. *Science*, 177:393–396.

Anthony, E. J., & Benedek, T., Eds. (1970), *Parenthood: Its Psychology and Psychopathology*. Boston: Little, Brown & Co.

Arlow, J. A. (1980), Thoughts on development of the superego. Presented at Hampstead Clinic, London, November.

Aserinsky, E., & Kleitman, N. (1953), Regularly occurring periods of eye motility and concomitant phenomena during sleep. *Science*, 118:273–274.

——— (1955), A motility cycle in sleeping infants as manifested by ocular and gross bodily activity. *J. Appl. Physiol.*, 8:11–18.

Baerends, G. P. (1950), Specialization in organs and movements with a releasing function. *Sympos. Soc. Exper. Biol.*, 4.

Bailey, P. (1933), *Intracranial Tumors*. Springfield, Ill.: Thomas.

Bakwin, H. (1942), Loneliness in infants. *Amer. J. Dis. Child.*, 63:30–40.

Barlow, J. S. (1964), Evoked responses in relation to visual perception and oculomotor reaction times in man. *Ann. N.Y. Acad. Sci.*, 112:432–467.

Bayley, N. (1969), *Bayley Scales of Infant Development*. New York: Psychological Corp.

Bell, C. (1806), *The Anatomy and Philosophy of Expression as Connected with the Fine Arts*. London: Murray.

Bell, R. Q., & Harper, L. V. (1977), *Child Effects on Adults*. Hillsdale, N.J.: Lawrence Erlbaum.

——— & Hertz, T. W. (1976), Toward more comparability and generalizability of developmental research. *Child Devel.*, 47:6–13.

Bell, S. (1970), The development of the concept of object as related to infant-mother attachment. *Child Devel.*, 41: 291–311.

Bender, L. (1939), Mental hygiene and the child. *Amer. J. Orthopsychiat.*, 9:574–580.
——— (1947), Childhood schizophrenia. *Amer. J. Orthopsychiat.*, 17:40–56.
——— & Yarnell, H. (1941), An observation nursery: A study of 250 children in the psychiatric division of Bellevue Hospital. *Amer. J. Psychiat.*, 97:1158–1174.
Bender, M. B. (1952), *Disorders in Perception, with Particular Reference to the Phenomena of Extinction and Displacement*. Springfield, Ill.: Thomas.
Benedek, T. (1953), Dynamics of the countertransference. *Bull. Menninger Clin.*, 17:201–208.
——— (1954), Countertransference in the training analyst. *Bull. Menninger Clin.*, 18:12–16.
Benjamin, J. D. (1959), Prediction and psychopathological theory. In: *The Psychopathology of Childhood*, ed. L. Jessner & E. Pavenstedt. New York: Grune & Stratton.
——— (1960), The innate and the experiential. *Pittsburgh Bicentennial Conference on Experimental Psychiatry*. Pittsburgh: University of Pittsburgh Press.
——— (1961), Some developmental observations relating to the theory of anxiety. *J. Amer. Psychoanal. Assn.*, 9:652–668.
Berger, H. (1929), Über das elektroenkephalogramm des menschen. *Arch. Psychiat. Nervenkr.*, 87:527–570.
Bergman, P., & Escalona, S. K. (1949), Unusual sensitivities in very young children. *The Psychoanalytic Study of the Child*, 3/4:333–352. New York: International Universities Press.
Bibring, E. (1943), The conception of the repetition compulsion. *Psychoanal. Quart.*, 12:486–519.
Blanton, M. G. (1917), The behavior of the human infant during the first thirty days of life. *Psychol. Rev.*, 24:456–483.
Bower, G. (1981), Mood and memory. *Amer. Psychologist*, 36:129–148.
Bowlby, J. (1944), Forty-four Juvenile Thieves: Their character and home life. *Int. J. Psychoanal.*, 25: 19–53, 107–128.
——— (1946), *Forty-Four Juvenile Thieves*. London: Ballière, Tindale & Cox.
——— (1951), *Maternal Care and Mental Health*. World Health Organization Monograph No. 2. Geneva: World Health Organization.
——— (1960), Grief and mourning in infancy and early childhood. *The Psychoanalytic Study of the Child*, 15:9–52.
Brainerd, P. P. (1927), Some observations of infant learning and instincts. *Pred. Sem.*, 34:231–254.
Brazelton, T. B. (1962), Crying in infancy. *Pediatrics*, 29:579–588.
——— (1973), *Neonatal Behavioral Assessment Scale*. Spastics International Medical Publications Monograph No. 50. Philadelphia: Lippincott.
——— & Als, H. (1979), Four early stages in the development of mother-infant interaction. *The Psychoanalytic Study of the Child*, 34:349–369. New Haven: Yale University Press.
——— Koslowski, B., & Main, M. (1974), The origins of reciprocity: The early mother-infant interaction. In: *The Effect of the Infant on Its Caregiver*, ed. M. Lewis & L. A. Rosenblum. New York: Wiley, pp. 49–76.
Brentano, F. (1874), *Psychologie vom Empirischen Standpunkt*.
Breuer, J., & Freud, S. (1895), Studies on hysteria. *Standard Edition*, 2. London: Hogarth Press, 1955.
Bridges, K. M. (1932), Emotional development in early infancy. *Child Devel.*, 3:340.

Broad, C. D. (1925), *The Mind and Its Place in Nature*. London: Kegan Paul.
Bühler, C. (1927), Die ersten sozialen verhaltungsweisen des kindes. *Quellen und Studien zur Jugendkunde*, Jena: Heft 5.
———— (1931), *Kindheit und Jugend*. Leipzig: Hirzl.
———— (1933), The social behavior of children. In: *A Handbook of Child Psychology*. Worcester, Mass.: Clark University Press, pp. 374–417.
———— (1937a), *The First Year of Life*. London: Kegan Paul.
———— (1937b), *From Birth to Maturity*. London: Kegan Paul.
———— & Hetzer, H. (1932), *Kleinkinder Tests*. Leipzig: Barth.
———— ———— & Mabel, F. (1928), Die affektwirksamkeit von fremdheitseindrücken im ersten lebensjahr. *Ztschr. f. Psychol.*, 107:21–38.
Bühler, K. (1918), *Die Geistige Entwicklung des Kindes*, 4th ed. Jena, 1942.
———— (1934), *Sprachtheorie*. Jena: Fischer.
Calhoun, J. B. (1962), Population density and social pathology. *Sci. Amer.*, 206:139–148.
Campos, J., & Stenberg, C. (1981), Perception, appraisal, and emotion: The onset of social referencing. In: *Infant Social Cognition*, ed. M. E. Lamb & L. R. Sherrod. Hillsdale, N.J.: Lawrence Erlbaum.
Canestrini, S. (1913), Ueber das Sinnesleben des Neuge Borenen. *Monogr. a. d. Geb. d. Neur. Psychiat.*, No. 5.
Cannon, W. B. (1934), *Bodily Changes in Pain, Hunger, Fear and Rage*. New York: Appleton-Century.
Casler, L. (1961), Maternal deprivation: A critical review of the literature. *Soc. Res. Child Devel.*, No. 2, 1–64.
Chapin, H. D. (1915a), Are institutions for infants necessary? *JAMA*, 64:1–3.
———— (1915b), A plea for accurate statistics in infants' institutions. *Arch. Peds.*, 32:724–726.
Clark, L. P. (1932), A contribution to the early development of the ego. *Amer. J. Psychiat.*, 11:1161–1180.
Clarke, A. M., & Clarke, A. D. B. (1977), *Early Experience: Myth and Evidence*. New York: Free Press.
Clarke-Stewart, K. A. (1977), The father's impact on mother and child. Paper presented at the biennial meeting of the Society for Research in Child Development, New Orleans.
Cobb, W. A. (1963), The normal adult EEG. In: *Electroencephalography*, ed. D. Hill & G. Pharr. New York: Macmillan.
Cobliner, W. G. (1955), Intra-communication and attitude: A methodological note. *J. Psychol.*, 39.
Compayré, G. (1893), *L'évolution Intellectuelle et Morale de l'Enfant*. Paris: Hachette.
Craig, W. (1918), Appetites and aversions as constituents of instinct. *Biol. Bull.* 34:91–107.
Cushing, H. (1932), *Papers Relating to the Pituitary Body, Hypothalamus, and Parasympathetic Nervous System*. Springfield, Ill.: Thomas.
Danziger, L., & Frankl, L. (1934), Zum Problem der Funktionsreifung. *J. Kinderforsch.*, 43.
Darwin, C. (1872), *The Expression of Emotions in Man and Animals*. New York: Philosophical Library, 1955.
David, M., & Appel, G. (1961), Études des facteurs de carence affective dans une pouponnière. *Psychiat. Enfant*, 4.

Davis, K. (1940), Extreme social isolation of a child. *Amer. J. Sociol.*, 45:554–565.
——— (1947), Final note on a case of extreme isolation. *Amer. J. Sociol.*, 53:432–437.
Davison, C., & Selby, N. E. (1935), Hypothermia in cases of hypothalamic lesions. *Arch. Neurol. Psychiat. Chicago,* 33:570–591.
Dawson, G. D. (1958), The central control of sensory inflow. *Proc. Roy. Soc. Med.*, 51:531–535.
De Ajuriaguerra, J. (1965), Paper presented at the vingtièmes Rencontres Internationales de Genève.
Dearborn, G. V. N. (1897), The emotion of joy. *Psychol. Rev. Monogr.*, No. 2.
——— (1900), The nature of the smile and laugh. *Science,* 11:851–855.
Décarie, T. Gouin (1962), *Intelligence and Affectivity in Early Childhood.* New York: International Universities Press.
Déjérine, J., and Roussy, G. (1906), Le syndrome thalamique. *Rev. Neur.*, 14:512–532.
Dement, W. C. (1955), Dream recall and eye movements during sleep in schizophrenics and normals. *J. Nerv. Ment. Dis.*, 122:263–269.
——— (1960), The effect of dream deprivation. *Science,* 131:1705–1707.
——— & Kleitman, N. (1957), Cyclic variations in EEG during sleep and their relation to eye movements, body motility, and dreaming. *EEG Clin. Neurophysiol.*, 9:673–690.
Denny-Brown, D. (1929), On the nature of postural reflexes. *Proc. Roy. Soc. Med.*, 104: 371–411.
Dollard, J. (1939), *Frustration and Aggression.* New Haven: Yale University Press.
Drillien, M. (1948), Studies in prematurity. Part 4: Development and progress of the prematurely born child in the pre-school period. *Arch. Dis. Childhood,* 23:69–83.
Durfee, H., & Wolf, K. M. (1933), Anstaltspflege und Entwicklung im ersten Lebensjahr. *Ztschr. f. Kinderforsch.*, 42:273–320.
Dusser de Barenne, J. D. (1937), Sensory motor cortex and thalamus opticus. *Amer. J. Physiol.*, 38:913–926.
Economo, C. von (1929), *Die Encephalitis Lethargica.* Berlin: Urban & Schwarzenberg.
——— (1931), *Encephalitis Lethargica, Its Sequelae and Treatment.* London.
——— & Poetzel, O. (1929), Der schlaf. *J. f. Aezlt. Fb.*
Eibl-Eibesfeldt, I. (1957), Ausdrucksformen der Säugetiere. *Handbuch der Zoologie.* Berlin: Walter de Gruyter.
Ekman, P., & Oster, H. (1979), Facial expression of emotion. *Annual Review of Psychology,* 30.
Ellingson, R. J. (1967), The study of brain electrical activity in infants. In: *Advances in Child Development and Behavior,* Vol. 3, ed. L. P. Lipsitt & C. C. Spiker. New York: Academic Press, pp. 53–97.
Emde, R. N. (1970), Endogenous and exogenous smiling in early infancy. Paper presented at the American Psychiatric Association, San Francisco, May 13, 1970.
——— (1980a), Levels of meaning for infant emotions: A bi. social view. In: *Development of Cognition, Affect, and Social Relations,* ed. W. A. Collins. Minnesota Symposia on Child Psychology, Vol. 13. Hillsdale, N.J.: Lawrence Erlbaum, pp. 1–37.

——— (1980b), Towards a psychoanalytic theory of affect: I. The organizational model and its propositions. II: Emerging models of emotional development in infancy. In: *The Course of Life: Psychoanalytic Contributions toward Understanding Personality Development*, ed. S. Greenspan & G. Pollock. Vol. 1: *Infancy and Early Childhood*. Washington, D.C.: U.S. Government Printing Office, pp. 63–83, 85–112.

——— Gaensbauer, T., & Harmon, R. J. (1976), *Emotional Expression in Infancy: A Biobehavioral Study*. [Psychological Issues, Monogr. 37] New York: International Universities Press.

——— Harmon, R. J., Metcalf, D. R., Koenig, K. L., & Wagonfeld, S. (1971), Stress and neonatal sleep. *Psychosom. Med.*, 33:491–497.

——— & Koenig, K. L. (1969a), Neonatal smiling and rapid eye movement states. *J. Amer. Acad. Child Psychiat.*, 8:57–67.

——— ——— (1969b), Neonatal smiling, frowning, and rapid eye movement states. *J. Amer. Acad. Child Psychiat.*, 8:637–656.

——— McCartney, R. D., & Harmon, R. J. (1971), Neonatal smiling in REM states: IV. Premature Study. *Child Devel.*, 42:1657–1661.

——— & Metcalf, D. R. (1970), An electroencephalographic study of behavioral rapid eye movement states in the human newborn. *J. Nerv. Ment. Dis.*, 150:376–386.

Engel, G. L. (1962), Anxiety and depression-withdrawal. *Internat. J. Psychoanal.*, 43:89–97.

——— & Reichsman, F. (1956), Spontaneous and experimentally induced depression in an infant with a gastric fistula: A contribution to the problem of depression. *J. Amer. Psychoanal. Assn.*, 4:428–452.

English, H. B., & English, A. C. (1958), *A Comprehensive Dictionary of Psychological and Psychoanalytical Terms*. New York: David McKay.

Erikson, E. H. (1950), *Childhood and Society*. New York: Norton.

Federn, P. (1912), *Die Onanie: Vierzehn Beiträge zu einer Diskussion der Wiener Psychoanalytischen Vereinigung*. Wiesbaden: I. F. Bergmann.

Fenichel, O. (1926), Identification. *The Collected Papers of Otto Fenichel*, Vol. 1. New York: Norton, 1953, pp. 97–112.

——— (1945), *The Psychoanalytic Theory of Neurosis*. New York: Norton.

——— (n. d.), Theoretical implications of the didactic analysis. Topeka: Topeka Institute for Psychoanalysis.

Ferenczi, S. (1913), Stages in the development of the sense of reality. In: *Sex in Psychoanalysis*. New York: Basic Books, 1950, pp. 213–239.

Fisher, C. (1965), Psychoanalytic implications of recent research on sleep and dreaming. *J. Amer. Psychoanal. Assn.*, 13:197–303.

——— & Dement, W. C. (1962), Manipulation expérimentale du cycle rêve-sommeil par rapport aux états psychopathologiques. *Rev. Méd. Psychosomatique*, 4:5–12.

——— Gross, J., & Zuch, F. (1965), A cycle of penile erection synchronous with dreaming (REM) sleep: Preliminary report. *A.M.A. Arch. Gen. Psychiat.*, 12:29–45.

Foerster, O. (1936), The motor cortex in men in the light of Hughling Jackson's doctrines. *Brain*, 59:135–159.

Fraiberg, S. (1968), Parallel and divergent patterns in blind and sighted infants. *The Psychoanalytic Study of the Child*, 23:264–300. New York: International Universities Press.

———— (1969), Libidinal object constancy and mental representation. *The Psychoanalytic Study of the Child*, 24:9–47. New York: International Universities Press.

———— & Freedman, D. A. (1964), Observations on a congenitally blind child with severe ego deviations. *The Psychoanalytic Study of the Child*, 19:113–169. New York: International Universities Press.

Frankl, L., & Rubinow, O. (1934), Die erste dingauffassung beim säugling. *Ztschr. f. Psychol.*, 133:1–71.

French, T. M. (1929), Psychogenic material related to the function of the semicircular canals. *Int. J. Psycho-Anal.*, 10:398–410.

Freud, A. (1936), *The Ego and the Mechanisms of Defense*. New York: International Universities Press, 1966.

———— (1952a), The mutual influences in the development of ego and id. *The Psychoanalytic Study of the Child*, 7:42–50. New York: International Universities Press.

———— (1952b), The role of bodily illness in the mental life of children. *The Psychoanalytic Study of the Child*, 7:69–81.

———— (1965), *Normality and Pathology in Childhood*. New York: International Universities Press.

Freud, S. (1895a), On the grounds for detaching a particular syndrome from neurasthenia under the description "anxiety neurosis." *Standard Edition*, 3:87–117. London: Hogarth Press, 1962.

———— (1895b), Project for a Scientific Psychology. *Standard Edition*, 1:283–397. London: Hogarth Press, 1966.

———— (1900), The Interpretation of Dreams. *Standard Edition*, 4 & 5. London: Hogarth Press, 1953.

———— (1901), The Psychopathology of Everyday Life. *Standard Edition*, 6. London: Hogarth Press, 1957.

———— (1905a), Jokes and Their Relation to the Unconscious. *Standard Edition*, 8. London: Hogarth Press, 1950.

———— (1905b), Three Essays on the Theory of Sexuality. *Standard Edition*, 7:125–243. London: Hogarth Press, 1953.

———— (1909), Notes upon a case of obsessional neurosis. *Standard Edition*, 10:153–318. London: Hogarth Press, 1955.

———— (1911), Formulations on the two principles of mental functioning. *Standard Edition*, 12:213–226. London: Hogarth Press, 1958.

———— (1913), Totem and Taboo. *Standard Edition*, 13:131–162. London: Hogarth Press, 1955.

———— (1914), On Narcissism: An introduction. *Standard Edition*, 14:67–102. London: Hogarth Press, 1955.

———— (1915a), Instincts and their vicissitudes. *Standard Edition*, 14:109–140. London: Hogarth Press, 1957.

———— (1915b), The unconscious. *Standard Edition*, 14:159–215. London: Hogarth Press, 1957.

———— (1916–17), Introductory Lectures on Psycho-Analysis. *Standard Edition*, 16. London: Hogarth Press, 1963.

———— (1917a), A metapsychological supplement to the theory of dreams. *Standard Edition*, 14:217–235. London: Hogarth Press, 1957.

———— (1917b), Mourning and melancholia. *Standard Edition*, 14:237–260. London: Hogarth Press, 1957.

————— (1919), The "uncanny." *Standard Edition,* 17:218–256. London: Hogarth Press, 1955.

————— (1920), Beyond the Pleasure Principle. *Standard Edition,* 18:7–64. London: Hogarth Press, 1961.

————— (1921), Group psychology and the analysis of the ego. *Standard Edition,* 18:67–143. London: Hogarth Press, 1955.

————— (1923), The ego and the id. *Standard Edition,* 19:3–66. London: Hogarth Press, 1961.

————— (1924), The economic problem of masochism. *Standard Edition,* 19:157–170. London: Hogarth Press, 1961.

————— (1925a), Negation. *Standard Edition,* 19:235–239. London: Hogarth Press, 1961.

————— (1925b), A Note upon the "Mystic Writing-Pad." *Standard Edition,* 19:227–232. London: Hogarth Press, 1961.

————— (1926), Inhibitions, symptoms and anxiety. *Standard Edition,* 20:77–174. London: Hogarth Press, 1959.

————— (1930), Civilization and its Discontents. *Standard Edition,* 21:59–145. London: Hogarth Press, 1961.

————— (1933), New Introductory Lectures on Psycho-Analysis. *Standard Edition,* 22:3–182. London: Hogarth Press, 1964.

Fulton, J. F. (1938), *Physiology of the Nervous System.* New York: Oxford University Press.

————— & Bailey, P. (1935), Tumors in the region of the third ventricle. *J. Nerv. Ment. Dis.,* 69.

Furer, M. (1972), The history of the superego concept in psychoanalysis: A review of the literature. In: *Moral Values and the Superego Concept,* ed. S. C. Post. New York: International Universities Press, pp. 11–62.

Gaensbauer, T. J., Mrazek, D., & Emde, R. N. (1979), Patterning of emotional response in a playroom laboratory situation. *Infant Behavior and Development,* 2:163–178.

————— & Sands, K. (1979), Distorted affective communications in abused/neglected infants and their potential impact on caretakers. *J. Amer. Acad. Child Psychiatrists,* 18:236–250.

Gelb, A., & Goldstein, K. (1920), *Psychologische Analysen Hirnpathologischer Faelle.* Leipzig.

Gesell, A., & Amatruda, C. S. (1941), *Developmental Diagnosis.* New York: Harper.

————— & Ilg, F. L. (1937), *Feeding Behavior of Infants.* Philadelphia: Lippincott.

————— & Thompson, H. (1934), *Infant Behavior: Its Genesis and Growth.* New York: McGraw-Hill.

Gewirtz, J. L. (1965), The course of infant smiling in four child-rearing environments in Israel. In: *Determinants of Infant Behavior,* Vol. 3, ed. B. M. Foss. New York: Wiley, pp. 205–248.

Gifford, S. (1960), Sleep, time and the early ego: Comments on the development of the 24-hour sleep-wakefulness pattern as a precursor of ego functioning. *J. Amer. Psychoanal. Assn.,* 8:5–42.

————— (1965), Individual differentiation in twins. Paper presented at the Twenty-fourth International Psycho-Analytic Congress, Amsterdam.

Gitelson, M. (1952), The emotional position of the analyst in the psycho-analytic situation. *Internat. J. Psycho-Anal.,* 33:1–10.

Glover, E. (1927), *The Technique of Psychoanalysis*. New York: International Universities Press, 1955.

———— (1943), The concept of dissociation. In: *On the Early Development of Mind*. New York: International Universities Press, 1956, pp. 307–323.

———— (1950), Functional aspects of the mental apparatus. In: *On the Early Development of Mind*. New York: International Universities Press, 1956, pp. 364–378.

Goldfarb, W. (1943), Effects of early institutional care on adolescent personality. *J. Exper. Educ.*, 12:106–129.

———— (1944a), Effects of early institutional care on adolescent personality: Rorschach data. *Amer. J. Orthopsychiat.*, 14:441–447.

———— (1944b), Infant rearing as a factor in foster home placement. *Amer. J. Orthopsychiat.*, 14:162–167.

———— & Klopfer, B. (1944), Rorschach characteristics of institutional children. *Rorschach Res. Exchange*, 8:92–100.

Goldstein, K. (1928), Beobachtungen über die veränderung des gesamtverhaltens bei gehirnschädigung. *Mschr. Psychiat. Neurol.*, No. 68.

———— (1936), The significance of the frontal lobes for mental performances. *J. Neurol. Psychopath.*, 17:27–40.

Greenacre, P. (1941), The predisposition to anxiety. *Psychoanal. Quart.*, 10:66–94, 510–638.

———— (1944), Infant reactions to restraint. *Amer. J. Orthopsychiat.*, 14:204–218.

———— (1945), The biological economy of birth. *The Psychoanalytic Study of the Child*, 1:31–51. New York: International Universities Press.

———— (1954), The role of transference. *J. Amer. Psychoanal. Assn.*, 2:671–684.

———— (1958), Toward an understanding of the physical nucleus of some defense reactions. *Internat. J. Psycho-Anal.*, 39:69–76.

Greenson, R. (1954), About the sound "mm. . . ." *Psychoanal. Quart.*, 23:234–239.

Greenspan, S. I. (1975), *A Consideration of Some Learning Variables in the Context of Psychoanalytic Theory: Toward a Psychoanalytic Learning Perspective.* [Psychological Issues, Monogr. 33.] New York: International Universities Press.

Grinker, R. (1937), *Neurology*. Springfield: Charles C Thomas.

———— (1939), Hypothalamic functions in psychosomatic interrelations. *Psychosom. Med.*, 1:19–47.

Guernsey, M. (1928), Eine genetische studie über nachahmung. *Ztschr. f. Psychol.*, 107.

Haeckel, E. (1867), *Naturliche Schopfungs Geschichte*.

Haith, M. M., & Campos, J. J. (1977), Human infancy. *Annual Review of Psychology*, 28:251–293.

Halverson, H. M. (1937), Studies of the grasping responses of early infancy, I, II, III. *J. Genet. Psychol.*, 51.

Hammett, F. S. (1922), Studies of the thyroid apparatus. *Endocrinology*, 4.

Harlow, H. F. (1958), The nature of love. *Amer. Psychologist*, 13:673–685.

———— (1959), Love in infant monkeys. *Sci. American*, 200:68–74.

———— (1960a), Affectional behavior in the infant monkey. In: *Central Nervous System and Behavior*, ed. M. A. B. Brazier. New York: Josiah Macy, Jr., Foundation.

————— (1960b), Development of the second and third affectional systems in Macaque monkeys. Manuscript.

————— (1960c), The maternal and infantile affectional patterns. Manuscript.

————— (1960d), Nature and development of the affectional systems. Manuscript.

————— (1960e), Primary affectional patterns in primates. *Amer. J. Orthopsychiat.*, 30:676–684.

————— (1962), The heterosexual affectional system in monkeys. *Amer. Psychologist*, 17:1–9.

————— & Harlow, M. K. (1964), The effects of early social deprivation on primates. Paper presented and discussed by René Spitz at the Clinique Psychiatrique de l'Université de Genève, on Déafferentation Expérimentale et Clinique.

————— & Zimmerman, R. (1959), Affectional responses in the infant monkey. *Science*, 130:421–432.

Harmon, R. J., & Emde, R. N. (1971), Spontaneous REM behaviors in a microcephalic infant: A clinical anatomical study. *Perceptual and Motor Skills*, 34:827–833.

————— & Morgan, G. A. (1975), Infants' reactions to unfamiliar adults: A discussion of some important issues. Paper presented at the Biennial Meeting of the Society for Research in Child Development, Denver. ERIC Document Reproduction Service No. PS 008 221.

Harnik, J. (1932), Introjection and projection in the mechanism of depression. *Internat. J. Psycho-Anal.*, 13:425–432.

Hartmann, E. (1967), *The Biology of Dreaming*. Springfield, Ill.: Thomas.

Hartmann, H. (1939), *Ego Psychology and the Problem of Adaptation*. New York: International Universities Press, 1958.

————— (1948), Comments on the psychoanalytic theory of instinctual drives. *Psychiat. Quart.*, 17:368–388.

————— (1950), Comments on the psychoanalytic theory of the ego. *The Psychoanalytic Study of the Child*, 5:74–96. New York: International Universities Press.

————— (1952), The mutual influences in the development of ego and id. *The Psychoanalytic Study of the Child*, 7:9–30.

————— Kris, E., & Loewenstein, R. M. (1946), Comments on the formation of psychic structure. *The Psychoanalytic Study of the Child*, 2:11–38. New York: International Universities Press.

————— ————— ————— (1949), Notes on the theory of aggression. *The Psychoanalytic Study of the Child*, 3/4:9–36.

Head, H. (1908), Sensation and the cerebral cortex. *Brain*.

Hebb, D. O. (1946), On the nature of fear. *Psychol. Rev.*, 31.

————— & Riesen, A. H. (1943), The genesis of irrational fears. *Bull. Canad. Psychol. Assn.*, 3:49–50.

Hendrick, I. (1942), Instinct and the ego during infancy. *Psychoanal. Quart.*, 11:33–58.

Hess, W. R. (1924, 1925), Über die Wechselbeziehungen zwischen psychischen und vegetativen Funktionen. *Schweiz. Arch. Neurol. Psychiat.*, 15:260–277; 16:36–55, 285–306.

Hetzer, H., & Ripin, R. (1930), Frühestes lernen des Säuglings in der Ernährungssituation. *Ztschr. f. Psychol.*, 118:82–127.

————— & Wislitzky, S. (1930), Experimente ueber Erwartung und Erinneurung beim Kleinkind. *Ztschr. f. Psychol.*, 118.

————— & Wolf, K. M. (1928), Baby tests. *Ztschr. f. Psychol.*, 107:62–104.

Hoffer, W. (1949), Mouth, hand and ego-integration. *The Psychoanalytic Study of the Child*, 3/4:49–56.
———— (1950), Oral aggressiveness and ego development. *Internat. J. Psycho-Anal.*, 31:160–168.
Hoffman, E. P. (1935), Projektion und ichentwicklung. *Internat. Ztschr. f. Psychoanal.*, 21:342–373.
Hooker, D. (1942), Fetal reflexes and instinctual processes. *Psychosom. Med.*, 4.
———— (1943), Reflex activities in the human fetus. In: *Child Behavior and Development*, ed. R. G. Barker, J. S. Kounin, and H. F. Wright. New York: McGraw-Hill.
Hull, J. (1943), *Principles of Behavior: An Introduction to Behavior Theory*. New York: Appleton-Century.
Isakower, O. (1938), A contribution to the pathopsychology of phenomena associated with falling asleep. *Internat. J. Psycho-Anal.*, 19:331–345.
———— (1954), Spoken words in dreams. *Psychoanal. Quart.*, 23:1–6.
Izard, C. (1977), *Human Emotions*. New York: Plenum Press.
Jackson, E., Campos, J.J., & Fischer, K. W. (1978), The question of decalage between object permanence and person permanence. *Child Devel.*
Jacobson, E. (1943), Depression: The Oedipus conflict in the development of depressive mechanisms. *Psychoanal. Quart.*, 12:541–560.
———— (1954), The self and the object world. *The Psychoanalytic Study of the Child*, 9:75–127. New York: International Universities Press.
———— (1964), *The Self and the Object World*. New York: International Universities Press.
James, W. (1890), *Principles of Psychology*, Vol. 2. New York: Henry Holt.
Jensen, K. (1932), Differential reaction to taste and temperature in newborn infants. *Genet. Psychol. Monogr.*, 12:361–479.
Jersild, A. T., & Holmes, F. B. (1935), Children's fear. *Child Devel. Monogr.*, 20.
Jones, E. (1955), *The Life and Work of Sigmund Freud*, Vol. 2. New York: Basic Books.
Jones, H. E. (1940), Personal reactions of the yearbook committee. *Thirty-Ninth Yearbook, National Society for the Study of Education*, 1:454–456.
Jones, M. C. (1926), The development of behavior patterns in young children. *Ped. Sem.*, 33:537–585.
Kagan, J. (1971), *Change and Continuity in Infancy*. New York: Wiley.
———— Kearsley, R. B., & Zelazo, P. R. (1978), *Infancy: Its Place in Human Development*. Cambridge, Mass.: Harvard University Press.
Kaila, E. (1932), Die reaktionen des säuglings auf das menschliche gesicht. *Ann. Univ. Aboensis*, 17:1–114.
Kardiner, A. (1932), The bio-analysis of the epileptic reaction. *Psychiat. Quart.*, 1:3–4.
———— (1941), *The Traumatic Neuroses of War*. New York: Hoeber.
Kempf, E. J. (1921), *The Autonomic Functions and the Personality. Nerv. Ment. Dis. Monogr.* No. 28.
Kestenbaum, A. (1930), Zur entwicklung der augenbewegungen und des optokinetischen nystagmus. *Arch. f. Opthalmol.*, 124:115.
Kety, S. S. (1972), Progress in neurobiology and its implications for society. Challenge of life: biomedical progress and human value. *Roche Annual Symposium*. Basel.
Klein, M. A. (1932), *The Psycho-Analysis of Children*. London: Hogarth Press.

———— (1935), Contributions to the Psychogenesis of manic-depressive states. In: *Contributions to Psychoanalysis, 1921–1945*. London: Hogarth Press, 1948.

———— (1940), Mourning and its relation to manic-depressive states. *Internat. J. Psycho-Anal.*, 21:125–153.

———— (1944), Emotional life and the ego of the infant with special reference to the depressive position. Controversial Series of the London Psychoanalytic Society, IV, *Discussion*, March 1944.

———— (1945), The Oedipus complex in the light of early anxieties. *Internat. J. Psycho-Anal.*, 26:11–33.

———— (1948), *Contributions to Psychoanalysis, 1921–1945*. London: Hogarth Press.

Kleitmann, N. (1929), Sleep. *Physiol. Rev.*, 9:624–665.

———— (1939), *Sleep and Wakefulness*. Chicago: University of Chicago Press.

Kohut, H. (1971), *The Analysis of the Self*. New York: International Universities Press.

———— (1977), *The Restoration of the Self*. New York: International Universities Press.

Kris, E. (1944), Art and regression. *Trans. N.Y. Acad. Sci.*, 6:236–250.

———— (1952), The psychology of caricature. In: *Psychoanalytic Explorations in Art*. New York: International Universities Press, pp. 173–188.

Kubie, L. S. (1934), The physical basis of personality. *Child Study*, 11:131–160.

———— (1941a), The ontogeny of anxiety. *Psychoanal. Rev.*, 28:78–85.

———— (1941b), A physiological approach to the concept of anxiety. *Psychosom. Med.*, 3:263–276.

———— (1952), A research project in community mental hygiene: A fantasy. *Ment. Hyg.*, 36:220–226.

———— (1953), The distortion of the symbolic process in neurosis and psychosis. *J. Amer. Psychoanal. Assn.*, 1:59–86.

Kueppers, E. (1923), Grundplan des Nervensystems und die Lokalisation des Psychischen. *Ztschr. f. d. ges. Neur. & Psych.*, 72.

———— (1931), Weiteres zur lokalisation des psychischen. *Ztschr. f. d. ges. Neur. & Psych.*, 83.

Laforgue, R. (1926), Verdrängung und Skotomisation. *Internat. Ztschr. f. Psychoanal.*, 12:54–65.

Lagache, D. (1952), Le problème du transfert. *Rev. Franç. de Psychanal*, 16:5–22.

———— (1953), Some aspects of transference. *Internat. J. Psycho-Anal.*, 34.

———— (1954), La doctrine Freudienne et la théorie du transfert. *Acta Psychother., Psychosom. Orthopaed.*, 2:228–249.

Lamb, M. E. (1978), The father's role in the infant's social world. In: *Mother/Child, Father/Child Relationships*, ed. J. E. Stevens, Jr., & M. Mathews. Washington, D.C.: National Association for the Education of Young Children.

Lampl-de Groot, J. (1950), On masturbation and its influence on general development. *The Psychoanalytic Study of the Child*, 5:153–174. New York: International Universities Press.

Lashley, K. S. (1951), The problem of serial order in behavior. In: *Cerebral Mechanisms in Behavior*, ed. L. A. Jeffres. New York: Wiley.

Lebovici, S., & McDougall, J. (1960), *Un Cas de Psychose Infantile: Étude Psychanalytique*. Paris: Presses Universitaires de France.

Levine, M. T., & Bell, A. I. (1950), The treatment of "colic" in infancy by use of the pacifier. *J. Ped.*, 37.

464 References

Levy, D. (1943), *Maternal Overprotection.* New York: Columbia University Press.

Lewin, B. D. (1946), Sleep, the mouth and the dream screen. *Psychoanal. Quart.,* 15:419–434.

——— (1948), Inferences from the dream screen. *Internat. J. Psycho-Anal.,* 29:224–231.

——— (1953a), The forgetting of dreams. In: *Drives, Affects, Behavior,* Vol. 1, ed. R. M. Loewenstein. New York: International Universities Press, pp. 191–202.

——— (1953b), Reconsideration of the dream screen. *Psychoanal. Quart.,* 22:174–199.

Lewis, M., & Brooks-Gunn, J. (1979), *Social Cognition and the Acquisition of the Self.* New York: Plenum.

Lichtenstein, H. (1963), The dilemma of human identity. *J. Amer. Psychoanal. Assn.,* 11:173–223.

Lindner, S. (1934), Das Saugen an den Fingern, Lippen, etc. bei den Kindern. *Ztschr. f. Psychoanal. Päd.,* 8:117–138.

Linn, L. (1953), Psychological implications of the "activating system." *Amer. J. Psychiat.,* 110:61–65.

——— (1955), Some developmental aspects of the body image. *Internat. J. Psycho-Anal.,* 36:36–42.

Loewald, H. W. (1960), On the therapeutic action of psycho-analysis. *Internat. J. Psycho-Anal.,* 41:16–33.

——— (1978), *Psychoanalysis and the History of the Individual.* New Haven: Yale University Press.

Lorand, S., & Asbot, J. (1952), Ueber die durch Reizung der Brustwarze angeregten reflektorischen Uteruskontraktionen. *Zentralbl. f. Gynänkol.,* 74.

Lorenz, K. (1950), The comparative method in studying innate behavior patterns. *Symposia Soc. Exper. Biol.,* 4.

——— (1963), *Das Sogenannte Böse: Zur Naturgeschichte der Aggression.* Vienna: Borotha Schoeler. Published in English as *On Aggression.* New York: Harcourt Brace, 1966.

Lowrey, L. G. (1940), Personality distortion and early institutional care. *Amer. J. Orthopsychiat.,* 10:576–585.

Macalpine, I. (1950), The development of the transference. *Psychoanal. Quart.,* 19:501–519.

Mahler, M. S. (1952), On Child Psychosis and Schizophrenia: Autistic and symbiotic infantile psychoses. *The Psychoanalytic Study of the Child,* 7:286–305. New York: International Universities Press.

——— (1957), On two crucial phases of integration concerning problems of identity: Separation-individuation and bisexual identity. Abstracted in Panel: Problems of Identity, rep. D. Rubinfine. *J. Amer. Psychoanal. Assn.,* 6:131–142, 1958.

——— (1958), Autism and symbiosis: Two extreme disturbances of identity. *Internat. J. Psycho-Anal.,* 39:77–83.

——— (1960), Perceptual de-differentiation and psychotic "object relationship." *Internat. J. Psycho-Anal.,* 41:548–552.

Margolin, S. (1953), On the psychological origin and function of symbols. Paper presented at the Meeting of the New York Psychoanalytic Society.

Marquis, D. P. (1931), Can conditioned responses be established in the new-born infant? *Ped. Seminary Genet. Psych.,* 39.

McBride, A. F., & Hebb, D. O. (1948), Behavior of the captive bottlenose dolphin, *tursips truncatus. J. Comp. Physiol. Psychol.,* 41:111–123.

McCall, R. (1979), The development of intellectual functioning in infancy and the prediction of later I.Q. In: *Handbook of Infant Development*, ed. J. D. Osofsky. New York: Wiley.

————— & McGhee, P. (1977), The discrepancy hypothesis of attention and affect in infants. In: *The Structuring of Experience*, ed. I. Uzgiris & F. Weizman. New York: Plenum.

McGraw, M. B. (1935), *Growth: A Study of Johnny and Jimmy*. New York: Appleton-Century.

Mead, G. H. (1934), *Mind, Self, and Society from the Standpoint of a Social Behaviorist*. Chicago: University of Chicago Press.

Mead, M., & Macgregor, F. (1951), *Growth and Culture: A Photographic Study of Balinese Childhood*. New York: Putnam.

Menninger, K. (1954), Psychological aspects of the organism under stress. *J. Amer. Psychoanal. Assn.*, 2:67–106, 280–311.

Metcalf, D. R. (1969), Effect of extrauterine experience on ontogenesis of EEG sleep spindles. *Psychosom. Med.*, 31:393–399.

————— & Emde, R. N. (1969), Ontogenesis of sleep in early human infancy. *Psychophysiology*, 6:264.

————— Mondale, J., & Butler, F. K. (1971), Ontogenesis of spontaneous K. complexes. *Psychophysiology*, 8:340–347.

Minkowski, M. (1924-1925), Zum gegenwärtigen Stand der Lehre von den Reflexen in entwicklungsgeschichtlicher und anatomisch-physiologischer Beziehung. *Schweiz. Arch. Neurol. Psychiat.*, 15/16.

————— (1928), Neurobiologische studien am menschlichen foetus. In: *Abderhaldens Handbuch d. Biol. Arbeitsmethoden*, 5. Berlin: Urban.

Montagu, M. F. A. (1950), Constitutional and prenatal factors in infant and child health. In: *Problems of Infancy and Childhood*, ed. M. J. E. Senn. New York: Josiah Macy, Jr., Foundation.

————— (1953), The sensory influences of the skin. *Texas Reports on Biol. & Med.*, 11:291–301.

Moore, B. (1958), Isolation, object relations and acting out. Unpublished paper.

Moore, K. C. (1896), The mental development of a child. *Psychol. Rev. Monogr.*, No. 3.

Moro, E. (1918), Das erste Trimenon. *München Med. Wchnschr.*, 65:1147–1150.

Murchison, C. (1933), *Handbook of Child Psychology*. Worcester, Mass.: Clark University Press.

Murphy, G., & Murphy, L. B. (1931), *Experimental Social Psychology*. New York: Harper.

Needham, J. (1931), *Chemical Embryology*. New York: Macmillan.

Nunberg, H. (1951), Transference and reality. *Internat. J. Psycho-Anal.*, 32:1–9.

Oppenheimer, R. (1956), Analogy in science. *Amer. Psychologist*, 11:127–135.

Orlansky, H. (1949), Infant care and personality. *Psychol. Bull.*, 46: 1–48.

Orr, D. W. (1954), Transference and countertransference. *J. Amer. Psychoanal. Assn.*, 2:621–670.

Osofsky, J. D. (1979), *Handbook of Infant Development*. New York: Wiley.

Oswald, I. (1962), *Sleep and Waking*. New York: Elsevier.

Papez, J. W. (1937), A proposed mechanism of emotion. *Arch. Neurol. Psychiat., Chicago*, 38.

————— (1939), Cerebral Mechanisms. *J. Nerv. Ment. Dis.*, 90.

Paradise, J. (1966), Maternal and other factors in the etiology of infantile colic. *JAMA*, 197:191–199.

Pavlov, I. P. (1927), *Conditioned Reflexes*. London: Oxford Univ. Press.

―――― (1928), *Lectures on Conditioned Reflexes*. New York: Liveright.

Piaget, J. (1936a), La Construction du Réel. Paris: Neuchâtel.

―――― (1936b), *Origins of Intelligence in Children*. New York: International Universities Press, 1952.

―――― (1950), *The Psychology of Intelligence*. New York: Harcourt Brace.

―――― (1973), The affective unconscious and the cognitive unconscious. *J. Amer. Psychoanal. Assn.*, 21:249–261.

Pichon, E. (1936), *Le Développement psychique de l'Enfant et de l'Adolescent*. Paris: Masson.

Pinneau, S. R. (1955), The infantile disorders of hospitalism and anaclitic depression. *Psychol. Bull.*, 53:429–452.

Polak, P. R., Emde, R. N., & Spitz, R. A. (1964a), The smiling response. I. Methodology, quantification, and natural history. *J. Nerv. Ment. Dis.*, 139:103–109.

―――― ―――― ―――― (1964b), The smiling response. II. Visual discrimination and the onset of depth perception. *J. Nerv. Ment. Dis.*, 139:407–415.

Racker, H. A. (1953), A contribution to the problem of counter-transference. *Internat. J. Psycho-Anal.*, 34:313–324.

Rado, S. (1927), Das Problem der Melancholie. *Internat. Ztschr. f. Psychiat.*, 13:439–455.

Rank, B., Putnam, M. C., & Rochlin, G. (1948), The significance of the "emotional climate" in early feeding difficulties. *Psychosom. Med.*, 1:279–283.

Rank, O. (1924), *Das Trauma der Geburt und seine Bedeutung für die Psychoanalyse*. Vienna: Internationaler Psychoanalytischer Verlag.

Rapaport, D. (1942), *Emotions and Memory*. New York: International Universities Press, 1950.

Reich, A. (1951), On counter-transference. *Internat. J. Psycho-Anal.*, 32:3–7.

Reich, W. (1925), *Der triebhafte Charakter: Eine psychoanalytische Studie zur Pathologie des Ich*. Leipzig: Internationaler Psychoanalytischer Verlag.

Reyniers, J. A. (1946, 1949), Germ-free life studies. *Lobund Reports*, Nos. 1 and 2.

Rheingold, H. A. (1956), The modification of social responsiveness in institutional babies. *Monogr. Soc. Res. Child Devel.*, 21.

Ribble, M. A. (1938), Clinical studies of instinctive reaction in new-born babies. *Amer. J. Psychiat.*, 95:149–160.

―――― (1939), The significance of infantile sucking for the psychic development of the individual. *J. Nerv. Ment. Dis.*, 90:455–463.

―――― (1941), Disorganizing factors of infant personality. *Amer. J. Psychiat.*, 98:459–463.

Riesen, A. H. (1965), Effects of visual deprivation on perceptual function and the neural substrate. *Symposium Bel-Air II, Genève 1964: Déafferéntation Expérimentale et Clinique*, ed. J. de Ajuriaguerra. Geneva: Georg, pp. 275–280.

Ripin, R. (1930), A study of the infant's feeding reactions during the first six months of life. *Arch. Psychol.*, 116.

―――― & Hetzer, H. (1930), Frühestes lernen des säuglings in der ernährungssituation. *Ztschr. f. Psychol.*, 118:82–127.

Riviere, J. (1936), On the genesis of psychical conflict in earliest infancy. *Internat. J. Psycho-Anal.*, 17:395–422.

Rubinow, O., & Frankl, L. (1934), Die erste Dingauffassung beim Saugling. *Ztschr. f. Psychol.*, 133:1–72.

Rutter, M. (1979), Maternal deprivation, 1972–1978: New findings, new concepts, new approaches. *Child Devel.*, 50:283–305.

Rycroft, C. (1951), A contribution to the study of the dream screen. *Internat. J. Psycho-Anal.*, 32.

———— (1953), Some observations on a case of vertigo. *Internat. J. Psycho-Anal.*, 34:241–247.

Sameroff, A. J., & Cavanaugh, P. L. (1979), Learning in infancy: A developmental perspective. In: *Handbook of Infant Development*, ed. J. D. Osofsky. New York: Wiley, pp. 344–392.

———— & Harris, A. E. (1979), Dialectical approaches to early thought and language. In: *Psychological Development from Infancy: Image to Intention*, ed. M. H. Bornstein & W. Kessen. Hillsdale, N.J.: Lawrence Erlbaum, pp. 339–372.

Sandler, J. (1960a), The background of safety. *Internat. J. Psycho-Anal.*, 41:353–356.

———— (1960b), On the concept of superego. *The Psychoanalytic Study of the Child*, 15:128–162. New York: International Universities Press.

Schilder, P. (1928), *Introduction to a Psychoanalytic Psychiatry*. *Nerv. Ment. Dis. Monogr.* No. 50.

Schlossman, A. (1920), Zur Frage der Säuglingssterblichkeit. *Münchner Med. Wochenschrift*, 67.

Scott, W. C. M. (1948), Some embryological, neurological, psychiatric and psychoanalytic implications of the body scheme. *Internat. J. Psycho-Anal.*, 29:141–155.

Searl, M. N. (1933), The psychology of screaming. *Internat. J. Psycho-Anal.*, 14:193–205.

Sherrington, C. S. (1906), *The Integrative Action of the Nervous System*. New Haven: Yale University Press, 1947.

Shinn, M. W. (1900), *The Biography of a Baby*. Boston: Houghton Mifflin.

Shirley, M. M. (1933), *The First Two Years: A Study of Twenty-Five Babies*, Vol. 2. Minneapolis: Minnesota Press.

Sigismund, B. (1856), *Kind und welt: I. Die fünf ersten Perioden des Kindesalters*. Braunschweig: Vieweg.

Silberer, H. (1911), Symbolik des Erwachens und Schwellensymbolik überhaupt. *Jahrb. f. Psychoanal. Psychopathol. Forschungen*, 3:621–660.

Simmel, E. (1948), Alcoholism and addiction. *Psychiat. Quart.*, 17:6–31.

Simpson, B. R. (1939), The wandering I.Q. *J. Psychol.*, 7:351–367.

Skeels, H. M. (1938), Mental development of children in foster homes. *J. Consult. Psychol.*, 2:33–43.

———— (1940), Some Iowa studies of the mental growth of children in relation to differentials of the environment: A summary. *Thirty-Ninth Yearbook, National Society for the Study of Education*, 2:281–308.

———— Updegraff, R., Wellman, B. L., & Williams, H. M. (1938), A study of environmental stimulation: An orphanage preschool project. *University of Iowa Studies in Child Welfare*. 15, No. 4.

Skodak, M. (1939), Children in foster homes. *University of Iowa Studies in Child Welfare*, 16, No. 1.

Soto, R. (1937), Porque en la casa de cuna no hay dispepsia transitoria? *Rev. Mexicana de Puericultura,* 8.

Sperling, O. (1944), On appersonation. *Internat. J. Psycho-Anal.,* 25:128–132.

Spiegel, L. A. (1959), The self, the sense of self, and perception. *The Psychoanalytic Study of the Child,* 14:81–109. New York: International Universities Press.

Spielrein, S. (1922), Die entstehung der kindlichen worte papa und mama. *Imago,* 8:345–367.

Spitz, R. A. (1936), Differentiation and integration. Paper presented at the Vienna Society for Psychoanalysis.

———— (1945a), Diacritic and coenesthetic organization. *This Volume.*

———— (1945b), Hospitalism: An inquiry into the genesis of psychiatric conditions in early childhood. *This Volume.*

———— (1946a), Anaclitic depression: An inquiry into the genesis of psychiatric conditions in early childhood, II. *This Volume.*

———— (1946b), Hospitalism: A follow-up report. *This Volume.*

———— (1946c), Profilaxis versus tratamiento en las neurosis traumaticas. *Rev. Psicoanál.,* 4:35–47.

———— (1946d), The smiling response: A contribution to the ontogenesis of social relations. *This Volume.*

———— (1947), Emotional growth in the first year. *Child Study,* Spring.

———— (1948), La perte de la mère par le nourrisson. *Enfance,* 1: 373–391.

———— (1949), Autoeroticism: Some empirical findings and hypotheses on three of its manifestations in the first year of life. *This Volume.*

———— (1950a), Anxiety in infancy: A study of its manifestations in the first year of life. *Internat. J. Psycho-Anal.,* 31:138–143.

———— (1950b), *Digital Extension Reflex. Arch. Neurol. & Psychiat.,* 63.

———— (1950c), Experimental design and psychoanalytic concepts. Paper presented to the Fifty-Eighth Meeting of the American Psychological Association, Symposium on Experimental Approach to Psychoanalytic Theory.

———— (1950d), Psychiatric therapy in infancy. *This Volume.*

———— (1951a), Eczema. Manuscript.

———— (1951b), Psychogenic diseases in infancy: An attempt at their etiological classification. *This Volume.*

———— (1951c), Purposive grasping. *J. Personality,* 1:141–148.

———— (1952), Authority and masturbation: Some remarks on a bibliographical investigation. *Psychoanal. Quart.,* 21:113-145.

———— (1953), Aggression: Its role in the establishment of object relations. *This Volume.*

———— (1954), La genèse des premières relations objectales. *Rev. Franç. Psychanal.,* 18:479–575.

———— (1955a), Childhood development phenomena: 1. The influence of the mother-child relationship and its disturbances. 2. The case of Felicia. In: *Mental Health and Infant Development,* ed. K. Soddy. New York: Basic Books, pp. 103–116.

———— (1955b), A note on the extrapolation of ethological findings. *Internat. J. Psycho-Anal.,* 36:162–165.

———— (1955c), The primal cavity: A contribution to the genesis of perception and its role for psychoanalytic theory. *This Volume.*

———— (1955d), Reply to Dr. Pinneau. *Psychol. Bull.,* 54:453–462.

———— (1956a), Countertransference: Comments on its varying role in the analytic situation. *This Volume.*

———— (1956b), Transference: The analytical setting and its prototype. *This Volume,* pp. xxx–xxx.

———— (1957), *No and Yes: On the Beginnings of Human Communication.* New York: International Universities Press.

———— (1958a), On the genesis of superego components. *This Volume.*

———— (1958b), *La Première Année de la Vie de l'Enfant.* Paris: Presses Universitaires de France.

———— (1959), *A Genetic Field Theory of Ego Formation: Its Implications for Pathology.* New York: International Universities Press.

———— (1961), Some early prototypes of ego defenses. *This Volume.*

———— (1962), Autoerotism re-examined: The role of early sexual behavior patterns in personality formation. *This Volume.*

———— (1963a), Life and the dialogue. *This Volume.*

———— (1963b), Ontogenesis: The proleptic function of emotion. *This Volume,* pp. xxx–xxx.

———— (1964), The derailment of dialogue: Stimulus overload, action cycles and the completion gradient. *This Volume.*

———— (1965a), The evolution of dialogue. *This Volume.*

———— (1965b), *The First Year of Life: A Psychoanalytic Study of Normal and Deviant Object Relations.* New York: International Universities Press.

———— (1966), Metapsychology and direct infant observation. *This Volume.*

———— (1971), The adaptive viewpoint: Its role in autism and child psychiatry. *J. Autism and Childhood Schizophr.,* 1:239–245.

———— (1972), Bridges: On anticipation, duration and meaning. *This Volume.*

———— & Wolf, K.M. (1947), Environment vs. race: Environment as an etiological factor in psychiatric disturbances in infancy. *Arch. Neur. Psychiat.,* 57, No. 1.

Sroufe, A. (1979), Socioemotional development. In: *Handbook of Infant Development,* ed. J. Osofsky. New York: Wiley, pp. 463–516.

Steele, B. F. (1976), Violence within the family. In: *Child Abuse and Neglect,* ed. R. Helfet & C. H. Kempe. Cambridge, Mass.: Ballinger.

Stenberg, C., Campos, J., & Emde, R. N. (1982), Facial expression of anger in seven-month olds. *Child Devel.,* 53.

Stern, A. (1924), On the countertransference in psychoanalysis. *Psychoanal. Rev.,* 11:166–174.

Stern, C., & Stern, W. (1907), *Die Kindersprache.* Leipzig: Barth.

Stern, D. N. (1974), The goal and structure of mother infant play. *J. Amer. Acad. Child Psychiat.,* 13:402–421.

———— (1977), *The First Relationship: Mother and Infant.* Cambridge, Mass.: Harvard University Press.

Stern, W. (1930), *Psychology of Early Childhood up to the Sixth Year of Age,* 2nd ed. New York: Henry Holt.

Stewart, A., Weiland, J., Leider, A., Mangham, C., & Ripley, H. (1953), Excessive infant crying in relation to parent behavior. *Amer. J. Psychiat.,* 110:687–694.

Stoddard, G. D. (1940), Intellectual Development of the Child: An answer to the critics of the Iowa studies. *School & Society,* 51:529–536.

Stone, L., Smith, H., & Murphy, L., Eds. (1973), *The Competent Infant: Research and Commentary.* New York: Basic Books.

Strachey, A. (1943), *A New German-English Vocabulary.* Baltimore: Williams & Wilkins.

Sylvester, E. (1947), Pathogenic Influence of Maternal Attitudes in the Neonatal Period. In: *Problems of Early Infancy.* New York: Josiah Macy, Jr., Foundation.

Tennes, K., Emde, R. N., Kisley, A. J., & Metcalf, D. R. (1972), The stimulus barrier in early infancy: An exploration of some formulations of John Benjamin. In: *Psychoanalysis and Contemporary Science,* ed. R. R. Holt & E. Peterfreund. New York: Macmillan, pp. 206–234.

Thorndike, E. L. (1913), *The Psychology of Learning.* New York: Teacher's College.

Tiedmann, D. (1927), Beobachtungen über die entwicklung der seelenfähigkeiten bei kindern. *Ped. Sem.,* 34:205–230, 1927.

Tilney, F., & Kubie, L. S. (1931), Behavior and its relation to the development of the brain. *Bull. Neurol. Inst., New York,* 1:229–313.

Tinbergen, N. (1950), The hierarchical organization of nervous mechanisms underlying instinctive behavior. *Sympos. Soc. Exper. Biol.,* 4.

——— (1951), *The Study of Instincts.* London: Oxford University Press.

Tolman, E. C. (1932), *Purposive Behavior.* New York: Century.

Tower, L. E. (1956), Countertransference. *J. Amer. Psychoanal. Assn.,* 4:224–255.

Updegraff, R. (1932), The determination of a reliable intelligence quotient for the young child. *J. Genet. Psychol.,* 41:152–166.

Vogt, C., & Vogt, O. (1920), Zur lehre der erkrankungen des striaeren systems. *J. Psychol. Neurol.,* 25.

Volkelt, H. (1929), Neueuntersuchungen über die kindliche auffassung und wiedergabe von formen. *Bericht über den 4. Kongress für Heilpädagogik.* Berlin: Springer.

von Holst, E., & Mittelstaedt, H. (1950), Das reafferenzprinzip. *Naturwiss.,* 37.

von Senden, M. (1932), *Space and Sight.* London: Methuen, 1960.

Waddington, C. H. (1940), *Organizers and Genes.* Cambridge: Cambridge University Press.

Wallon, H. (1925), *L'Enfant Turbulent.* Paris: Alcan.

Washburn, R. W. (1929), A study of the smiling and laughing of infants in the first year of life. *Genet. Psychol. Monogr.,* 6:399–537.

Watson, J. B. (1924), *Behaviorism.* New York: Norton.

Weiss, P. (1939), *Principles of Development.* New York: Holt.

Weissman, P. (1954), Ego and superego in obsessional character. *Psychoanal. Quart.,* 23:529–543.

Werner, H. (1948), *Comparative Psychology of Mental Development.* New York: International Universities Press.

——— & Kaplan, B. (1963), *Symbol Formation: An Organismic-Developmental Approach to Language and the Expression of Thought.* New York: Wiley.

Wessel, M., Cobb, J., Jackson, E., Harris, S., & Detwiler, A. (1954), Paroxysmal fussing in infancy, sometimes called colic. *Pediatrics,* 15:421–434.

Wildernberg-Kantrow, R. (1937), An investigation of conditioned feeding responses and concomitant adaptive behavior in young infants. *Iowa University Child Welfare Research Station.*

Winnicott, D. W. (1953), Transitional objects and transitional phenomena. *Internat. J. Psycho-Anal.,* 34:89–97.

Wolff, G. (1944), Maternal and infant mortality in 1944. *U.S. Children's Bureau Statistics Series*, No. 1. Washington, D. C.: Social Security Administration.

Wolff, P. H. (1967), Cognitive considerations for a psychoanalytic theory of language acquisition. In: *Motives and Thought: Psychoanalytic Essays in Honor of David Rapaport*, ed. R. Holt. [Psychological Issues Monogr. 18/19.] New York: International Universities Press.

Woodworth, R. S. (1941), Heredity and environment. *Social Science Research Council*, Bulletin No. 47, p. 95.

Zajonc, R. B. (1979), Feeling and thinking: Preferences need no inferences. Distinguished Scientific Contribution Award Address, presented at a Meeting of the American Psychological Association, New York, September 2.

Zeigarnik, B. (1927), Über das behalten von erledigten und unerledigten handlungen. *Psychol. Forsch.*, 9:1–85.

Index